What People Are Saying About the Award-Winning *Let's Eat Out!*

"Invaluable resource and comprehensive guide for eating out whether at home or abroad"
Allergic Living Magazine

"Excellent for helping celiacs / coeliacs & those on special diets regain their quality of life"
Sue Shepherd PhD, Author & Dietitian

"Empowers readers to safely dine out anywhere"
Gluten Intolerance Group

"Essential reference for celiac / coeliac and food allergy clients that eat in restaurants and travel… great for dietitians counseling clients or for those working in food service"
Dietitians of Canada

"Prepares prospective diners for everything that is likely to come their way"
Foods Matter, UK

"Visa to the world of eating out for people who normally have to worry constantly about their children"
All About Kids Magazine

"Aids both consumers and food service staff in better collaborating on dealing with allergies and the likelihood of more arising"
Food Service Magazine

"At last, a book that gives allergy sufferers the freedom to eat out safely"
Allergy New Zealand

"Fantastic presentation of invaluable material for those with special dietary needs… even chefs and restaurant owners could learn something about the food they serve"
Writer's Digest, US

"Consumers, food service owners, operators, chefs and staff will find this book extremely helpful and a tremendous resource"
College Services Magazine

"Must read for anyone with food sensitivities or celiac / coeliac disease and the hospitality industry" *Shelley Case, BSc, RD & Author*

"Helps communicate food requirements when dining out locally or travelling abroad" *Canadian Living Magazine*

"Important for travelers who may be trying all sorts of new cuisines and don't know what to be on the lookout for in menus and food items" *Los Angeles Times*

"First of its kind... makes you hungry and gives you the power to protect yourself from food allergies at the same time... well-written, professionally researched and gorgeous book" *BookReview.com*

"Extremely helpful... great reference tool for families" *Food Allergy Initiative*

"Thorough guide to worry-free foods, with advice for diners who love foods that don't love them back" *US Airways Magazine*

"Pioneering effort for safe eating experiences" *Celiac Sprue Association*

"True lifesavers of the allergic and intolerant" *GoDairyFree*

"Defensive guide identifying hundreds of often unexpected sources of food allergens in restaurant meals" *The Nutrition Reporter, US*

"Instructs travelers with food sensitivities or allergies how to eat what they want, where they want and when they want" *Canadian Travel Press Magazine*

"Detailed advice to what ingredients are in traditional restaurant dishes, rather than particular places for eating out" *Manawatu Standard*

Enhanced and Revised

Let's Eat Out

with Celiac/Coeliac & Food Allergies!

A Timeless Reference for Special Diets

Kim Koeller & Robert La France

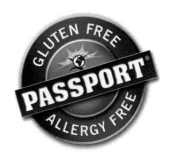

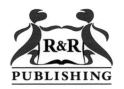

R&R
PUBLISHING

Library of Congress Control Number: 2005929744

GlutenFree Passport®, AllergyFree Passport® and its logo are trademarks of AllergyFree Passport®, LLC

First Edition 2005
Enhanced Edition 2009

[handwritten: QDV. K819L 2009]

Koeller, Kim.
    Let's eat out : with celiac / coeliac & food allergies!
: a timeless reference for special diets / Kim Koeller &
Robert La France. -- Enhanced and rev.
    p. cm. -- (Allergy free passport)
    Includes index.
    ISBN-13: 978-0-9764845-5-4
    ISBN-10: 0-9764845-5-2

    1. Food allergy--Diet therapy. 2. Gluten-free diet.
I. La France, Robert. II. Title. III. Title:
Celiac / coeliac & food allergies! IV. Title: Celiac,
coeliac and food allergies. V. Series: Allergy free
passport.

    RC588.D53K635 2009   616.97'50654
                        QBI09-600013

Front Cover photos: Jupiter Images® (left); Getty Images® (middle and right)

Interior photos provided by: Brand X Pictures™, Creatas Images, Digital Vision, Getty Images®, Ingram, Istockphoto™, MedioImages™, Photodisc®, Shutterstock™, Jupiter Images® and Thinkstock™ Images.

Book design: Emily Brackett/Visible Logic, Inc., Portland, ME

Published by:
R & R Publishing, LLC
Chicago, IL 60606
United States of America
info@rnrpublishing.com
http://www.rnrpublishing.com

ISBN 978-0-9764845-5-4

Printed in Canada

Dedication

To our parents—

Vivi	Norma
&	&
Ed	Roland

To Robbie, Robert and our team of angels

To our supporters, advocates and nay-sayers alike

To dreams, synchronicities and driving change around the world

Acknowledgements

Thank you to our core team in collaborating to deliver the enhanced edition of *Let's Eat Out!* including: Katie Mayer, Emily Brackett, Cara Swider, Julie Brink, Apphia Parsons and of course, our loyal and tireless shipper. Sincere appreciation to our supporters in helping to make this a reality: Lori Rennie, Maureen Boudreau, Deb McDonald, Michelle Somkovic, Scott Myers, Graham Price, Katie Koeller, Richard La France, Eriks Jekabsons, Jennifer Cadden, Fernando Cardao, Sione Jongstra, Georgia Cavvouras, Austen Huigens, Christi Holston, Kim Aung, Courtney Lane and our focus group teams. A very special thanks to our trusted Quality Assurance advisor for your enthusiasm, dedication and continuous attention to detail: check, double-check, triple-check...we couldn't have done it without you!

We are also grateful for the expertise and insights of Grant Landis, Ben Carnevale, Carol Kats, Janet Bass, Bennett Berg, Ronni Alicea, Faris Aoun, Claire Kett, John Thornborrow, our clients and global business network. Thank you for helping us envision new horizons, conquer uncharted territories and drive change throughout the world.

Once again, our gratitude to the culinary advisors and chefs who validated our restaurant cuisine content which stands the test of time: Crystal Crawley, Arber Murici, Lumi Devine, Freddy Sanchez, Billy Wilcoxen, Sueson Vess, Lisa Artz, Tim Gannon, Laura Cherry, domenica catelli, Tariq Zaman, Samir Majmudar, Pam Panyasiri, Nicolas Bergerault, Stephane Tremolani, Alfredo Rosiv and Jeff Dattilo.

From Kim—special thanks to Cory Van Wolvelaere, Dale Renner and Paul Cameron for believing in me and my "out-of-the-box" ideas which built the foundation for our pioneering initiatives. Also, my deep appreciation to the health professionals who assist me throughout this adventure of life: Alan Wolf, Leslie Stevenson, Christine Davis, Roger Hughes, Neung Khunsri, Danny Odroniec, Patty Hare, Luis Bracamonte, Dr. Dean Politis, Dr. Erin Arnold, Dr. John Hefferon and Dr. John Hicks.

Last, but certainly not least, cheers to our family and friends for your never-ending encouragement and love—thanks for everything! To everyone—we wish you the freedom of safe eating anywhere.

—Kim and Robert

Intention of Book

This 5-time award-winning book—*Let's Eat Out with Celiac / Coeliac & Food Allergies!* is intended to provide information useful to people living with celiac / coeliac, food allergies and special diets. AllergyFree Passport®, LLC and GlutenFree Passport® as the authors, R & R Publishing, LLC as the publisher, the contributors and reviewers of this book (collectively "we") have made reasonable efforts to make sure that the information provided is accurate and complete. We believe that factual information contained in this book was correct to the best of our knowledge at the time of publication. However, we do not warrant or guarantee that any of the information is accurate or complete. It is not possible for us to have gathered all the information available or independently analyzed or tested the information.

We assume no responsibility for errors, inaccuracies, omissions or typographical errors contained in this book. We expressly disclaim responsibility for any adverse effects arising from the use or application of the information contained herein, as well as responsibility for any liability, injury, loss or damage, whether it be actual, special, consequential, personal or otherwise, which is incurred or allegedly incurred as a direct or indirect consequence of the use and application of any of the contents of this book or for references made within it.

The information contained in this book should not be viewed as medical advice. Questions regarding celiac / coeliac, food allergies, special diets, drug and food interactions and anything related to a specific individual should be addressed to a doctor or other medical practitioner.

We are not responsible for any goods and/or services referred to in this book. By providing this information, we do not endorse any business or advocate the use of any products or services referred to in this book, and the owners or operators of the businesses referred to in this book do not endorse AllergyFree Passport®, LLC, GlutenFree Passport® or R & R Publishing, LLC. We expressly disclaim any liability relating to the use of any goods and/or services referred to in this book.

Although the authors and the publishers of this book are appreciative of the support and information received, AllergyFree Passport®, LLC, GlutenFree Passport® and R & R Publishing, LLC are not affiliated with (and have not received any compensation from or related to) any of the individuals, products, organizations, associations, airlines, restaurants or businesses identified in this book.

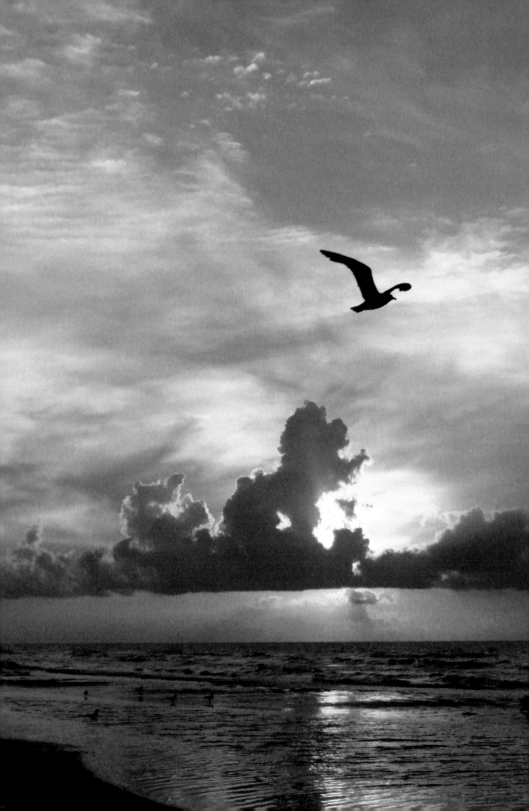

Award-Winning *Let's Eat Out!* Table of Contents

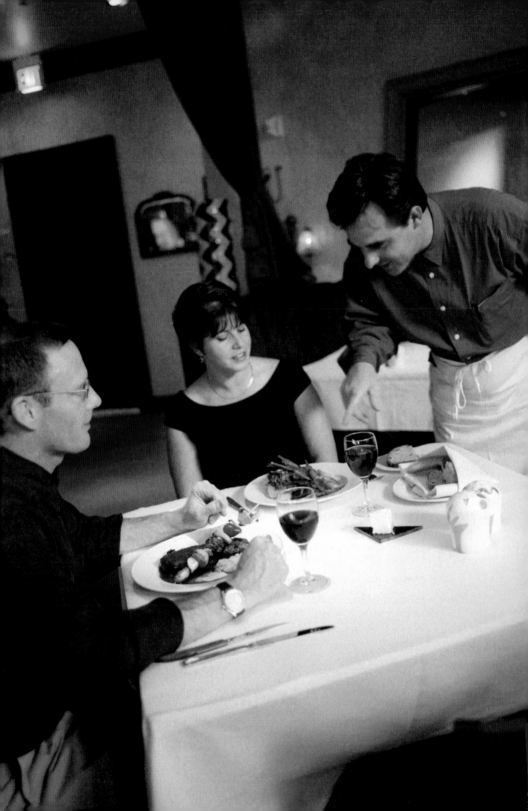

One can say everything best over a meal.
—George Elliot

Introduction

Overview

Eating out in restaurants, around the corner or anywhere around the world, is truly one of life's greatest pleasures. It needs to be enjoyed by all including those managing gluten and allergen-free lifestyles. Food also has tremendous power in our lives. It gives us physical nourishment and provides us with the opportunity to socialize with friends, family and business associates.

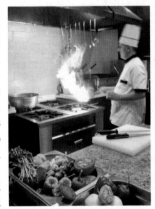

The collaborative effort between guests and eating establishments has been a tradition for hundreds of years, dating back to the 18th century. At that time, Mathurin Roze de Chantoiseau opened the first restaurant in Paris which claimed to serve "only those foods that either maintain or re-establish health". Little did he know that the objective for the world's first documented restaurant would mean so much to the hundreds of millions of people impacted by special diets across the globe.

Eating out in restaurants, at social gatherings and while traveling are key concerns for those on special diets, greatly impacting each individual's quality of life. Cutting edge global market research from AllergyFree Passport® and its affiliate GlutenFree Passport® reveals that the primary factors which influence special diet guests when eating away from home include:

- Safety of gluten and allergen-free meals

- Knowledgeable restaurant and food service personnel

- Fear of an anaphylactic, allergic or gluten reaction

In addition, individuals are also concerned about traveling, which includes eating out in restaurants, finding snacks, flying, choosing accommodations and communicating in foreign languages. At the same time, many restaurants and travel providers around the world are expanding their gluten and allergen-free offerings due to increased customer demand.

Let's Eat Out with Celiac / Coeliac and Food Allergies! is a first-of-its-kind "how-to" book designed to address these considerations by providing an in-depth understanding about eating out and traveling with special dietary requirements for reader audiences such as:

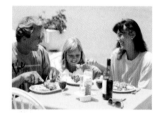

1. Individuals managing celiac / coeliac disease, food allergies and other special diets

2. Family, friends, schoolmates and business colleagues supporting those living gluten & allergen-free lifestyles

3. Industry professionals from restaurants, food service and hospitality serving individuals on special diets

4. Healthcare practitioners advising and counseling individuals impacted by dietary considerations

The book facilitates safe eating experiences by empowering individuals and businesses alike with detailed knowledge about common food allergens such as corn, dairy, eggs, fish, gluten, peanuts, shellfish, soy, tree nuts and wheat. Focused on ingredients, food preparation techniques, hidden allergens, cross-contamination and travel, this book can be used as a daily resource, a reference guide, an educational tool and/or a training manual depending upon your specific perspective.

We hope it meets your diverse needs and empowers you with the knowledge to achieve your desired gluten and allergen-free objectives. This introductory chapter describes:

- Book scope and approach
- Background of authors
- Inspiration for book series
- Book design and methodology

Book Scope and Approach

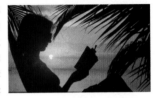

Let's Eat Out with Celiac / Coeliac and Food Allergies! is the enhanced and revised book edition for the *Let's Eat Out!* series which also includes three convenient cuisine-specific guides and one multi-lingual phrase book as described in the Appendix. It should be noted that celiac / coeliac disease is an auto-immune disorder with a permanent intolerance to gluten, the protein found in wheat, rye and barley. Spelled celiac in North America and coeliac throughout the rest of the world, it can only be treated and controlled by the strict adherence to a 100% gluten-free diet. In addition, some individuals managing food allergies may be at risk to anaphylaxis which is a life threatening condition requiring immediate medical attention.

This award-winning book series provides easy-to-use resources that are succinct and flexible to meet the various readers' needs. The scope of the book is the result of years of extensive global market research, consultations, analysis and personal experiences. The content approach and structure are based upon focus group testing/feedback by hundreds of individuals impacted by gluten and allergen-free diets, in-depth hospitality industry assessments and proven results with safe eating experiences worldwide.

The majority of the book content encompasses seven international cuisines which can be found in many cities and countries around the world. This innovative initiative focuses on what can be safely eaten when ordering meals in restaurants based upon a "cuisine-specific" approach.

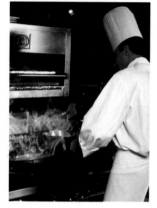

Each cuisine details suggested dishes, meal descriptions and potential food allergen considerations. To determine the 175-plus menu items provided in these chapters, thousands of menus and recipes from all over the world were researched to identify which items were most commonly found in each cuisine. Once established, each was then reviewed to determine which had the highest likelihood of being gluten and wheat-free. The selection was further narrowed down by which dishes had the highest likelihood of not including the eight other food allergens including corn, dairy, eggs, fish, peanuts, shellfish, soy and tree nuts. Then, ingredients, food preparation techniques, hidden allergens and cross-contamination concerns were defined for each menu item.

To ensure accuracy, rigorous quality assurance testing was also conducted with chefs, restaurants and culinary schools worldwide to confirm each of the descriptions, considerations and traditional/non-traditional culinary practices.

Other sections of the book focus on additional eating out and travel guidelines including the proven guest and restaurant approach to safe eating experiences, the learning curve for special diets and the collaborative process. Snack, breakfast and beverage suggestions help individuals safely travel on-the-road with confidence and ease. Applicable checklists detailing considerations for airlines, snacks, hotels, cruise lines and foreign travel are also included for guests and travel providers.

The book is organized in a manner that allows you to use the information in a number of different ways. As with any book, it can be read cover to cover as a reference guide or, if preferred, you can skip around by chapter depending upon what topics you are most interested in learning about. Each chapter stands on its own. It's all about your needs, preferences and areas of concern.

For example, if you're planning to go to an Italian restaurant either close to home or while traveling, you may want to learn about Italian cuisine, potential menu items, associated guidelines and how to communicate your needs. If you work in a French restaurant and want to understand the ingredients, hidden allergens and food preparation techniques, refer to the French cuisine chapter. If you need to re-familiarize yourself on menu items or want a "cheat sheet" to help you navigate the various dishes, review the appropriate cuisines by item in the Allergen-Free or Gluten-Free Preparation Checklists.

If you're going to purchase special dietary products, you can flip to the snack section and reference applicable suggestions. If you are booking airline tickets and want to request a gluten or allergen-free meal, refer to the list of special meal codes in the airline section. The list goes on and on...

Armed with the critical questions to ask, appropriate knowledge and preparation checklists, guests have the opportunity and freedom to safely eat in any restaurant. At the same time, eating establishments can ensure that potentially problematic ingredients, preparation techniques and cross-contamination concerns are addressed when preparing and serving special diet guests.

Background of Authors

Kim Koeller and Robert La France are co-authors of the award-winning *Let's Eat Out!* series and authoritative experts on eating out and traveling with special diets. As internationally recognized speakers, Kim and Robert have presented at celiac / coeliac, food allergy and product industry conferences across Australia, Canada, Europe, New Zealand, United States and other parts of the world. Collectively, they have worked with clients on four continents, traveled over 2.5 million miles, dined-out in 35-plus countries and have conversational skills in 5 languages.

Kim personally manages celiac / coeliac disease as well as over a dozen food related allergies and intolerances including dairy, seafood, fish, pork, preservatives and chemicals. As an international business consultant, she has spent the last 25-plus years eating the majority of her meals in restaurants around the world.

In 2005, Kim founded AllergyFree Passport® and GlutenFree Passport®, global health consulting firms, to drive change worldwide for gluten and allergen-free

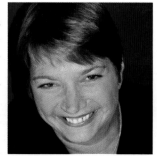

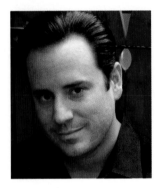

lifestyles. Prior to this, she was a partner with Accenture, the world's leading management consulting firm. Focused on global customer relationship management (CRM) and cutting edge technologies, Kim collaborated with cross-industry Fortune 500 clients delivering innovative sales and service project solutions worldwide for over 17 years. She earned her Masters degree in International Management from the Thunderbird School of Global Management and her Bachelors degree in the French Language from Purdue University.

As a restaurant industry veteran, Robert has spent over 15 years in the hospitality and food service business across all aspects of operations. His international expertise has ranged from small single restaurants to large publicly traded companies with 100-plus locations. Robert's first-hand experiences have afforded him the opportunity to develop deep insights into guest requirements, concerns of cross-contamination and hidden allergens in food preparation.

With a passion for the culinary arts, Robert has been responsible for training hundreds of restaurant personnel, working extensively with Asian, European and North American cuisines. He graduated cum laude from Arizona State University with a Bachelor of Music in Vocal Performance.

Inspiration for Book and Series

The inspiration to create the original *Let's Eat Out!* book and associated series evolved from a number of events, factors and experiences including:

1. Kim's diagnosis with celiac / coeliac disease and food allergies

2. Void in global market place for educational resources about safe eating out experiences

3. Combination of Kim and Robert's areas of expertise

4. Desire to share proven results with hundreds of millions of people impacted by special diets worldwide

After years of misdiagnosis, in 2002, Kim was diagnosed with celiac / coeliac disease and dozens of food allergies as detailed in Chapter 1—Our Personal Journeys from Both Sides of the Table. At that time, she was a partner with Accenture, working with clients across the globe which required her to travel the majority of the time. After tremendous research and effort, she discovered that information about eating outside the home with special diets was practically non-existent. Consequently, she was unsure about what dishes were safe for her to eat while eating out away from home and traveling to various destinations.

Robert, on the other hand, as a restaurant industry professional, had a deep understanding of culinary practices in most international cuisines. When Kim and Robert began going out to eat, he would help expand her choices of eating options either by knowing what was in the dish or by asking the waiter or chef a series of questions to ensure that the meal was safe. Through trial and error, they developed the "cuisine-specific" approach to eating out. After years of research and effort, coupled with overwhelming excitement, they decided to share this invaluable knowledge to improve overall quality of life and give the gift of freedom to others around the world.

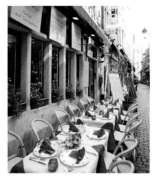

Due to Kim's expertise with delivering industry-leading solutions and her love for pioneering projects, she teamed up with Robert to create this first-of-its-kind book series educating individuals and businesses on safe eating out and traveling with special diets.

Initially published in 2005, the book has been recognized by various publishing industry organizations with awards such as Best Health & Diet, Best Health & Wellness, Best Travel, Best First Non-Fiction and Best Classic Reference. In addition, the *Multi-Lingual Phrase Passport* has also received Best Language and Best Travel Guide awards. The *Let's Eat Out!* book series has been featured in hundreds of magazines, newspapers, radio and TV shows as well as endorsed by celiac / coeliac and food allergy associations across the globe.

While presenting at hundreds of conferences worldwide, Kim and Robert received tremendous positive feedback about the book series and its impact on special diet lifestyles. At the same time, individuals and businesses requested even more detailed information specific to cuisines, menu items, eating out and traveling. After years of extensive research and testing, the new, extremely detailed *Gluten and Allergen-Free Preparation Checklists* in Chapters 11 and 12 now address this demand. Additionally, in-depth travel checklists have also been developed based upon thousands of discussions, to further increase the comfort level with airlines, hotels, cruises and foreign travel.

Voilà! The enhanced and revised edition was created and published!

Book Design and Methodology

Sold in 25-plus countries, this innovative series reflects the collaborative efforts of hundreds of individuals and organizations around the world. The book chapters are categorized into the following six areas for your reference:

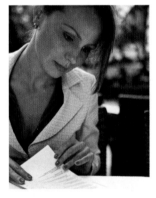

- Personal journeys from both sides of the table
- Approach to safe eating experiences
- Ingredient and preparation technique guidelines
- Seven international cuisines
- Preparation checklists by cuisine
- On-the-road travel suggestions

Personal Journeys from Both Sides of the Table—Chapter 1
Each co-author shares their personal insights from managing a gluten and allergen-free lifestyle to dealing with special diets in restaurants, ultimately providing you with this "how-to" cuisine-specific reference.

Approach to Safe Eating Experiences—Chapter 2
The chapter outlines the learning curve associated with special dietary needs as well as two distinct approaches to dining out from both the guest and

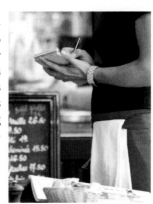

restaurant perspectives. The guest approach to eating outside the home and the restaurant approach to handling special diets detail specific "how-to" steps for each respective party. In addition, suggested questions are provided to help assess your level of preparedness along the way. The collaborative process then outlines the key components required for mutually safe eating experiences from the planning effort to table-side communications.

Ingredient and Preparation Technique Guidelines—Chapter 3

The guidelines describe worldwide product labeling regulations, the Codex Alimentarius, gluten-free labeling, ingredient sourcing and manufacturing processes to be aware of around the world. A Quick Reference Guide is provided outlining key ingredients, food preparation techniques, hidden allergens and cross-contamination concerns by each of the 10 food allergens including corn, dairy, eggs, fish, gluten, peanuts, shellfish, soy, tree nuts and wheat. Each key ingredient is further detailed with traditional and non-traditional culinary practices that highlight areas of consideration. Sample questions are included to help facilitate awareness and understanding for both guest and restaurant staff.

Seven International Cuisines—Chapters 4 through 10

The cuisine chapters detail over 175 menu items from seven of the most common international cuisines found around the world including American Steak and Seafood, Chinese, French, Indian, Italian, Mexican and Thai. The format is standardized across the cuisines, allowing you to easily recognize each section. This design has proven to be effective across the globe in disseminating the necessary information for each cuisine and their respective menu items.

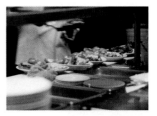

The chapter begins with an overview, explaining background information on the history and culture that are indicative of each cuisine. This information gives you a better understanding of the factors involved in the evolution of the cuisine and the development of traditional practices.

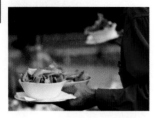

Each cuisine highlights the following:

Traditional Ingredients outline the most common types of foods and beverages that are found in the cuisine such as vegetables, meats, seafood, sides and seasonings.

Gluten Awareness details the areas of food preparation that must be considered for gluten-free meals. These areas of food preparation are explained in detail and a series of requests are presented to help simplify the ordering process. Many of these considerations are identical from chapter to chapter, while others may vary slightly based upon cuisine.

Other Allergy Considerations identify potential sources of hidden food allergens that may be present based upon both traditional and non-traditional culinary practices. Through extensive research, a common theme was discovered across all cuisines: practicality. There are many reasons why restaurants may incorporate non-traditional culinary practices into their cuisine. Lack of availability, associated costs of importing special ingredients and regular customers' preferences can influence an establishment's approach to cooking.

Dining Considerations outline relevant service styles for each cuisine and what to expect from a dining experience based on meal schedules and cultural customs. Specific information about restaurant menus is also presented.

Sample Cuisine Menus identify the name of each dish in its native language along with the English equivalent. In the case of cuisines from countries that do not use the Latin alphabet, such as India and Thailand, the names of each dish are provided phonetically. International cuisines often present each menu item in the language of the country you are in as well as the native language.

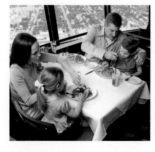

Cuisine Menu Item Descriptions summarize each dish's ingredients and the culinary preparation techniques involved in their creation. Specific areas of food preparation are detailed to show what items need to be confirmed with the restaurant for a gluten/wheat-free meal. Each description also identifies common food allergens that could potentially be included as well as areas of food preparation that must be questioned to ensure safe gluten and allergen-free eating experiences. After each description, the following concerns are outlined:

Gluten-Free Decision Factors:

- "Ensure" an ingredient is not present as part of the food preparation

Food Allergen Preparation Considerations:

- "Contains" an allergen from an ingredient in alphabetical order

- "May contain" an allergen from an ingredient in alphabetical order

Preparation Checklists by Cuisine— Chapters 11 and 12

The *Allergen-Free and Gluten-Free Preparation Checklists* are designed to quickly identify ingredients, food preparation techniques, hidden allergens and cross-contamination concerns by menu item. This significantly simplifies the ordering process between guests and restaurants by quickly identifying questions to ask so that meals are gluten and allergen-free. These comprehensive "cheat sheets" also provide guidelines on key areas of concern to consider for each of the dishes within the seven international cuisine chapters.

In Chapter 11, *Allergen-Free Preparation Checklists*, over 130 considerations are detailed to address areas where you may potentially encounter the 10 common food allergens. Each of these food allergens are also color coded for easy reference.

In Chapter 12, *Gluten-Free Preparation Checklists*, 25-plus key areas of concern are identified for each of the menu items which have the potential to contain gluten or wheat.

Armed with these detailed checklists at your fingertips, one can effectively communicate special dietary needs to ensure that the menu items have been prepared without the specific allergen(s) of concern and are safe to eat.

Color Key for the Preparation Checklists

Corn–dark brown
Soy–light brown
Gluten/Wheat–dark yellow
Dairy–light yellow
Fish–dark blue
Shellfish–light blue
Peanuts–dark green
Tree Nuts–light green
Eggs–pink

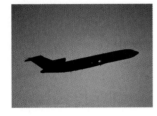

On-The-Road Travel Suggestions—Chapters 13 and 14

These suggestions are designed to assist you while eating outside the home and traveling across the globe. *Snack, Breakfast and Beverage Suggestions* focus on snack tips, breakfast alternatives and non-alcoholic and alcoholic beverage options either at home or on-the-road. The three types of snacks that are described include no preparation, hot water preparation and cooler required. In addition to a breakfast meal overview, a list of common ingredients found in beverages is outlined. Also, suggested non-alcoholic beverages are detailed as well as a list of alcoholic beverages with their associated distillation process.

Airline, Hotel, Cruise and Travel Tips provide detailed checklists to jump start planning efforts for safe gluten and/or allergen-free travels anywhere around the world. The airline-specific guidelines address carry-on snack considerations and over 25 standard airline meal codes based on medically prescribed lifestyles, recommended lifestyles, age, religious considerations and health preferences. Two additional checklists detail how to effectively order airline meals and how to travel by air while at risk to anaphylaxis.

The hotel and accommodations checklist address how to safely travel when exploring new destinations by land or sea. International travel tips and sample translation cards are also provided to help increase your comfort level while staying in English or foreign-speaking destinations.

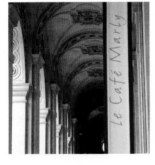

The gluten and allergen-free translation cards provide key phrases integral to communicating specific food concerns while traveling in foreign-speaking countries. Even if you do not know how to pronounce the words, the format is designed so that you may point directly to the card to express your concerns and/or provide it to the staff and chef. Available in a downloadable format, these phrases have been translated by a professional translation service and quality assurance tested with native speakers to ensure accuracy and applicability based upon contemporary cultural idioms.

Additional Gluten and Allergen-Free Resources—Appendix

The appendix outlines extensive on-line resources to further assist in your search for information about eating outside the home as well as catering to guests with special dietary requirements. These resources include thousands of global gluten and allergen-free organizations, eating establishments, reading materials, stores, manufacturers, airlines, products, labeling regulations, translation cards and websites around the world.

Closing Remarks

Knowledge is power! Our mission is to drive change worldwide for gluten and allergen-free lifestyles. Specifically our vision is to empower individuals with celiac / coeliac, food allergies and special diets to safely eat out whether around the corner or around the world. We also educate businesses to recognize and expand their offerings to address special dietary needs.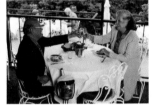

From our own experiences, we realize that knowledge alone, however, is not enough to avoid encountering food allergens while eating out and traveling. This requires due diligence, collaborating with restaurant and travel professionals, educating yourself and reading labels to facilitate safe eating experiences. By addressing this process ourselves, we feel confident that posing the right questions, combined with understanding the cuisines and suggestions will help alleviate some of the stress associated with managing celiac / coeliac disease, food allergies and special diets.

And remember,

> **"Life loves to be taken by the lapel and told, 'I am with you kid. Let's go!'"**
> —Maya Angelou

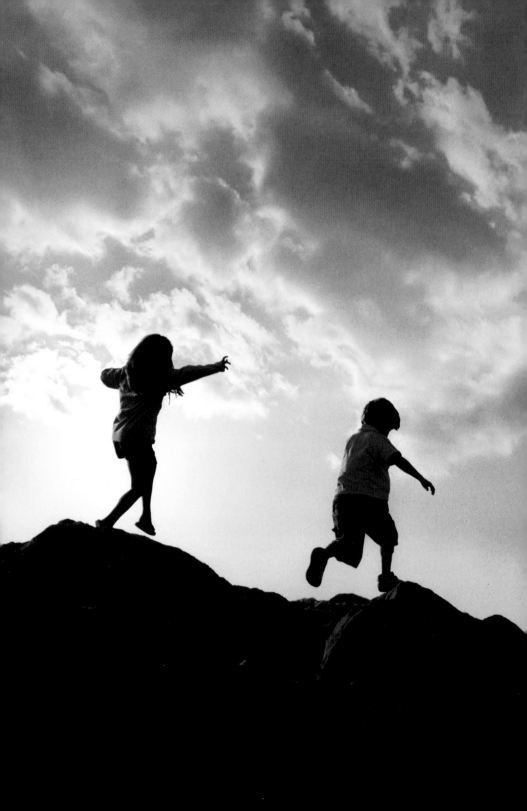

Do not follow where the path may lead.
Go instead where there is no path and leave a trail.
—Ralph Waldo Emerson

1

Chapter 1

Our Personal Journeys from Both Sides of the Table

Chapter Overview

We view life as a series of journeys which lead to new adventures. Every journey has its ups and downs, from positive moments that you always want to savor to those so painful that you may want to forget. Most journeys and adventures typically take unexpected twists and turns which give us the opportunity to learn something about ourselves, others and life in general.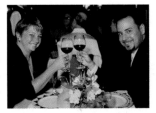

From our perspective, the only failures in life are when we do not learn from these opportunities. As the saying goes, every education has its tuition. We would like to share our journeys with you, the reader, to provide our first hand insights reflecting:

- Kim's journey to embracing the gluten and allergen-free life

- Robert's journey in dealing with special diets: The other side of the table

Kim's Journey to Embracing the Gluten and Allergen-Free Life

1

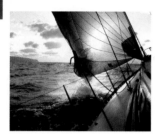

I've definitely had my fair share of twists and turns with their accompanying lessons along the path called life. Writing our first book as well as this enhanced edition has forced me to summarize my experiences and make sense of them. It's amazing how much I had forgotten or blocked out of my mind.

My health concerns over the years include 12 orthopedic surgeries, multiple broken bones and over 3 years of physical therapy, combined with 9-plus years of digestive disorders, skin conditions, fatigue, joint inflammation and misdiagnosis. It finally all made sense in 2002, when I was diagnosed with celiac / coeliac disease as well as dozens of food allergies and environmental intolerances. Then in 2008, I was diagnosed with osteopenia.

Although many of my health lessons have been extremely challenging, I think of them as gifts and something to be appreciated. I did sometimes question how I was going to get through all of them in one piece. Sometimes, that light at the end of the tunnel did seem like it had been turned off, yet in the end they were each unusual learning opportunities!

Looking back, I am now very thankful for each of these experiences which have led to my current path in life. Despite my health challenges, I continue to enjoy being as athletic as possible while having fun with family and friends. I am very grateful that I traveled extensively prior to my diagnosis of celiac / coeliac and food allergies, and still love exploring the world to this day. I also appreciate all of the opportunities, both personal and professional, that I have had to live, work and experience local cultures first-hand on four continents as an international management consultant. Working with global clients and traveling while safely eating outside my home continues to be an integral part to embracing my gluten and allergen-free lifestyle.

I would like to share my story with you, in the hope that it may help with your unique adventures. My journeys are organized within the following six areas:

- Early evidence of allergies and intolerances

- Adventures in traveling

- My journey with sports and health

- Discovery and diagnosis

- The road to empowerment

- Thanks to family, friends and restaurants

Early Evidence of Allergies and Intolerances

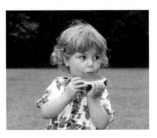

Ever since I was a young girl, I've been allergic to cats, fish and seafood. My throat starts to close, my eyes water and breathing is difficult. Sometimes, I feel nauseous, start sneezing and wheezing. In my teenage years, after experiencing skin reactions, it was determined through the process of elimination that I was allergic to goose feathers, down and wool. I also had reactions to various chemicals and additives in detergents, soaps, creams and make-up.

In my mid 20's, I had swollen and blood shot eyes. Again, through the process of elimination, my optometrist determined that this was an allergic reaction to thimersol, a chemical in some saline solutions for contact lenses. It still makes me laugh thinking about the questions I received from friends concerning my appearance during that time!

In my late 20's, I experienced bladder issues which were extremely rare for my age. After visiting numerous specialists and extensive testing, I consulted with my general physician. Based on her recommendation, I removed caffeine as the first part of my elimination diet. My condition improved slightly; however, the symptoms were still occurring. Next, she identified another potential culprit—aspartame. After eliminating all foods with aspartame from my diet, the issues were immediately resolved. I was so relieved that we had finally figured it out. I am eternally grateful to this physician for identifying the causes of these symptoms.

A few months later, I realized that I had the tendency to get sick within 30 to 60 minutes after eating Chinese food. Once again, through the process of

1

elimination and investigation, we determined that Monosodium Glutamate (MSG) was the cause of my reactions.

Another situation occurred within a few minutes of receiving anesthesia for one of my surgeries. My throat started to close up and my breathing became extremely labored. Realizing that I was having an allergic reaction, I found out that they had given me penicillin. Luckily, I remembered that my great aunt had died from a shot of penicillin, so I was grateful that they immediately counteracted my reaction with an injection. Looking back, these may have been early warning signs of things to come. I just wasn't aware of my level of sensitivities at the time. In hindsight, there was a definite pattern emerging which unfortunately took over 15 years to fully decipher.

Adventures in Traveling

I've always been very fascinated by new places, people and cultures. The first time I realized my love for traveling was when I was five years old and my family drove from Chicago to my Aunt Greta's farm in Ohio. Throughout my childhood, for two weeks every summer, my family and I trekked throughout the United States and Canada in a camper trailer, exploring different destinations and experiencing new adventures. I loved it! For my 8th grade graduation present, my parents gave me the choice of flying to New York to visit relatives or a new bicycle. I chose the trip, of course, and still remember where I was sitting on the plane to this day!

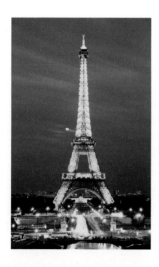

Hearing my grandparents occasionally recite phrases in French and German always intrigued me. I started taking French lessons at the age of 13 and adored learning languages. One of my teachers in high school even taught me Spanish in her spare time after class. My first trip to Europe was at the age of 16 with my French class as an early high school graduation present. After falling in love with Paris, my new criteria for choosing a university focused on two areas: a study abroad program and a Big 10 sports program.

During my third year of college, I lived in Strasbourg, France and studied all of my courses in French. My diet primarily consisted of baguettes (French bread), petit pains au chocolat (chocolate croissants), yogurt and cheese. I backpacked through Europe, played tour guide when friends and family came to visit and felt great physically. To this day, I still meet friends in Paris every year to enjoy the culture and, of course, the outdoor cafés.

After graduating from Purdue University with a Bachelor of Arts Degree in the French language with a minor in business, I worked with domestic corporate clients for six years. I then earned my Masters in International Management at the Thunderbird School of Global Management and met lots of excellent friends along the way.

For the next 17 years, as a global business consultant with Accenture, the world's leading management consulting firm, I worked with clients all over the world. Leveraging my expertise in customer interaction solutions, I managed diverse project teams across global customer relationship management (CRM), worldwide technologies and business integration practices. We collaborated with cross-industry Fortune 500 clients delivering innovative sales and service engagements on four continents, including 12 first-ever industry leading implementations.

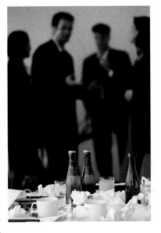

Discovering life and cultures in South America, Europe and Australia was also extremely rewarding, both personally and professionally. I lived in Sao Paulo for seven months, Sydney for five months, Turin for three months and numerous European locations such as Geneva, London, Munich and Prague for one to two months. While living in these countries, I learned conversational skills in Italian and Portuguese. Throughout this time, I continued to avoid foods that I knew did not agree with me and managed my knee-related problems.

Working in North America, my travel typically involved flying two to eight times a week. I consulted with clients from New York to San Francisco, Dallas to Toronto, Los Angeles to Washington DC, Montreal to Mexico City and everywhere in between.

Working my way up the corporate ladder to Partner, I loved my clients, my career and almost every minute of my personal and business travel. Since establishing GlutenFree Passport® and AllergyFree

1

Passport®, I have continued working with clients and organizations across the globe enabling me to travel to Australia, Europe, New Zealand and throughout North America on a regular basis. Over the past 25-plus years, I have flown almost 2 million miles to more than 30 countries and have eaten the majority of my meals in restaurants.

As glamorous as this may sound, it required a lot of energy, especially during my recuperation from six knee surgeries and four stress fractures. While traveling from continent to continent, I was in more planes and taxis with crutches and pushed in wheelchairs through airports than I ever care to remember!

My Journey with Sports and Health

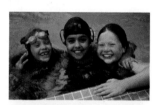
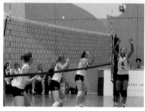

Since childhood, the two things that I've been most passionate about are traveling and sports. From a sports perspective, I was a healthy athletic child, teenager and young adult who loved volleyball, tennis, cheerleading, softball, basketball, swimming, diving, surfing and yes, even baton twirling! I experienced my fair share of broken bones including my elbow, collarbone, fingers and wrist. These were all typical injuries due to athletics and I took each of them in stride.

In celebration of our 30th birthdays, my friends and I completed our first team relay triathlon. Swimming in Lake Michigan for a mile was a challenge for me since I already had overcome two knee surgeries due to skiing and volleyball, as well as four forearm reconstructive surgeries as a result of a severe car accident. Over the next few years, our teams of family and friends accomplished a total of three team relay triathlons and had lots of fun in the process!

By my mid 30's, due to continuous pain and instability, I was required to have three more knee surgeries within three and a half years just to be able to walk. My first was arthroscopic to repair my cartilage. The second was an Anterior Cruciate Ligament (ACL) reconstruction requiring 6 ½ hours of surgery and 10 months of physical therapy to walk again. I gained weight and felt continuous abdominal bloating. Unfortunately, I never regained the energy level that I had before this surgery.

1

During this time, I began experiencing acid reflux, cramping, diarrhea, flatulence, vomiting, heartburn and indigestion. On top of all this, my third knee surgery was an ACL on the other knee, requiring three hours of surgery and five months of physical therapy. In hindsight, these traumas may have potentially triggered my celiac / coeliac disease, which was yet to be diagnosed.

Based upon my surgeries and injuries, I began an in-depth exploration of Eastern and alternative healing practices. These included acupuncture, Chinese medicine, herbs, reiki, reflexology and massage therapy. The combination of Eastern and Western practices with health professionals helped me recover from these injuries. However, no matter what we tried, I couldn't regain my energy level or lose the excess weight. My only "exercise" was physical therapy, restricted swimming and minimal walking. If that wasn't enough, I had to have one more knee surgery to remove the screws from my previous reconstruction requiring more anesthesia and physical therapy.

By this time, I had grown weary of recuperating from surgeries and physical therapy. I chose boxing as my new fitness challenge to jumpstart my metabolism and increase flexibility. Thanks to the patience of my boxing coach, my endurance, strength and agility improved with each lesson—all without boxing an opponent in the ring! Finally, my first new sport in years and a great change of pace from all the injuries. Hoorah!

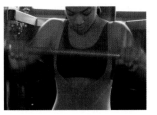

My excitement was short-lived as a year and a half later I lost the range of motion in my arm and could only lift it a few inches from my body. After a month of testing, the doctors determined that I actually needed two rotator cuff surgeries in a matter of 4 ½ months caused by bone spurs. I was also still experiencing stiffness, muscle cramps and inflamed joints throughout the rest of my body. So back to physical therapy, walking and swimming once again.

A few years later, I was diagnosed with celiac / coeliac disease and dozens of allergies. Finally, after following a strict gluten and allergen-free diet, I started feeling as though my body was repairing itself and getting stronger. Being an athlete, I wanted to test myself

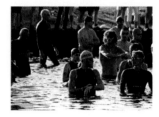

from a health perspective. Could I complete another mile swim in Lake Michigan as part of a relay triathlon team after all of my surgeries, physical therapy and latest diagnoses?

My friends and I decided to go for it. Just two years after my diagnosis, I finished the mile swim in the largest triathlon in the US. I wish that I could say that my finishing time was stellar—unfortunately, that was not the case. I was one of the last people out of Lake Michigan in Chicago that day. Nevertheless, the sense of accomplishment was incredible. I had achieved my goal!

For the next two years, I continued to enjoy swimming, boxing lessons and weight training supported by my healthy and strong body! Then, the next few years became rather challenging from a fitness perspective again due to bone issues as described later. Once resolved, I again set out to train for triathlons and get back to being physically fit, flexible and balanced. Finally, my road to health was coming full circle after 20-plus years of challenges, pain and great struggle. As my Dad always said, "You can accomplish anything you set your mind to as long as you're willing to work for it. It's just a matter of attitude and how determined you are to succeed to the best of your ability."

Discovery and Diagnosis

Throughout my surgeries and recuperation, my digestion, respiratory and skin related issues continued to escalate. After constant abdominal pain and diarrhea, I was so weak that I had to be driven to the doctor who immediately scheduled me for a colonoscopy. The doctor found polyps in my colon and diagnosed me with ulcerative colitis, leaky gut and Crohn's disease.

After careful analysis, I found health professionals who specialized in digestive disorders. Based upon more testing, a strict regimen of a bland diet, protein drinks, sulphasalazine, herbs and various supplements were recommended. My insides were finally starting to repair themselves and my energy level was improving slightly. I still felt as though my food was not being processed appropriately, but at least my body was getting somewhat better with my symptoms occurring less frequently.

My acupuncturist, who was also an MD, began assessing the cause of my joint pain and bone spurs. She asked about my consumption of dairy, which I ate on a daily basis. Needless to say, I loved milk, yogurt, cheese and cottage cheese. Upon her recommendation, I eliminated dairy from my diet and immediately began to feel a difference in my joints and my throat. I felt better and decided to avoid dairy since I never wanted to endure another surgery again!

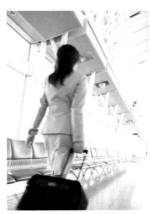

While traveling, I was also getting sick within 30 to 60 minutes after eating airplane meals and snacks due to preservatives. I started to eliminate various foods from my diet and focus on listening to how my body responded to different foods. I followed some rotation diet recommendations including vegetables, fruits, pastas and meats. Unfortunately, at this point, I was totally unaware of any hidden allergens in foods. Although I thought I had eliminated specific potential allergens from my diet, in reality, I had not.

During this time, I lived in Italy. I ate incredible pasta, Italian bread, salamis and salads. My favorite meals were Veal Milanese, Chicken Parmigiana and Beef Medallions with sauce. While home in the States for a week at a time, I would avoid these foods because I enjoyed them so much more in Italy. By the end of each week in the States, I realized that I felt a bit better. Back in Italy, I continued eating my favorite foods and experienced bloating, cramping, flatulence and indigestion again. I remember thinking that my reactions were a bit unusual and maybe I just needed to reduce the amount of pasta I ate, which I did.

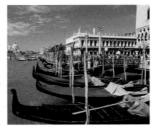

I also found myself taking Mylanta, ginger, turmeric and other digestive aids on a daily basis. I was still experiencing very low energy, fatigue and lethargy. All of a sudden, extremely dark circles appeared under my eyes, my skin turned a pale grey and my nails became brittle. My headaches escalated to migraines. My nausea escalated into vomiting. My gums started bleeding and a couple of my teeth were loose. I started having palpitations and sensitivity to cold. I was unable to sleep for longer than two hours at a time and keeping foods in my body was a challenge.

1

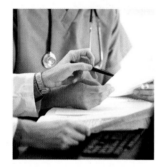

What was going on with me? I attributed these reactions to my increased stress level due to working extremely long hours on more high-profile client projects after my promotion to Partner at Accenture. I just couldn't believe how bad I felt physically. Luckily, my two friends, Kelly and Allison, approached me in "the bunkroom" and insisted I investigate these symptoms with a doctor. I can still hear their words, "Kim, something is definitely not right and you have to check it out now." I am forever thankful to my friends for their encouragement and persistence in convincing me to seek medical attention.

As you can imagine, after 12 orthopedic surgeries and over 3 years of physical therapy, coupled with a high tolerance for pain, I tried to avoid doctors at all costs (nothing personal to those of you who are doctors!). I contacted numerous healthcare professionals for referrals and suggested that maybe, just maybe, this had to do with allergies. A multitude of medical tests were conducted by different medical teams. Although there were discrepancies between the various test results, they confirmed my allergic reactions to dairy, fish, shellfish, chemicals and cats. After years of misdiagnosis, I was told that I had celiac / coeliac disease as well as allergies to other food and environmental allergens. These included pork, preservatives, sodium nitrate, fluoride, ammonia, bleach and food dyes to name a few.

Once I understood what needed to be eliminated from my diet, with commitment to strict adherence, I began to feel a difference immediately. It was truly amazing! After more than 10 years of chronic pain and over 8 years to be properly diagnosed, my team of specialists determined what I needed to do to feel better. I finally started to repair my body.

Following a gluten and allergen-free diet combined with exercise, herbs and detoxification, my quality of life began to increase significantly. The majority of my recovery took place during the next two years. I just kept feeling better and younger. My energy level continued to increase as my body focused on processing the proper nutrients rather than trying to protect me from intolerable foods. For the next four years, I was healthier, more energetic and happier than I had been in a very long time!

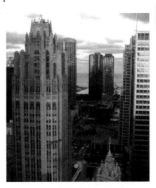

Then my next journey began. After a few months of unexplained pain in my right foot, I visited my orthopedic surgeon. I learned that I had a stress fracture and needed to wear an immobilizing boot for 2 months. Unfortunately for me, it took over 7 months to heal and finally be able to wear shoes on both feet again.

After this, I had my Bone Mineral Density (BMD) tested to assess the strength of my bones. The doctor stated that my Dual Energy X-ray Absorptiometry (DEXA) scan showed the BMD to be normal and that my next test should be in another 2–3 years. Based on this feedback, I started training for another team triathlon which unfortunately was short-lived.

Then, to make a very long story short, within 8 months, I had three more stress fractures. After lots of pain and immobilizers, my orthopedic doctor detected osteopenia in my left foot which describes a BMD which is lower than normal peak. How could this be the case if all of my tests were normal? I finally met with other specialists who determined that I had deficiencies in Vitamin D, calcium and magnesium to name a few. To keep my condition from progressing to osteoporosis, I started increasing my intake of specific supplements. I also focused on eating more safe gluten and allergen-free foods that supported good bone health coupled with exercise, acupuncture, reiki, Trager therapy and energy work to help heal my body once again.

After requesting my original DEXA scan test report, I discovered that I had originally been misinformed about my BMD results. In actuality, they had only indicated normal bone density for my lumbar spine and hip. For my femoral neck, the results showed, in plain black and white print, moderate osteopenia. To think, my situation could have been completely avoided if it had been addressed immediately instead of not knowing for over one year. Obviously, that doctor will *never* ever be consulted again!

I just keep telling myself that everything happens for a reason, so I hope that my experiences somehow help some of you avoid similar issues along your path. Yet again, I am back to enjoying my healthy adventures

1

wherever they may take me. I continue to be amazed at what our minds, bodies and spirits are capable of accomplishing once we have all of the facts and determine how to balance the needs of our bodies.

The Road to Empowerment

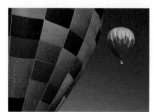

When I first received my life changing diagnosis of celiac / coeliac and food allergies, I felt relief that my team of specialists finally figured "it" out. I made the decision shortly thereafter that my health considerations were not going to limit me and that I was going to do what needed to be done to take back my freedom. However, a critical new question surfaced—"How do I live?"

At that time, I began yet another new phase of my journey which evolved into the foundation for Chapter 2—Approach to Safe Eating Experiences. The following are my four key stages of learning about special diets:

1. Awareness—What exactly have I been diagnosed with?

2. Information—What can I eat and what do I need to avoid?

3. Knowledge—Now that I have this information, how do I apply it to real life?

4. Empowerment—How do I live and enjoy myself while being diligent with foods anywhere in the world?

There was a lot of trial and error, a continuous learning curve and huge adjustments throughout the next few years. Going through each stage to eliminate all of the allergens as well as following a 100% gluten and allergen-free diet to become empowered was difficult to say the least. Yet it was all worth it in the end!

At the beginning of stage 1—awareness, I just remember sitting there dumbfounded, thinking, "Wow! What do I do? How do you even spell these words? What in the world do they mean? What exactly is my diagnosis? What is gluten? What are hidden allergens? More importantly, what can I eat when I'm at home in Chicago or away traveling in the States or overseas? How do I eat in airports, hotels and at client meetings?"

Most people recently diagnosed typically think just the opposite, "What meals can be prepared at home? What cookbooks can be purchased? How can my favorite recipes be modified? How do I ensure that my home is gluten and allergen-free? What items and brands can I purchase?" Eating outside the home and travel may or may not be at the top of the priority list for those newly diagnosed.

For me, learning to eat anywhere and traveling with celiac / coeliac and all of my allergies was priority number one. Global travel was an integral part of my personality and international business career. I was not willing to give up what I loved to do, both from a personal and professional standpoint. I had to figure out how to control my special diet instead of letting my special diet control me. In order to continue my lifestyle, I needed to quickly figure out how to eat safe gluten and allergen-free foods anywhere in the world, regardless of my location or destination.

As a result, I moved into stage 2—information gathering. I spent all of my free time researching what I could and could not eat outside and inside the home, both across the globe and in the US. I spent hours upon hours in grocery stores, diligently reviewing product lists and reading labels only to walk out completely exhausted. I reviewed cookbooks for ingredients trying to figure out how to order certain dishes when I was in restaurants.

I conducted extensive research to determine how to safely eat outside the home in restaurants located in both English and foreign language speaking countries. I scoured hundreds and hundreds of websites, subscribed to allergy-related publications and joined 20-plus international celiac / coeliac and allergy associations. With all of this information, I studied, took notes, memorized and felt like I was back at school again.

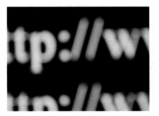

The focus of this literature was either on gluten and allergen-free cooking in the home or background information about coping with allergies. A very small percentage of these books discussed eating in restaurants and traveling with gluten and allergen-free diets. I was very surprised to realize that books devoted to these topics had not been written. There was a tre-

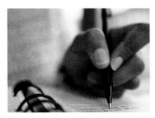

1

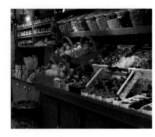

mendous void in the global marketplace for educating individuals and businesses about eating outside the home with special diets. I then contacted 100-plus global associations for information and researched various cities.

I began assimilating the information that I had gathered into knowledge which marked my progression into stage 3. I explored many cuisines, restaurants, stores and pharmacies first hand and even discovered the standard airline code to order a gluten-free meal (GFML). I created detailed spreadsheets identifying ingredients in various cuisines and dishes as well as lists of fast food chains and restaurants with potential foods to eat. I designed electronic and pocket-size paper tri-fold materials with foreign language phrases to communicate with restaurants overseas. I then downloaded all of these files to my mobile phone for easy access anywhere. What can I say, it's the consultant in me to always be prepared!

At the time, I was solely focused on plain and simple foods that I thought would be safe to eat, based upon my research, both in restaurants and at home. I just could not bear the thought of having any of my old symptoms occur again since it took me so long to get to this point. Unfortunately, regardless of my efforts, I still got sick while traveling, although infrequently. In the early days, while doubled over in pain and recuperating for days, I sometimes would wonder to myself, "Why exactly am I doing this? It would have been so much safer for me to cook my own meals and accept the situation." However, staying at home or preparing meals in a hotel room kitchenette while traveling is just not in my nature.

Then, I reached the stage that, although still in pain for days, I would wonder, "How did this happen?" instead of "Why did I do this?" I immediately would assess what could have caused me to get sick, how this could have been avoided and what I would change the next time around.

I started experimenting with what snacks made the most sense to carry with me on airplanes and to my destinations. I still laugh when I think about the security guard at a US airport who said, "Is that a hard boiled egg that I just saw in the carry-on luggage scanner?" I continued traveling to numerous destinations across the globe due to my client project commitments, learning about local cuisines, exploring stores and finding new snacks along the way.

Additionally, I started working on the multi-faceted 311 project for the City of New York. One of my friends from graduate school introduced me to Robert, a colleague of his from the restaurant business living in Manhattan. When we went out to dinner, I was still ordering plain everything and anything. With Robert's culinary experience and extensive restaurant background, he started convincing me that my food choices could expand from plain salad, chicken or broccoli to new things such as red wine reduction sauce.

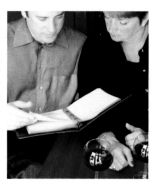

Based upon my dining experiences with Robert, we began to combine our knowledge of safe and unsafe ingredients. There was extensive trial and error determining what foods to eat in restaurants and what were the safest menu items. It took some time, but we began to discover what had the highest probability of having hidden allergens and where I might have issues with food preparation techniques.

We started to develop our own list of what questions to ask and what areas of food preparation may pose the biggest concerns. After identifying what could make things easier on the restaurant staff, we determined what could simplify the ordering process for both the guest and the server while still ensuring a safe dining experience. We started to cautiously experiment with various restaurants, cuisines and menu items.

My world began to open back up again. I started thinking that I could safely and confidently eat out like a normal person—just with special dietary considerations. Feeling empowered to live and enjoy myself while being diligent with foods anywhere in the world is truly incredible! I began to feel that I finally had the most difficult part of the learning curve behind me.

Realizing how valuable this research and knowledge could be for other individuals living with special diets as well as for businesses, my friends and family encouraged me to write a book that could potentially help millions on a global basis. Robert and I started to evaluate how

1

best to share our experiences with guests and restaurants around the world. We wanted to empower people with knowledge to safely eat outside the home, from a trip to your Grandmother's house to traveling internationally, as well as educate businesses on how to recognize and expand their gluten and allergen-free offerings.

I had the perspective of the individual impacted with celiac / coeliac and food allergies combined with my business consulting knowledge. Robert had the restaurant perspective of serving guests with special dietary requirements coupled with his culinary experiences. The combination of our backgrounds and expertise made the ideal atmosphere for collaboration on what eventually culminated into this internationally acclaimed 7-time award winning book series!

Thanks to Family, Friends and Restaurants

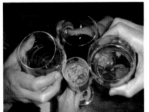

I am also very grateful for the support I received from family, friends and business colleagues over the years once they understood my situation. Thank you all for taking my dietary concerns into consideration and helping me when needed. Eating outside the home is a collaborative effort between the person impacted with special diets, their dining companions and the people preparing the food including restaurant professionals, food service and even relatives.

Sometimes, it gets a bit tiresome explaining special dietary requirements on a constant basis. Although I've only mentioned a few of you below, everyone's help, acknowledgment and understanding are much appreciated. These are also examples of how those of you readers can help family, friends and even customers with special diets while in restaurants, at social gatherings, school or your own home.

Mom - I'll always remember you perfecting your delicious gluten and allergen-free coffee cakes, Grandma's chocolate chip cookies, apple crisps and my angel food birthday cakes. Thank you so much for the many safe and tasty meals including the turkey at family parties. They will go down in history for me and when the grandkids want to eat my "special" food—you know it's good.

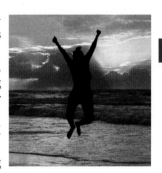

Bob - I very much appreciate your knowledge, diligence and expertise in helping to expand my options so I could confidently become a foodie again—yeah!

Club Girls including Shar, Hops, Cindy, Slukes, Karen, Kathy, Jody and Kathy - Thanks for considering my special diet concerns when preparing goodies for our fun get-togethers.

Ivanka - My appreciation for thinking about what I can potentially eat wherever we might be.

Faris - Thanks for your support and understanding from exploring fun restaurants to eating my portions at the cooking school to our wine-tasting adventures.

Brad - I appreciate your help when we go "spelunking" to discover new places and open up our choices of possibilities.

Betsy and Gary - Thanks for calling me to check what I can eat and what is safe when you're hosting your infamous dinner parties!

Consuelo and Dawn - My gratitude for thinking about my special diet when considering places to eat!

Lisa and Jan - Your research on newly-opened restaurants to check what dishes I might enjoy means so much to me—thanks for your pool parties, too!

Beth and Kathy - I appreciate you asking questions and thinking about what I could and could not eat at our various family gatherings.

Katinka - Changing plans to an allergen-friendly restaurant meant the world to me.

Todd - I still laugh thinking about the restaurant in Washington DC that wouldn't serve me and you politely asked, "Can't you just make her a salad?"

Camille and Eva - Thanks for your concern and diligence when ordering safe take-out for me on those long nights of work during our client project.

Bev - My gratitude for the pep talk a few days after my diagnosis, while I was still in shock and sitting on the floor at a closed O'Hare airport with my raw carrots and a bottle of water.

University of Chicago Celiac Disease Center - I'll always remember the welcome package that initially opened my eyes to the world of gluten-free foods!

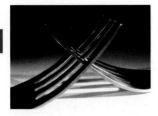

Highlights of my restaurant experiences are thanks to the respective waiters, waitresses, managers, room service staff, owners and chefs from all over the world. You may never realize just how much you may have impacted someone's life, health and memories while you were preparing our safe foods, taking our orders and listening to our needs!

I hope that you, the reader, also experience similar benefits and gifts on your journey to health, adventure and travel. A small sampling of my most memorable eating experiences that are safe from gluten and all of my other allergen concerns include:

- Ristoro Di Lamole in Tuscany for surprising me with gluten-free pasta

- Walt Disney World in Orlando for my "Mickey" meals

- Christchurch Cathedral Café in New Zealand for my first soup and bread lunch

- Matteos Pizza in Tennessee for my first personalized delivery order

- Chesterfield Beer Festival in the UK for bartending and taste testing 16 gluten-free beers

- In-N-Out Burger for my protein burgers wrapped in lettuce

- Café Marley in Paris for my first main dish served with an amazing sauce

- The Palm and Ruth's Chris for my mouth-watering salads and steaks

- Rotorua food stand in New Zealand for my first cake at an airport

- Il Bistro in Seattle for the first time I had three allergen-free dessert choices

- Gaucho Grill in London for delicious Argentinean dishes

I am also grateful for those amazing moments in time that can only be experienced outside your own home. Favorites that inspire me to explore new restaurants and places with friends and family around the world are the Enoteca in Montalcino, Rothschild Chateau and the Parisian cafés. I also remember those travel adventures in English-speaking destinations that are among the top of my list including the Ocean Spirit catamaran at the Great Barrier Reef, sunrise over the Grand Canyon, wine tasting in Martinborough New Zealand and my hideaways in Miami, Santa Monica and Sydney.

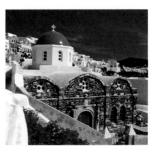

Even more challenging is safely eating in foreign-speaking countries, especially in cultures with different alphabets. Of course, more research, planning and education are required when you are on your own without the benefit of tour guides or translators. I will always cherish Paris, sailing the Greek Isles, New Years in Florence, the Baltic Sea in Latvia and exploring both Moscow and St. Petersburg in Russia. Experiencing local cultures, foreign cuisines and new restaurants are key and all part of the fun adventures even if it takes more effort and preparation!

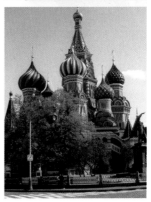

In closing, I want to share some of my first-hand insights throughout my journey:

- The amount of hard work, adjustments and frustrations are worth it

- Recovery is definitely possible and doable—it just takes a lot of effort and determination

- You are in charge of your health and always listen to your body

- Learn something new every day

- What goes around, comes around

- You *can* safely eat out anywhere—just educate yourself, be prepared and communicate your needs

- Live each day to the fullest: work hard, play hard and most importantly, have fun!

1

Robert's Journey in Dealing with Special Diets: The Other Side of the Table

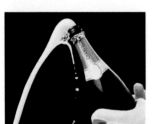

How did I get here? I mean here, in front of my computer finalizing what is the culmination of years of research and writing. I have spent the majority of my adult life in front of people, either in front of guests as a restaurant service industry professional or on stage as an actor.

Never in a million years did I think I would co-write a book, much less this enhanced edition, about eating outside the home and travel for people with special dietary requirements. In the end, it turns out that my life experiences were the perfect compliment to Kim's; one side knows the realities of living life while managing special dietary requirements and the other side knows the restaurant position on how to effectively serve those who must adhere to special diets. Without those two perspectives working in collaboration, this work could never have been accomplished.

Understanding guest requirements was a priority for me in my restaurant career. Looking back, I tried to determine what events in my life caused me to take this part of my job so seriously. After all, the restaurant business is transient to say the least. Many restaurants have a constantly revolving door of employees coming and going. Why was I one of those employees that stayed? The answer, I have come to believe, is that most of the establishments I worked in focused on making the guest happy. I found that aspect of the job particularly rewarding, especially when it came to guests who had special dietary needs.

To further describe my journey, I have organized my experiences into the three following sections:

- An introduction to food allergies

- In the trenches: The restaurant perspective

- Catering to gluten and allergen-free guests

- Supporting friends and family with special diets

An Introduction to Food Allergies

I vaguely remember the first time I heard the term "food allergy." I was very young, probably in about first or second grade. Those were the days when we had snack time as part of our daily routine. When snack time came around, we usually had cookies or nuts and always a pint of whole milk. At the time, we were all taught about the "food pyramid" through government materials and films, which had catchy tunes that entertained us and provided valuable information about a well balanced diet. Although it was many years ago, I can still remember those songs and some of their lyrics! "Milk group...meat group....fruit and vegetable group.... bread and cereal group."

There was a classmate of mine who was shorter in stature and looked frail compared to the other kids. His complexion seemed a bit pale and he was always very quiet and reserved. When he first joined our class, the teacher announced to everyone that this boy had "food allergies" and explained that he could not drink milk or eat chocolate or peanuts. I can still remember the look of sadness on his face as we were told this information.

All of the children looked forward to the mid-afternoon snack, as it was a break from the arduous tasks of coloring inside the lines and reading the advanced texts from the "Dick and Jane" books, as well as a chance to boost our blood sugar levels which were depleted from the post lunch recess. We received our

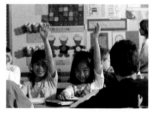

pints of milk and snacks, which were devoured with the utmost ferocity. This one boy, however, was set apart from the group and ate raw vegetables, special snack chips and drank fruit juice. I thought it was kind of neat that he got to eat something different than the rest of us, yet it was clear to me that he just wanted to be like the other kids and eat what we were eating.

He was only in my class a year. I believe his family moved to another town. His presence certainly impacted me though, so much so that I can remember it to this day. Half the time I can't remember what I did last week, so reminiscing about something that happened so long ago indicates to me that the experience opened my eyes to something new.

At the time, the general awareness of food allergies in the US was in its infancy. I only had a few friends diagnosed with food allergies. I did have family and friends who were very particular about what types of food they would eat. My father detested mushrooms, my sister Robbie hated peas and I would rather starve than eat fried liver and onions. It wasn't until I started working in restaurants in high school that I really got a sense of how many people had special dietary concerns or were living with food allergies.

In the Trenches: The Restaurant Perspective

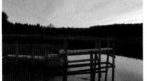

Working in the restaurant service industry is truly an adventure. Nowhere else can one come into contact with so many people on a personal level every day. One summer, I was working at a family resort in Maine on one of the most beautiful lakes in America (as rated by National Geographic Magazine). *Quisisana*, which is Italian for "a place where one heals one's self," was aptly named. It was a place where people could escape from the big cities of the East coast and enjoy a family "summer camp." Many of the guests were regular visitors, some returning to Lake Kezar and the woods of Maine every summer for 50 years.

At the time I was working as a front waiter, which is a glorified term for a busboy. We served three meals a day and it was my responsibility to fill water glasses, pour coffee and deliver bread and butter to every table. There was an elderly couple who had been coming to the resort for many years, probably decades, who sat in my section for two weeks. I learned very quickly that Mrs. Shapiro did not like butter. The look on her face, when I brought her a dish of individually wrapped pats of butter, was frightening. She exclaimed, "No butter at our table!" The panic stricken look on her face was enough to make me nervous for the rest of the meal. "What did I do wrong?" I thought. "It's just butter! It's not the end of the world." Some mistakes in life you make only once and this was certainly one of them. It was none of my business why she had such a dramatic response. It was my job to make her happy, so I was very conscious about only bringing margarine to their table after that.

1

Looking back, I wonder if she was lactose intolerant or maybe she was on a medically prescribed diet. I never asked them about her vehement response and they never offered an explanation. She certainly was a very picky eater. The choices she made for her meals were simple and basic, if not bland. My best friend Mike and I worked as a team for the Shapiros and we still have conversations about them from time to time. "How's your tuna sandwich, Mrs. Shapiro?" we would ask. Her daily apathetic response, "Eh....it's tuna." She was clearly frustrated with her food limitations. They were very nice people though and my experience with them taught me a valuable lesson as a person working in the restaurant industry: regardless of what I thought of a special request, even if I didn't understand it, my job was to make the guest happy during their dining experience. If you make the effort to accommodate people, they leave happy and want to return because they have had an enjoyable experience with someone who cared about their needs. By the middle of the first week, Mrs. Shapiro had us well trained. We knew exactly what she wanted and didn't want, which provided her with a certain sense of comfort. She was happy to see us and felt safe at the table knowing that we were fully aware of her special needs.

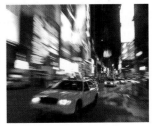

Most chefs and waiters I know truly care about their patrons and take individual dietary considerations very seriously. Unfortunately, accidents do happen. A number of years ago, a good friend of mine was working at a popular chain restaurant at Times Square in New York City. A married couple came in to eat with their young son who clearly stated to my waiter friend, "No onions, please." "No problem," he thought, as he had dealt with hundreds of special requests in the past. The boy wanted a simple pasta dish with marinara sauce. My friend submitted this order with the stipulation "no onions." Somewhere between placing the order in the computer and delivering the food to the table, this important detail was lost. Nevertheless, the family seemed to enjoy the meal and left satisfied.

Unfortunately, the parents never mentioned to my friend that the boy had a serious food allergy. The next day when he came back to work, the manager

1

asked him about the table with the special request of no onions. Apparently, the sauce contained onions and the child was sick. My friend felt horrible. He did what he was trained to do, by listing the request on the order. Should he have known the sauce had onions in it? If he didn't, shouldn't the cooks in the kitchen have known? That day, my friend realized the difference between a special order and serving a customer with a food allergy. Had he known that the child had a serious food allergy, rather than a special request, he would have been far more diligent in ensuring the proper meal was delivered. As a rule, it is extremely important to use the word "allergy" in restaurants. Failing to satisfy a simple special request has certain consequences. However, failing to deliver on an allergy request can have severe consequences. Today, restaurants know this and take it very seriously.

Catering to Gluten and Allergen-Free Guests

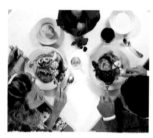

I witnessed a similar situation working at a popular upscale Chinese restaurant in Scottsdale, Arizona. We were very well trained on the menu and all the ingredients used in the restaurant. In fact, every server was given a mandatory test that required detailed knowledge of each dish that was served. This was not a minor hurdle or a joke—it was an absolute necessity to work on the floor of the restaurant. The tests were scrutinized so vigorously that to pass, one had to score above 85% just to work there! We were also instructed to inform the manager and chef of any guest that stated that they had a food allergy. This structure proved to be very efficient, as we had few complaints. The only flaw in this procedure was if a guest failed to declare that they had a food allergy.

One evening, a couple sat down in the section next to mine. Their food was delivered and they seemed to be enjoying the meal. Then it happened. The woman at the table turned red and was obviously going into some type of shock. The gentleman didn't know what to do; quite frankly, we didn't know what to do. Luckily, the manager did and called for an ambulance, which arrived almost immediately. After taking her vitals, they gave her a shot and she was stabilized in a short time. We were never told exactly what she had a reaction to, but we figured it was either the peanuts or the dried chili peppers that were in her meal. The event scared me. I knew that I never wanted to be responsible for someone having a severe reaction like that. From that night on, taking care of guests with food allergies and special requests became the most important part of my job.

In a very short time, regular guests with food allergies began to request seating in my section. They experienced a level of comfort when dining under my supervision and knew that I made every effort to ensure an allergen-free meal. I worked closely with each guest to determine what they could have on the menu. I would also be creative with them, "You can have this sauce, with that dish." or "Have you tried this dish? We can add this or omit that." It was actually fun and challenging for me. The kitchen didn't mind because every dish was made to order and we were encouraged to do everything possible to make the guests happy. My patrons really enjoyed it too, because they didn't have to eat the same thing every time they came to the restaurant, which can be a frustrating part of living with food allergies.

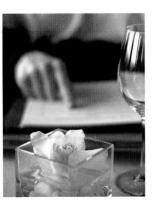

Mickey, a local helicopter pilot, was continually relieved to see me when she walked into the restaurant. If she came in on a night that I wasn't working, the next time she saw me, she would let me know about it. She was allergic to many things, including soy, poultry and wheat, which made it difficult to maneuver around a Chinese restaurant menu. She was very diligent in reminding me of exactly what she couldn't eat and how all the utensils needed to be cleaned before preparing her meal. This is so important, because no matter how often you think you've repeated yourself, it is best to remind the restaurant staff of your special dietary needs.

At first, Mickey only ordered steamed vegetables and rice. Her major concern was cross-contamination. So, as soon as I saw her, I would walk right back to the kitchen and tell the chef that our special guest had arrived and it was time to clean a wok and utensils in hot soapy water. It got to be such a regular occurrence that no one in the kitchen questioned the request. As Mickey's level of comfort with me and the restaurant increased, she

1

became more adventurous with her orders. When we would come up with something new and delicious for her that was safe, the look of excitement on her face was like a kid opening presents on Christmas!

Restaurants in New York City are wonderful in so many ways. As a city, New York is considered one of the best places in the world for dining. The pace of life in the Big Apple is so fast that the phrase "a New York minute" is not only a reality, it's a regular demand. People who live in the city just expect things to happen faster than people in most parts of the world. This includes restaurant owners, who want their tables "turned" or "served" as fast as possible, so they can afford to pay their ever-increasing rent. I worked for a few years at a popular Thai restaurant, where the staff was constantly pressured to turn their tables as fast as possible, and we did. Like most progressive establishments, we were also required to take a test on our menu knowledge so the staff was well educated on the cuisine. Much to the chagrin of the owners, the speed of my service always slowed down when I had a guest with food allergies. I felt it was more important to ensure an allergen-free dining experience for these guests than to hurry them through their meal. I always took the extra time and the regulars took notice. Once again, people requested seating in my section. They knew that if I didn't have the answer, I would take all the necessary time to discuss things with the chef.

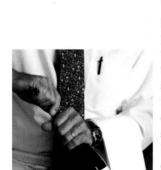

It may seem like a basic service, but it really gave me a sense of satisfaction to help people have an enjoyable dining experience. The look of excitement on a guest's face when you introduce a new dish to them that is safe to eat is extraordinary. Communication is the key to success. When you have food allergies, dining out is a collaborative effort between you and the restaurant staff. There isn't any way around it. It may not be the case with every restaurant, but there is a growing trend in the industry to accommodate guests with special dietary requirements. This is not just for financial gain, but also for the satisfaction that any guest can dine at their establishment and have a healthy, wholesome meal. From a restaurant perspective, this pursuit is extremely rewarding.

Supporting Friends and Family with Special Diets

In fall 2002, my dear friend Kim was diagnosed with celiac / coeliac disease. She was in town a few days a week over a seven month period working on delivering the enormous 3-1-1 project for the City of New York. We were enjoying a cocktail at my favorite neighborhood haunt when she told me she had celiac / coeliac disease. What disease? I had never heard of it and probably couldn't have spelled it if you asked.

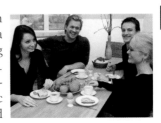

As we talked about it, I learned another new term I had no knowledge of...gluten. I was very aware of wheat allergies, as I came across them often in the business and was used to modifying orders for people on low carbohydrate diets. Gluten, however, was a detail that I never received the memo on. In fact, after hearing about it, I asked many of my friends in the restaurant business if they knew what gluten was. Most of them had never heard of it.

Kim was at a loss. She discovered she had a permanent intolerance to gluten, which is hidden in so many foods. I saw the frustration on her face, as she looked at the menu when we went out to dinner. "It has a sauce, I can't have that." "I don't know what's in that and I don't want to get sick." Soon I realized that she was living an extremely cautious life, which was completely out of character for her, because she didn't want to get sick. Who could blame her? I began to take a more active role in the ordering process with her and our collaboration yielded more choices for her to eat on a regular basis. After all, I'd worked in restaurants for a long time, cooking was a passion for me and I wasn't shy about asking questions.

As a team, we got very good at dining out together. Our meals were great, she had more options and she rarely got sick when we ate out. We developed an interesting approach to ordering by analyzing the menu and figuring out which questions to ask like, "Is there soy sauce in that marinade?" and "Do you have a designated fryer for the fries or do you use one fryer for everything?" It was a learning process for us as well as the servers who took our orders. They would say things like, "Wow, I would have never thought about that"

1

or "Soy sauce has wheat in it?" It was a fun challenge and it allowed us to enjoy our dining experiences more often without the fear of her getting sick.

About a year later, my brother discovered that he was allergic to wheat. He had struggled, like most people, for some time trying to figure out what he was eating that was making him sick. He went through the process of elimination diet and cut out various food allergens for periods of time to see if there was any improvement to his overall health.

When he finally got to wheat, the results were dramatic. He lost over twenty pounds and had more energy on a daily basis than he had had in years. His frequency of having hives decreased considerably and his skin looked so healthy that people often thought that he was younger than me! I don't know what that says about me, but he's my elder by a few years, so the visual change was amazing.

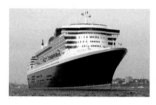

Rick and I are great friends. We have so much in common and are amazed that we are related. One of our shared passions is travel. We have had the opportunity to explore the Caribbean, Mexico and Central America together on a number of occasions. I was very excited to take him on a cruise through the Panama Canal, which is an experience I have been fortunate to enjoy a few times in my life.

One of my traditions is to get up at 5 a.m., have breakfast and be out on the deck to view the ship's passing through the first lock. Once through the first set of locks, the afternoon is spent drinking Bloody Marys or Bloody Caesars, depending on whether I was with Canadians or Americans. Rick and I stuck to tradition and had a wonderful afternoon, until he started to feel sick and his hives began to surface. Throughout the entire vacation we had been very diligent about ordering wheat-free meals, but we obviously missed something. Through the process of elimination, we determined there was only one possible culprit—the Bloody Mary mix. I went back to the bartender and asked to see the bottle of the mix and sure enough, printed in big letters, the label stated wheat as an ingredient.

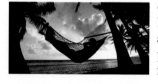

The next few days Rick felt terrible. He was sick to his stomach, often doubled over in pain and especially uncomfortable because of those huge itchy hives. His eyes and lips were also swollen. He ended up staying in his cabin for the next three days until he felt better and his symptoms went away. Twenty percent of our vacation was ruined because of that drink. We had no idea wheat could be a hidden allergen in Bloody Mary mix, but we certainly learned our lesson during that trip.

I consistently make an extra effort when I dine or travel with anyone with food allergies. I have found that having an extra watchful eye is both helpful and comforting to everyone at the table. Whether I am dining with my family or friends, I try to assist as much as I can by leveraging my knowledge of food and asking the right questions when appropriate.

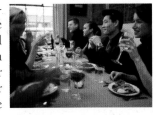

It is important to take a proactive role in the dining experience when you are out with people you care about, because the frustrations and fears associated with having food allergies can be a lot for one person to handle. That is why I feel this book is important for those individuals living with special diets. It is also for their loved ones, health professionals and people in the restaurant industry. At the end of the day, the more one knows about food preparation and the more the restaurant knows about your situation, the less likely you are to get sick. It's that simple!

Santé!   **Chin Chin!**

    ¡Salud!   **Cheers!**

        Chok-dee!

歡呼!   **चीयर्श**

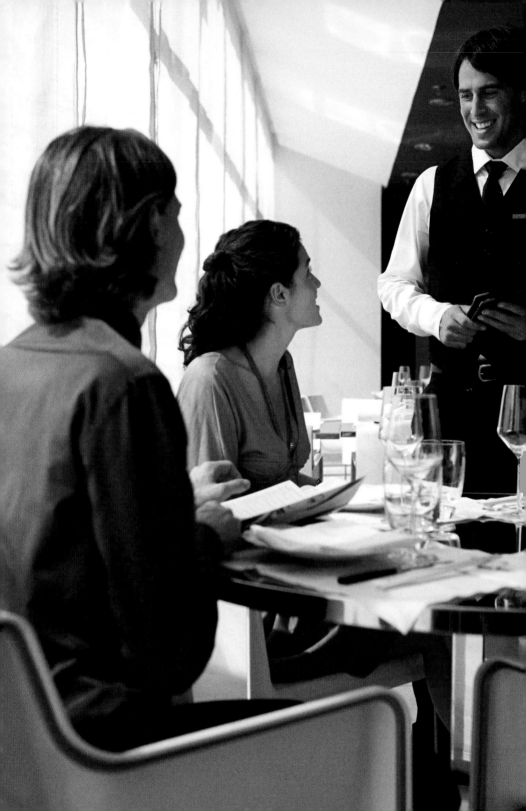

Food is our common ground, a universal experience.
—James Beard

2

Chapter 2
Approach to Safe Eating Experiences

Chapter Overview

Managing gluten and allergen-free diets increases the level of complexity involved in eating outside the home, particularly in restaurants. It requires a higher level of education, understanding and planning compared to the general public who, in most cases, can easily eat whatever they want, wherever they want. Knowing what foods are safe is of the utmost importance.

The suggestions outlined in this chapter are designed to give guests a greater sense of comfort when venturing beyond their front door to eat out while, at the same time, assisting restaurants in safely serving guests with special dietary concerns. Therefore, the approach to safe eating experiences entails an understanding of the:

• Learning curve associated with special diets

• Guest approach to eating outside the home

• Restaurant approach to handling special dietary requests

• Collaborative process of eating out

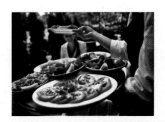

Learning Curve Associated with Special Diets

There is a learning curve for individuals who are guests in eating establishments managing gluten and allergen-free diets as well as for the restaurants who cater to them. The process of gaining the necessary knowledge to successfully handle special dietary requirements is similar for both parties.

The learning curve associated with special diets includes the following four key steps, for individuals and restaurant professionals alike:

- Awareness

- Information

- Knowledge

- Empowerment

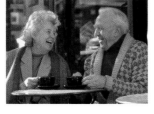

1. To gain awareness, you, as an individual, need to first educate yourself to understand exactly what you are allergic to or what special diet you are required to follow. You may be asking, "What have I been diagnosed with? Where do I begin my research? What resources are available to me and what do I do next?" These are all common questions associated with learning about your new way of life.

   On the other side of the table, restaurant professionals go through a similar experience. "What type of special diets may be required by our guests? What do we need to learn to better understand their needs? What resources are available to help us?"

2. The next step in the learning curve is information. As an individual, you must learn what you can and cannot eat on a fundamental level. Once this is understood, it is important to investigate where problematic allergens can be hidden in foods and what you need to do to adjust for this unexpected variable.

Likewise, restaurant professionals follow a similar thought process. "What can this guest eat and what is not allowable? What ingredients and food preparation techniques can be an issue and how can we adjust to suit their requirements?" The parallel is undeniable.

3. Once this understanding is accomplished, the third step is knowledge. Individuals need to apply what has been learned to safely eat in restaurants, as well as at home. Furthermore, you must learn to communicate your special requirements and determine an effective strategy for ordering safe meals in order to develop a comfort level with various cuisines and dishes.

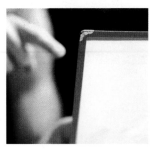

As a restaurant, you have a different set of concerns to address, such as how to train both front and back of the house staff. You also need to determine how to accurately convey this information between all employees involved in the process and identify what protocols need to be in operation.

Through effective training efforts, an establishment can teach their staff how to assist special diet guests by guiding them through the menu, taking into consideration ingredients, preparation techniques and hidden allergen concerns.

4. The final step of the learning curve is empowerment. As the guest, you need to know where and what you can eat, as well as what modifications can be made to easily accommodate your dietary requirements. Once this is achieved, you can focus on enjoying your eating experiences while remaining diligent about the foods you eat.

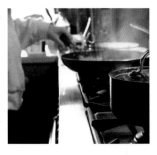

For the restaurant, the focus becomes how to simplify menu options to adjust for special dietary needs. This allows the restaurant to concentrate on providing safe and delicious meals for their guests, while ensuring a high standard of service, ultimately resulting in repeat and loyal business.

2

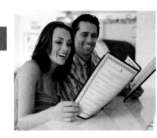

Guest Approach to Eating Outside the Home

Based upon years of research, personal experience and extensive discussions with hospitality professionals, the following approach is designed to help you, the person managing gluten and/or allergen-free lifestyles, eat out safely. The objective is to enjoy safe eating experiences regardless of your choice of restaurant, cuisine or location. These suggestions include eight key steps on how to safely eat outside the home:

1. Educate yourself about eating outside the home with special diets

2. Assess your dining comfort level for the meal

3. Identify your eating options and preferences

4. Determine desired level of pre-planning efforts

5. Communicate your special dietary needs with the restaurant

6. Order your meal

7. Receive order and appreciate your meal

8. Provide feedback on dining experience

Each of these eight key steps are described in detail to guide you in developing your own approach to eating outside the home. The questions to ask yourself, as the guest, may be helpful in assessing your level of preparedness along the way. If you are new to your diet, these ideas may give you some food for thought during the early stages of your learning curve.

For those who have been following a gluten and/or allergen-free diet for some time, you might find it interesting to reflect upon your previous experiences, correlate them to this recommended approach and, perhaps, learn something new in the process. These ideas are also provided for restaurants who want to understand the guest's perspective of how to handle special dietary needs.

On-Line Databases for Gluten-Free Restaurants

For the European Union, visit www.Gluten-Free-OnTheGo.com

For North and South America and other parts of the world, visit www.GlutenFreeOnTheGo.com

For additional eating out suggestions, visit www.GlutenFreePassport.com

1. Educate yourself about eating outside the home with special diets

a. Read applicable materials:

- Review books, publications, restaurant reviews and awareness programs

- Research the Internet, databases and other reference materials

b. Talk with other individuals managing gluten and/or allergen-free lifestyles

c. Attend educational sessions:

- Participate in associated conferences and cooking classes

- Hire a personal chef for consultation

Questions for Guests:
Do I have the information that I need to make informed choices and increase my comfort level in restaurants?

What additional research is required to expand my knowledge?

2

2. Assess your dining comfort level for the meal

a. Identify your safety factors:

- Determine how you feel physically

- Assess how safe you feel with eating out

b. Based upon your previous needs and experiences, evaluate what cuisines are low and high risk

c. Assess specific cuisines:

- Determine what type of cuisines satisfy your comfort level and tastes

- Identify your desired level of understanding about food preparation techniques

Questions for Guests:
How comfortable do I feel eating out in restaurants today?

What foods appeal to me?

How safe do I feel today with the food that I will be eating?

3. Identify your eating options and preferences

a. Determine the desired type of establishment:

- Fine dining or family-oriented restaurant

- Fast food/quick service or carry out/take away

Questions for Guests:
How much effort do I want to spend on deciding what to eat?

How comfortable am I with this restaurant, the cuisine and menu options?

b. Assess what type of cuisine you prefer:

- New and different

- Familiar with cuisine menu items

c. Determine important factors based on your comfort level:

- Recommended and new restaurant

- Familiar and where you have eaten before

- Features specific gluten and/or allergen-free menu

d. Select your restaurant

Questions for Guests:

What level of planning do I want to do prior to going to the restaurant?

What areas of food preparation need to be reviewed?

What hidden allergens do I need to be aware of?

Do I need to conduct more research to increase my comfort level about this cuisine and/or restaurant?

4. Determine desired level of pre-planning efforts

a. Conduct research as necessary on:

- Cuisine ingredients and preparation techniques

- Potential hidden allergens

- Restaurant menu options and items

b. Determine the best time for your meal:

- Decide to walk into a restaurant when convenient

- Reserve a desired time

- Reserve a time that is typically not crowded

c. Determine the level of communication necessary with the restaurant prior to your meal:

- None required

- Review menu on the Internet

- Call ahead to discuss your requirements

5. Communicate your special dietary needs with the restaurant

a. Determine your approach:

- Susceptible to anaphylaxis and life threatening conditions

- Have celiac / coeliac or food allergies

- On a special diet

b. Initiate your first contact with restaurant:

- Go to restaurant without prior communication

- Call ahead prior to walking in the door

- Pre-order your meal based upon your concerns

c. Discuss requirements with restaurant staff and potentially request manager or chef if needed

Questions for Guests:

How do I want to communicate the severity of my condition?

When and how do I want to explain my special dietary needs?

Are my requirements understood or do I need to speak with someone else to feel safe and comfortable?

2

6. Order your meal

a. Determine reference materials required to order meal:

- Assess if a dining card outlining dietary requirements is needed based upon your comfort level or language considerations

- Refer to your notes, books, quick reference guides, translation cards and foreign language phrase books as needed

b. Discuss the menu with the restaurant:

- Ask appropriate questions to determine meal choices based upon cuisine, dishes and preferences

- Explain your concerns to the restaurant

- Ask staff to verify and validate ingredients and preparation techniques as needed

Questions for Guests:

How do I want to communicate my needs to the restaurant—ask questions, give them materials outlining requirements or both?

What areas of food preparation need to be questioned?

What hidden allergens do I inquire about?

How comfortable do I feel that my order will be prepared as requested?

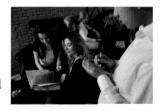

2

c. Place your order:

- Request special food preparation

- Confirm your order with restaurant

Questions for Guests:
Is my meal what I ordered?

If not, what needs to be modified to correct the order?

Would I return to this restaurant?

7. Receive order and appreciate your meal

a. Confirm your order upon delivery:

- Reiterate your special order request

- Receive dish and assess preparation

b. Enjoy your meal:

- Accept the dish

- Request dish be returned if special request is not met

c. Relax and appreciate the dining experience:

- Compliment the staff if your special requests are met

- Include a generous tip for good service, if appropriate

- Frequent the restaurant again based on experience

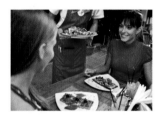

Questions for Guests:
What do I want to communicate to the staff regarding their service?

Would I recommend this establishment to others?

8. Provide feedback on dining experience

a. Provide constructive feedback to restaurant professionals on your eating experience

b. Recommend the establishment to your friends and family, as appropriate

c. Notify applicable on-line database resources and/or restaurant awareness programs about your experience

Restaurant Approach to Handling Special Dietary Requests

Knowledge and understanding coupled with clear table-side communication are the keys to ensuring safe, enjoyable gluten and/or allergen-free experiences for guests. Again, appropriate training on procedures for handling special diets needs to be in place. Establishing protocols for special dietary needs provides consistent dining experiences for each and every gluten and/or allergen-free guest.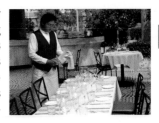

In order to achieve the optimal collaborative process with guests who have special dietary needs, there are seven important steps to take to prepare your operation for safe, happy and healthy guests.

1. Educate staff about special dietary requirements

2. Identify restaurant-specific ingredients and food preparation techniques to be potentially modified for special diets

3. Understand guest's dietary needs and discuss menu

4. Facilitate accurate understanding of order and concerns

5. Ensure fulfillment of gluten and/or allergen free-order

6. Deliver and confirm special meal

7. Follow-up with guests about service and ensure a satisfactory dining experience

Each of these suggestions are compiled into a checklist for restaurants to help ensure that the special dietary requirements of your guests are being addressed. The questions to ask yourself, as the restaurant, assess training effectiveness and the level of preparedness in handling special requests. These ideas are provided for eating establishments catering to gluten and/or allergen-free guests, as well as for those individuals who want to understand the restaurant's perspective to handling their special needs.

Questions for Restaurants:

Is the staff knowledgeable about special diets?

What are the current restaurant trends about special diets?

What training can we implement to improve awareness?

1. Educate staff about special dietary requirements

   a. Conduct training for management and staff on special diets

   b. Monitor training effectiveness and guest feedback

   c. Implement standard protocols for special diets

Questions for Restaurants:

What are the most common food allergens and ingredients?

Where are allergens hidden in our food preparation and menu items?

What can we offer that is safe for special diets?

How do we communicate and promote our efforts to guests?

2. Identify restaurant-specific ingredients and food preparation techniques to be potentially modified for special diets

   a. Identify common food allergens, ingredients and food preparation considerations

   b. Identify which menu items are naturally free of specific allergens

   c. Explore potential modifications to menu items based upon specific allergens and ingredients

   d. Determine possible cross-contamination and changes required in the kitchen

   e. Identify what ingredients and areas of food preparation cannot be modified

Questions for Restaurants:

What menu items can be modified based on specific allergens?

Does the staff, kitchen and chef understand these special dietary needs?

3. Understand guest's dietary needs and discuss menu

   a. Discuss guest's dietary conditions including:

     • Susceptible to anaphylaxis and life threatening conditions

     • Have celiac / coeliac, food allergies or on a special diet

   b. Discuss which menu items are safe based upon requirements and what dishes can be modified

   c. Discuss menu items that must be avoided

   d. Confirm menu items and preparation techniques with chef/kitchen based upon requirements

4. Facilitate accurate understanding of order and concerns

a. Determine if the special order is understood by the staff under the chef's supervision

b. Assess and factor in language considerations with the kitchen staff

c. Determine the feasibility of executing special requests based upon how busy the kitchen is

d. Assess if order can be prepared as requested

e. Follow-up with guest if order needs to be changed

Questions for Restaurants:

Does the kitchen understand the special meal?

What potential language barrier exists impacting communication?

How is the kitchen prepared for special requests?

Are any modifications to the order needed based upon chef feedback?

2

5. Ensure fulfillment of gluten and/or allergen-free order

a. Confirm that request can be handled

b. Monitor fulfillment of special request

c. Re-confirm order with kitchen prior to delivery

Questions for Restaurants:

Has the special order been prepared as requested?

Was the special request effectively addressed?

6. Deliver and confirm special meal

a. Deliver meal to guest

b. Confirm special meal meets requirements

c. Handle situation if meal does not meet guest's expectations and replace entire meal if needed

Questions for Restaurants:

Are we delivering the appropriate special meal to the guest?

Have we confirmed that the special order is prepared as requested?

7. Follow-up with guests about service and ensure a satisfactory eating experience

a. Ensure safe and satisfactory meal with guest

b. Provide guest feedback as needed

Questions for Restaurants:

Did we follow-up to confirm that the meal meet the guest's expectations?

What improvements can we implement to streamline our special order process?

Collaborative Process of Eating Out

The collaborative process between guests and restaurants is critical to a mutually positive eating experience with special dietary concerns. At the highest level, eating out is comprised of two components—the planning effort and the table-side communications between the two parties. As evidenced in the chart below, this process is similar for both guests and restaurants.

Collaborative Process Between Guests and Restaurants

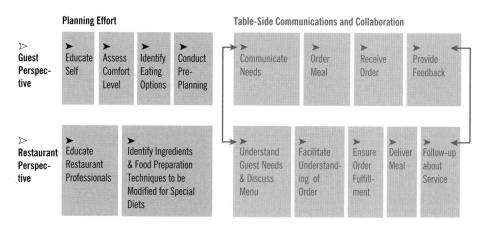

	Planning Effort				Table-Side Communications and Collaboration			
Guest Perspective	Educate Self	Assess Comfort Level	Identify Eating Options	Conduct Pre-Planning	Communicate Needs	Order Meal	Receive Order	Provide Feedback
Restaurant Perspective	Educate Restaurant Professionals	Identify Ingredients & Food Preparation Techniques to be Modified for Special Diets			Understand Guest Needs & Discuss Menu	Facilitate Understanding of Order	Ensure Order Fulfillment	Deliver Meal / Follow-up about Service

The planning effort for both parties focuses on education and should be completed prior to any interaction between the two. Based upon where guests and restaurants are in the learning curve, their approach to special diets may vary.

As the individual impacted by special diets, you need to understand how different eating establishments approach handling special request meals. It is also important for the restaurant to understand the spectrum of guests' knowledge about gluten and allergen-free diets.

Planning, table-side communications and collaboration are the critical success factors to ensuring that meals are safe for guests to eat. Each of the above steps in the collaborative process have been described within their respective approach sections. Remember, the guidelines and suggested questions to ask are intended to stimulate ideas prior to and during the collaborative process of eating out for each party.

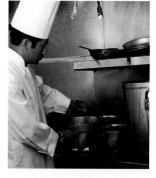

Summary

The level of awareness in the restaurant industry concerning special diets is continuing to improve across the globe, with higher levels of understanding in some geographic regions than in others. Also, the number of special menus and nutritional programs are expanding to more and more restaurants, with an increase in health conscious establishments worldwide. These trends can be directly tied to the relationships between restaurants and their guests.

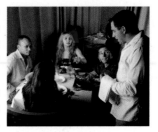

Due to the desire to provide quality service in a highly competitive market, restaurants typically have the best intentions when it comes to guest satisfaction. Many restaurants are flexible with special requests, and make the effort to serve safe and enjoyable meals based upon guests' specific dietary needs. Hospitality and food service professionals want you, as the guest, to be happy with your experience because they want you to come back often.

The collaboration between guests and restaurants has contributed to advancements across the global special diet communities. We learn from each other, so it is important to take note of any new knowledge that results from each eating experience from both perspectives. Going forward, our collective efforts will continue to increase the understanding of special diets resulting in improved quality of life for those managing gluten and/or allergen-free lifestyles.

Hopefully, reading this book assists you along your learning curve and makes the process easier whether eating out or serving guests around the corner or around the world. Remember, planning, communications and collaboration between guests and restaurants greatly improves safe eating experiences on a regular basis. Enjoy and have fun!

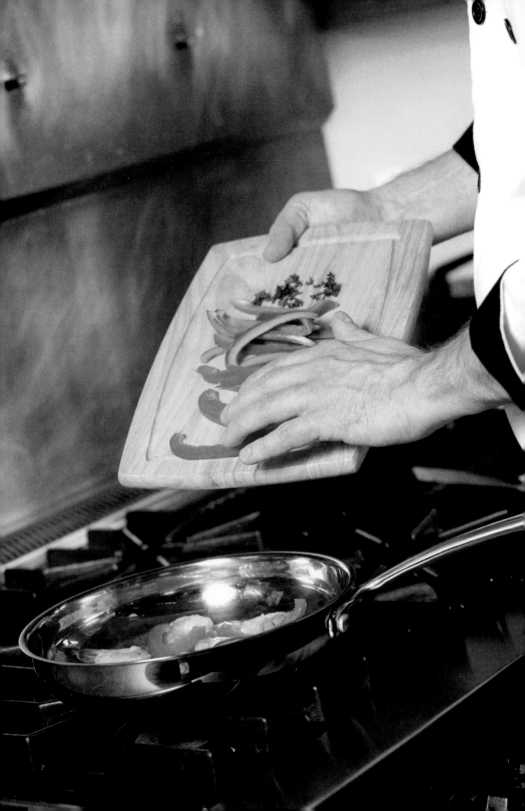

You don't have to cook fancy or complicated masterpieces—just good food from fresh ingredients.
—Julia Child

3

Chapter 3
Ingredient and Preparation Technique Guidelines

Chapter Overview

Although ingredients are labeled on packaged products, there is limited information available about nutrition and ingredients for menu items in restaurants and other eating establishments worldwide. Therefore, the best way to increase your comfort level as a guest eating outside the home or as a restaurant catering to those with special diets is to:

- Become knowledgeable about food ingredients
- Learn how food is prepared
- Discover what preparation techniques require your attention

You can learn to navigate through any menu by developing the ability to communicate the right questions and answers. Then, in time, you will become empowered with an understanding of common culinary practices. With a little bit of effort, guests and restaurants alike will be able to ensure safe and positive gluten and allergen-free dining experiences for all involved.

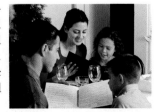

3

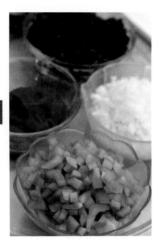

To accomplish this, guests and restaurants need to understand a few things about food ingredients and preparation techniques, which include:

- Areas of consideration

- Worldwide product labeling regulations

- Codex Alimentarius and gluten-free labeling

- Gluten and wheat-free grains/flours

- Ingredient sources and manufacturing processes

- Ingredient and preparation techniques: Quick Reference Guide

- Ingredient and preparation techniques by allergen

Areas of Consideration

Believe it or not, the areas that require your attention are very manageable. When it comes to common food allergens, there are three major areas to consider:

- Allergens as ingredients

- Allergens hidden in food preparation techniques

- Cross-contamination

Allergens as ingredients are typically much easier to identify and manage while eating outside the home. Obviously, if you are allergic to shrimp, you can request no shrimp on your salad. If you are allergic to dairy, you can request no cheese on your dish. If you are allergic to fish, do not order it. That is the straightforward approach.

Allergens hidden in food preparation techniques require a bit more investigation on your part. Are the french fried potatoes or chips fried in peanut oil? Is the chicken dusted with wheat flour prior to pan frying? Does the marinade for your meat contain soy sauce? As you can imagine, this can get complicated with unexpected surprises lurking around many corners. That being said, asking the right questions and having the right answers are extremely important.

Cross-contamination occurs in two primary instances and should be considered at any restaurant. One may occur when a meal is prepared in the same frying oil as other foods containing possible allergens. The second may occur when food particles are transferred from one food to another by using the same knife, cutting board, pan, grill or other utensils without washing the surfaces or tools in between uses.

To avoid cross-contamination, restaurants need to dedicate fryers for specific foods. Restaurants also need to wash all materials and cooking surfaces in hot, soapy water prior to preparing items for those with special dietary requirements. In the case of open flame grills, the intense heat typically turns most protein into carbon; however, scraping the grill may be required as a safety precaution. It is important to ensure that restaurants follow these procedures to avoid cross-contamination between foods.

Worldwide Product Labeling Regulations

In recent years, various geographic regions have instituted mandatory product labeling regulations and voluntary guidelines for manufacturers. Product labeling legislation across the globe varies by terms, definitions, food allergens covered, compound ingredients, substitutions, exemptions, placement and legibility. There are hundreds of pages detailing specific regulations and requirements based on the various geographic labeling laws.

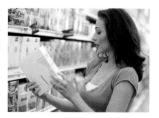

These regulations encompass various combinations of food allergens such as celery, dairy, eggs, fish, gluten, milk, mustard, peanuts, sesame, shellfish, soy, sulphur dioxide, tree nuts and wheat to name a few. These allergens are considered responsible for over 90% of allergic reactions to food on a worldwide basis.

It is mandatory to label ingredients derived from defined food allergens in most parts of the world. For example, since 2002, Food Standards Australia New Zealand (FSANZ) requires top food allergens to be named on ingredient lists. As of 2005, the European Union

3

Directive on product labeling requires manufacturers to identify specific allergens and their derivatives.

The US Food Allergen Labeling and Consumer Protection Act (FALCPA) has been in effect since 2006 with gluten-free guidelines detailed in 2009. Other countries and geographic regions have also instituted regulations on product labeling and voluntary guidelines for various food allergens and their derivatives.

It should be noted that labeling laws apply to the products manufactured in their country of origin. Imported products may or may not be required to adhere to the import country's labeling regulations. For example, FSANZ requires all imported products to label ingredients as defined by their standards whereas other geographic regions may differ in their requirements.

For the most up-to-date information on food allergen labeling around the world, visit the Reference Center at either www.GlutenFreePassport.com or www.Allergy FreePassport.com.

Codex Alimentarius and Gluten-Free Labeling

There are also differences in the definition of the term "gluten-free" and which foods are considered gluten-free on a worldwide basis. Some countries have specific gluten-free labeling regulations that define which ingredients and foods are acceptable and not acceptable. Some countries identify specific terminology and symbols which can be used on product labels while other countries do not.

The Codex Alimentarius Commission was created in 1963 by the Food and Agriculture Organization of the United Nations (FAO) and the World Health Organization (WHO). This international group develops mutually agreed upon food standards and guidelines to protect the health of consumers worldwide and to ensure fair trade practices. The Commission includes representatives from countries around the world, with some of the participating countries adopting the Codex Alimentarius standards while others develop their own standards and regulations.

As an example, the standard for gluten-free labeling in the European Union is guided by the Codex Alimentarius. Since the 1980s, the standard has been adopted for products to be labeled gluten-free with levels of 200mg gluten/kg or 200 parts per million (ppm).

As of 2008, the Codex standard on gluten-free labeling reflects two distinct categories:

- Products containing less than 20 ppm gluten can be labeled "gluten-free"

- Products containing gluten from 21 - 100 ppm can be labeled "very low gluten"

The European Commission is using the revised Codex standard as the basis for European Union legislation on gluten-free labeling which was published in 2009.

As another example, to be labeled gluten-free in Australia and New Zealand, a food must contain "No Detectable Gluten" by the most sensitive universally accepted test method. If gluten is not detected, then the food can be labeled "gluten-free".

For the most up-to-date standards and information on gluten-free labeling around the world, visit the Reference Center at www.GlutenFreePassport.com.

Gluten and Wheat-Free Grains/Flours

Gluten is the protein found in wheat, rye and barley. The following is a list of grains, flours and starches that are gluten-free and may be substituted for traditional gluten and wheat containing items:

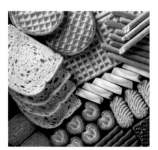

More restaurants are offering gluten and wheat-free bakery products to their special diet guests.

Amaranth	Nut Flours
Arrowroot	Pea
Beans	Pinto
Black Gram	Potato
Buckwheat	Quinoa
Chickpea (Besan)	Rice
Corn	Sorghum
Garbanzo	Soy
Garfava	Sweet Potato
Lentil	Tapioca (Manioc)
Millet	Teff
Montina™	

3

Testing shows that most oats have gluten levels beyond the acceptable range for those following gluten-free diets due to cross-contamination in the milling process. There are numerous manufacturers around the world that produce tested and certified gluten-free oats. Unless you are eating certified gluten-free oats, it is recommended that you avoid oats when managing a gluten-free diet.

It should be noted that an individual can have allergies, intolerances or sensitivities to wheat without having the dietary concerns for other grains that contain gluten.

Three grains that are wheat-free are kamut, spelt and triticale. However, they do contain gluten and must be avoided if managing a gluten-free diet.

Other grains and flours that contain gluten and wheat include:

Barley	Farro
Bulgur	Graham
Couscous	Matzoh Meal
Durum	Rye
Einkorn	Semolina
Emmer	Wheat Germ
Farina	Wheat Starch

Ingredient Sources and Manufacturing Processes

In addition to labeling regulations and definition of terms, sources of ingredients and manufacturing processes for products vary on a worldwide basis. For example, although gluten-containing ingredients [malt syrup (barley) and starch hydrolysates] can be used in the production of caramel color, they are not used according to food processors in North America. Corn is used most often, as it produces a longer shelf life and a much better product.

In Australia and New Zealand, caramel color is considered gluten-free since no residual gluten can be detected. In other areas of the world, caramel color may contain gluten (from barley) or soy and therefore needs to be questioned at your restaurant of choice depending upon your geographic location.

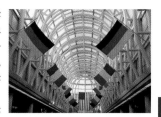

Global regulations differ in how they define the term colors or flavors. Our extensive global research indicates that colors or flavors may contain the majority of the common food allergens including: corn, dairy, eggs, gluten/wheat, peanuts, soy or tree nuts, and are identified as such throughout this book.

The only way to be certain of the contents of the colors or flavors in manufactured or pre-fabricated food items is to refer to the product label and understand the labeling regulations of the country of origin for the respective product.

As an example, according to industry and government experts, gluten-containing grains are not commonly used in flavorings. However, there are two exceptions:

1. Barley malt can be used as a flavoring agent and may or may not be listed on the label depending upon the country of origin's regulations. It might be listed as barley malt, barley malt extract or barley malt flavoring. Some companies may list it as "flavor (contains barley protein)" or occasionally may declare it only as "flavor".

2. Hydrolyzed wheat, corn and/or soy protein can be used as "flavor" or "flavor enhancers" in a variety of foods. However, in various parts of the world, they must be declared as "hydrolyzed proteins" and not hidden on the label as "flavor" or "natural flavor".

For purposes of this book, we have categorized "colors or flavors" as a term to encompass the possibility that manufactured or pre-fabricated products used in restaurants may contain common food allergens.

Ingredient and Preparation Techniques: Quick Reference Guide

Based upon the 175-plus menu items across seven international cuisines outlined in this book, the following represent the most common ingredients and preparation techniques that you may encounter while

3

eating out or serving guests anywhere in the world . It is acknowledged that this is not a complete list of every possible culinary practice. However, our research and discussions with many culinary professionals indicates that these are the most common culinary practices associated with each allergen.

These practices are mapped by the 10 most common food allergens which are color-coded in an easy-to-use format and include:

- Brown for corn and soy

- Yellow for gluten/wheat and dairy

- Blue for fish and shellfish

- Green for peanuts and tree nuts

- Pink for eggs

**Color Key for the
Quick Reference Guides**

| Corn–dark brown |
| Soy–light brown |
| Gluten/Wheat–dark yellow |
| Dairy–light yellow |
| Fish–dark blue |
| Shellfish–light blue |
| Peanuts–dark green |
| Tree Nuts–light green |
| Eggs–pink |

The 65-plus potential ingredients and techniques, listed in alphabetical order, identify where each allergen may be found. This is indicated by "typically contains allergen – ●" or "may contain allergen – ○", recommending that you check with the restaurant professional to ensure the absence of your specific food allergen.

At first, the level of detail included may seem overwhelming. Keep in mind that every effort has been made to incorporate both traditional and non-traditional culinary techniques. For example, the slim possibility that you may find soy sauce in a Mexican restaurant, while remote, has nonetheless been proven by our research. Although unusual to the cuisine, the question must be asked when there is a possibility that a culinary practice may be used. In addition, refer to product labels and associated ingredients, if applicable based upon the menu item ordered, to ensure that the dish is safe for eating.

Ingredient and Preparation Techniques:
Quick Reference Guide

	Corn	Dairy	Eggs	Fish	Gluten/Wheat	Peanuts	Shellfish	Soy	Tree Nuts
Almonds or Almond Extract	O								●
Anchovies				●					
Artificial Bacon Bits	O				O			O	
Artificial Mashed Potato Mix	O	O			O	O		O	
Batter	O		●		●				
Beans					O				
Bean Curd								●	
Bouillon	O				O			O	
Bread or Bread Crumbs	O	O	O		●	O		O	O
Breading	O	O	O		●			O	
Butter		●							
Cakes, Cookies or Biscuits		O	O		●	O		O	O
Calamari					O		●		
Cashews or Cashew Powder									●
Cheese	O	●						O	
Chocolate		●						O	
Clean Water					O				
Colors or Flavors	O	O	O		O	O		O	O
Corn Flour or Corn Meal	●								
Corn Starch	●								
Corn Syrup	●								
Crab							●		
Cream, Sour Cream or Whipped Cream		●							
Croutons	O	O	O		●	O		O	O

Ensure no cross-contamination in food preparation

● Typically contains allergen   O May contain allergen

Ingredient and Preparation Techniques: Quick Reference Guide

	Corn	Dairy	Eggs	Fish	Gluten/Wheat	Peanuts	Shellfish	Soy	Tree Nuts
Dedicated Fryer					O				
Dumpling Skins			O						
Egg Sealer			●						
Egg Yolks			●						
Escargot (Snails)							●		
Fish Sauce				●	O				
Fluffing Agent					O				
Garnishes					O	●			O
Imitation Crabmeat or Seafood	O		O	●	●			O	
Ketchup								O	
Lobster							●		
Malt	O				●				
Malt Vinegar					●				
Marinades					O				
Masa	●							O	
Mayonnaise			●		O			O	
Milk or Buttermilk		●							
Mussels							●		
Noodles or Pasta			O		●				
Oil	O				O	O		O	
Oysters							●		
Peanut Oil						●			
Pistachios									●
Prosciutto		O							
Salad Dressing	O	O	O	O	O			O	

Ensure no cross-contamination in food preparation

● Typically contains allergen   O May contain allergen

Ingredient and Preparation Techniques: Quick Reference Guide

3

	Corn	Dairy	Eggs	Fish	Gluten/Wheat	Peanuts	Shellfish	Soy	Tree Nuts
Salmon				●					
Sauce	O	O	O		O	O		O	O
Seasonings	O	O			O			O	
Shrimp							●		
Sides or Accompaniments	O	O	O		O	O		O	O
Soy Sauce					O			●	
Stabilizers					O				
Stocks and Broths				O	O		O		
Thickening Agent					O				
Tofu								●	
Tortillas or Tortilla Chips	O				O			O	
Tuna				●					
Vanilla Extract	O								
Vegetable Oil	O						O		O
Walnuts									●
Wheat Flour					●				
Wheat Flour Dusting					●				
Yogurt, Curd or Sauce		●			O				

Ensure no cross-contamination in food preparation

● Typically contains allergen   O May contain allergen

3

Ingredient and Preparation Techniques by Allergen

The allergens detailed in this section include: corn, dairy, eggs, fish, gluten/wheat, peanuts, shellfish, soy and tree nuts. Each allergen description outlines:

- Basic information on the allergen

- List of ingredients and food preparation techniques specific to the allergen

- Specific ingredients and techniques on how to manage the consideration and a sample question to ask the restaurant professional to ensure its absence in dishes

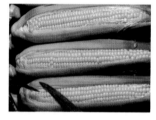

Corn

Corn, in its natural form, can obviously be detected as an ingredient in many dishes. In some parts of the world, it is referred to as maize. Additionally, hominy is another term for corn primarily found in North America.

The following potential ingredients and preparation techniques represent areas of concern while managing sensitivities to corn and its derivatives:

- Almond Extract
- Artificial Bacon Bits
- Artificial Mashed Potato Mix
- Batter
- Bouillon
- Bread or Bread Crumbs
- Breading
- Cheese
- Colors or Flavors
- Corn Flour or Corn Meal
- Corn Starch
- Corn Syrup

- Croutons
- Imitation Crabmeat or Seafood
- Malt
- Masa
- Salad Dressing
- Sauce
- Seasonings
- Sides or Accompaniments
- Tortillas or Tortilla Chips
- Vanilla Extract
- Vegetable Oil

Almond Extract is used in many cuisines and found primarily in breads, desserts and pastries. Almond extract typically contains corn and tree nuts.

- Sample question: *"Is there almond extract in the crème brulée (baked custard)?"*

Artificial Bacon Bits are used as substitutes for bacon primarily in North America and may contain corn, gluten/wheat and soy, as well as other ingredients. They are typically offered with baked potatoes and in salads.

- Sample question: *"Is the bacon included in this salad real or artificial?"*

Artificial Mashed Potato Mix is often used as a time saving and inexpensive solution for mashed potatoes in North America and may contain corn, dairy, gluten/wheat, peanuts and soy.

- Sample question: *"Are the mashed potatoes included with this dish real or artificial?"*

Batter may contain corn or gluten/wheat flour combined with eggs and is used in many types of international cuisines.

- Sample question: *"Is corn flour used to batter the chicken?"*

Bouillon is often used as a time saving and inexpensive solution for soup bases and sauces. It often contains corn, gluten/wheat and soy, as well as other ingredients.

- Sample question: *"Is this soup made with fresh chicken stock?"*

Bread or Bread Crumbs may contain corn, dairy, eggs, gluten/wheat, peanuts, soy and tree nuts, as well as other ingredients, and are used in many types of international cuisines.

- Sample question: *"Do you make your bread with corn oil?"*

Breading may contain corn, dairy, eggs, gluten/wheat and soy and is used in many international cuisines.

- Sample question: *"Is the petti di pollo (Italian chicken breast) breaded with corn meal?"*

3

Cheese contains dairy. Pasteurized processed cheese may also contain corn or soy depending upon the manufacturer. It is used as an ingredient in sauces, salads, dishes, sides and desserts.

- Sample question: *"Is this salad topped with pasteurized processed cheese containing corn syrup?"*

Colors or Flavors can be made from a variety of ingredients some of which contain corn, dairy, eggs, gluten/wheat, peanuts, soy and tree nuts. These may be included in prefabricated frozen desserts, beverages and food coloring.

- Sample question: *"Do you make your ice cream fresh in the restaurant or is it from a container that identifies corn or its derivatives as an ingredient on the label?"*

Corn Flour or Corn Meal may be used for battering, breading or flour dusting in many international cuisines.

- Sample question: *"Do you flour dust your chicken with corn flour?"*

Corn Starch may be used as a flour dusting for meats or fish and as a thickening agent for sauces and soups.

- Sample question: *"Is the chicken dusted in corn starch prior to frying?"*

Corn Syrup is a common ingredient in commercially produced sauces and dressings, as well as a sweetener for beverages.

- Sample question: *"Do you make your cocktail sauce with ketchup containing corn syrup?"*

Croutons may contain corn, dairy, eggs, gluten/wheat, peanuts, soy and tree nuts, as well as other ingredients, and are used in salads and soups in many types of international cuisines.

- Sample question: *"Is the salad topped with croutons?"*

Imitation Crabmeat or Seafood is also known as surimi and is commonly used in Asian cuisines. It is made of fish paste and a number of additives, then molded into a shape, usually resembling crabmeat. In addition to fish, surimi typically contains gluten/wheat and may contain corn, eggs and soy.

- Sample question: *"Do you use imitation crabmeat in your seafood bisque?"*

Malt may be made from corn or barley. Barley contains gluten and is commonly used in commercially produced beverages, confectionery products and frozen desserts.

- Sample question: *"Does the ice cream container identify malt or corn as an ingredient on the label?"*

Masa is made from corn meal and lard or vegetable oil, which may be made with corn and soy. It is used primarily in Central and South American cuisine.

- Sample question: *"Are the tortillas made with corn flour or corn meal?"*

Salad Dressing that is commercially produced may contain ingredients derived from corn, dairy, eggs, fish, gluten/wheat and soy. Vinaigrettes made fresh in restaurants with vegetable oil may also include corn and soy. If used in a fresh vinaigrette, olive oil that does not state 100% on the container may be mixed with vegetable oil.

- Sample question: *"Is this vinaigrette made with 100% olive oil?"*

3

Sauce may contain corn as an ingredient and corn starch as a thickening agent, as well as dairy, eggs, gluten/wheat, peanuts, soy and tree nuts. Commercially produced sauces may contain a number of different corn derivatives.

- Sample question: *"Do you use corn starch to thicken the sauce?"*

Seasonings that are commercially produced sometimes contain ingredients derived from corn, dairy, gluten/wheat and soy.

- Sample question: *"What type of seasonings do you use to flavor the chicken?"*

Sides or Accompaniments may contain corn, as well as other ingredients and their derivatives such as dairy, eggs, gluten/wheat, peanuts, soy and tree nuts.

- Sample question: *"Are the refried beans made with corn oil?"*

Tortillas or Tortilla Chips may contain corn, gluten/wheat or soy and are common in Central and South American cuisines. They can be made from either corn or wheat flour and lard or vegetable oil containing corn and soy.

- Sample question: *"What type of tortilla is the taco salad bowl made from?"*

Vanilla Extract may contain a corn derivative as an ingredient and is primarily used in desserts.

- Sample question: *"Do you use fresh vanilla beans in your rice pudding?"*

Vegetable Oil can be a blend of corn, peanuts, soy and other types of oils.

- Sample question: *"Can I have the asparagus sautéed in butter rather than vegetable oil?"*

Dairy

Dairy products are commonly used in many international cuisines and have many forms. In the case of product labels, dairy products can be represented using alternative names such as casein, caseinates, ghee, hydrolysates, lactalbumin, lactoglobulin, lactose and whey.

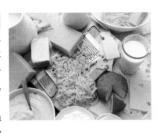

The following potential ingredients and preparation techniques represent areas of concern while managing sensitivities to dairy and its derivatives:

- Artificial Mashed Potato Mix
- Bread or Bread Crumbs
- Breading
- Butter
- Cakes, Cookies or Biscuits
- Cheese
- Chocolate
- Colors or Flavors
- Cream, Sour Cream or Whipped Cream
- Croutons
- Milk or Buttermilk
- Prosciutto
- Salad Dressing
- Sauce
- Seasonings
- Sides or Accompaniments
- Yogurt, Curd or Sauce

Artificial Mashed Potato Mix is often used as a time saving and inexpensive solution for mashed potatoes in North America and may contain dairy, corn, gluten/wheat, peanuts and soy.

- Sample question: *"Are the mashed potatoes included with this dish real or artificial?"*

Bread or Bread Crumbs may contain dairy, corn, eggs, gluten/wheat, peanuts, soy and tree nuts, as well as other ingredients, and are used in many types of international cuisines.

- Sample question: *"Are your dosas (South Indian bread) made with butter?"*

Breading may contain dairy, corn, eggs, gluten/wheat and soy and is used in many international cuisines.

- Sample question: *"Does the breading for the chicken breast contain butter?"*

3

Butter contains dairy and is often used as an ingredient or to sauté foods.

- Sample question: *"Can you sauté the haricots verts (French green beans) in vegetable oil?"*

Cakes, Cookies or Biscuits can contain dairy, eggs, gluten/wheat, peanuts, soy and tree nuts. They are included as ingredients or accompaniments to desserts in many international cuisines.

- Sample question: *"Is there any butter in the wafer?"*

Cheese contains dairy. Pasteurized processed cheese may also contain corn or soy depending upon the manufacturer. It is used as an ingredient in sauces, salads, dishes, sides and desserts.

- Sample question: *"Is this salad topped with cheese?"*

Chocolate contains dairy if it is identified as milk chocolate or listed on the label. It may also contain soy if made in the United States. It is used as an ingredient in desserts and some sauces.

- Sample question: *"Is this dessert prepared with milk chocolate or dark chocolate?"*

Colors or Flavors can be made from a variety of ingredients some of which contain dairy, corn, eggs, gluten/wheat, peanuts, soy and tree nuts. These may be included in prefabricated frozen desserts, beverages and food coloring.

- Sample question: *"Do you make your sherbet fresh in the restaurant or is it from a container that identifies dairy or its derivatives as an ingredient on the label?"*

Croutons may contain dairy, corn, eggs, gluten/wheat, peanuts, soy and tree nuts, as well as other ingredients, and are used in salads and soups in many types of international cuisines.

- Sample question: *"Is the salad topped with croutons?"*

Cream, Sour Cream or Whipped Cream contains dairy and can be used in many different areas of food preparation. Cream and sour cream are often used in sauces, while whipped cream is typically used for desserts.

- Sample question: *"Do you top your fresh berries with whipped cream?"*

Milk or Buttermilk contains dairy and is often used as an ingredient in sauces, soups, dishes and desserts.

- Sample question: *"Is there milk in your green chile sauce?"*

Prosciutto may contain dairy as an ingredient.

- Sample question: *"Does the prosciutto with the melon contain dairy?"*

Salad Dressing that is commercially produced may contain ingredients derived from dairy, corn, eggs, fish, gluten/wheat and soy.

- Sample question: *"Does this salad dressing identify dairy or its derivatives as an ingredient on the label?"*

Sauce may contain dairy as an ingredient, as well as corn, eggs, gluten/wheat, peanuts, soy and tree nuts. Commercially produced sauces may contain a number of different dairy derivatives.

- Sample question: *"Is there Parmesan cheese in your marinara sauce?"*

Seasonings that are commercially produced sometimes contain ingredients derived from dairy, corn, gluten/ wheat and soy.

- Sample question: *"What type of seasonings do you use to flavor the chicken?"*

Sides or Accompaniments may contain any number of dairy products including butter, cheese or cream, as well as other ingredients and their derivatives such as corn, eggs, gluten/wheat, peanuts, soy and tree nuts.

- Sample question: *"Are the refried beans topped with cheese?"*

Yogurt, Curd or Sauce typically contains dairy as an ingredient and is commonly used in Mediterranean, Middle Eastern and Indian cuisines.

- Sample question: *"Is there yogurt in this curry?"*

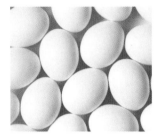

Eggs

Eggs are used in most international cuisines and are commonly found in commercially made food products. In the case of product labels, products derived from eggs can be represented using alternative names such as albumin (albumen), conalbumin, globulin, lecithin (from egg), livetin, lysozyme, ovalbumin, ovamucin, ovoglobulin, ovolactohydrolyze proteins, ovomacroglobulin, ovomucoid, ovotransferrin, ovovitellin, silco-albuminate and vitellin.

The following potential ingredients and preparation techniques represent areas of concern while managing sensitivities to eggs and its derivatives:

- Batter
- Bread or Bread Crumbs
- Breading
- Cakes, Cookies or Biscuits
- Colors or Flavors
- Croutons
- Dumpling Skins
- Egg Sealer

- Egg Yolks
- Imitation Crabmeat or Seafood
- Mayonnaise
- Noodles or Pasta
- Salad Dressing
- Sauce
- Sides or Accompaniments

Batter typically contains eggs combined with either corn or gluten/wheat flour and is used in many types of international cuisines.

- Sample question: *"Is the veal in this dish battered?"*

Bread or Bread Crumbs may contain eggs, corn, dairy, gluten/wheat, peanuts, soy and tree nuts, as well as other ingredients, and are used in many types of international cuisines.

- Sample question: *"Are the cozze al vapor (Italian steamed mussels) topped with bread crumbs that contain eggs?"*

Breading may contain eggs, corn, dairy, gluten/wheat and soy and is used in many international cuisines.

- Sample question: *"Does the breading on the chicken contain eggs?"*

Cakes, Cookies or Biscuits can contain eggs, dairy, gluten/wheat, peanuts, soy and tree nuts. They are included as ingredients or accompaniments to desserts in many international cuisines.

- Sample question: *"Are there any eggs in the almond cookie?"*

Colors or Flavors can be made from a variety of ingredients some of which contain eggs, corn, dairy, gluten/wheat, peanuts, soy and tree nuts. These may be included in prefabricated frozen desserts, beverages and food coloring.

- Sample question: *"Do you make your gelato fresh in the restaurant or is it from a container that identifies egg or its derivatives as an ingredient on the label?"*

Croutons may contain eggs, corn, dairy, gluten/wheat, peanuts, soy and tree nuts, as well as other ingredients, and are used in salads and soups in many types of international cuisines.

- Sample question: *"Is the salad topped with croutons?"*

Dumpling Skins are common in Asian cuisines and typically contain eggs.

- Sample question: *"Does the dumpling skin for the kanom jeeb (Thai shrimp dumplings) have eggs in it?"*

Egg Sealer is a term used for the process of sealing dumplings and parchment bags used for cooking.

- Sample question: *"Is egg used to seal the parchment paper bag in the saumon en papillote (French baked salmon)?"*

Egg Yolks are often used as an ingredient in sauces, dishes and desserts.

- Sample question: *"Does this sauce contain egg yolks?"*

Imitation Crabmeat or Seafood is also known as surimi and is commonly used in Asian cuisines. It is made of fish paste and a number of additives, then molded into a shape, usually resembling crabmeat. In addition to fish, surimi typically contains gluten/wheat and may contain eggs, corn and soy.

- Sample question: *"Do you use imitation crabmeat in your seafood bisque?"*

Mayonnaise contains eggs and is used as an ingredient in sauces, as well as a condiment. Commercially produced mayonnaise may also include soy.

- Sample question: *"Can I have my hamburger without mayonnaise?"*

Noodles or Pasta may contain eggs and gluten/wheat as ingredients.

- Sample question: *"Do the rice noodles contain eggs?"*

Salad Dressing that is commercially produced may contain ingredients derived from eggs, corn, dairy, fish, gluten/wheat and soy. Fresh Caesar dressing is typically made with eggs and some fresh French vinaigrettes may contain hard boiled eggs.

- Sample question: *"Does the dressing in the asperge à la vinaigrette (French asparagus salad) contain eggs or its derivatives?"*

Sauce may contain eggs as an ingredient, as well as corn, dairy, gluten/wheat, peanuts, soy and tree nuts. Commercially produced sauces may contain a number of different egg derivatives.

- Sample question: *"Can I have my filet mignon without béarnaise sauce?"*

Sides or Accompaniments may contain eggs, as well as other ingredients and their derivatives such as corn, dairy, gluten/wheat, peanuts, soy and tree nuts.

- Sample question: *"Is the pasta in the side salad made with eggs?"*

3

Fish

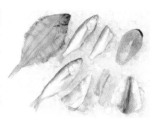

Fish is an easier allergy to manage, since it is used primarily as a main ingredient in most dishes. There are some commercially produced sauces that contain fish.

The following potential ingredients and preparation techniques represent areas of concern while managing sensitivities to fish:

- Anchovies
- Fish Sauce
- Imitation Crabmeat or Seafood
- Salad Dressing
- Salmon
- Stocks and Broths
- Tuna

Anchovies contain fish and are a common ingredient in European style salads and some commercially produced sauces.

- Sample question: *"Does your salade niçoise (French nice style salad) contain anchovies?"*

Fish Sauce is a common sauce in Southeast Asian cuisine and may also contain gluten/wheat based upon manufacturing processes outside of Thailand.

- Sample question: *"Is there fish sauce in your thom kha gai (Thai chicken and coconut soup)?"*

Imitation Crabmeat or Seafood is also known as surimi and is commonly used in Asian cuisines. It is made of fish paste and a number of additives, then molded into a shape, usually resembling crabmeat. In addition to fish, surimi may contain corn, eggs, gluten/wheat and soy.

- Sample question: *"Do you use imitation crabmeat in your seafood bisque?"*

3

Salad Dressing that is commercially produced may contain ingredients derived from fish, corn, dairy, eggs, gluten/wheat and soy. Fresh Caesar salad dressing typically contains anchovies.

- Sample question: *"Does the Caesar salad dressing contain anchovies?"*

Salmon contains fish and may be found in starters and dishes in many international cuisines.

- Sample question: *"Do you grill your steaks on the same side of the grill as your salmon and other fish?"*

Stocks and Broths may contain fish and shellfish if they are used in the preparation of seafood dishes.

- Sample question: *"Is your risotto ai funghi (Italian arborio rice and mushroom dish) made with fish stock?"*

Tuna contains fish and may be found in starters and dishes in many international cuisines.

- Sample question: *"Does this salad contain tuna?"*

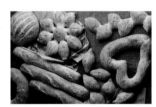

Gluten/Wheat

Gluten is the protein found in wheat, rye and barley. It is a composite name representing gliadin in wheat, hordein in barley and secalin in rye. Gluten can also be the name given for avenin, a slightly different protein found in oats. It should be noted that oats without measurable contamination from wheat, rye and barley may be referred to as certified gluten-free oats in some parts of the world. Individuals that experience a reaction to pure uncontaminated oats are reacting to the oat avenin.

Individuals can also have allergies, intolerances or sensitivities to wheat without having the dietary concerns for other grains that contain gluten. Gluten-free, wheat-free and gluten-containing grains are detailed earlier in this chapter.

The following potential ingredients and preparation techniques represent areas of concern while managing celiac / coeliac disease or sensitivities to gluten/wheat and their derivatives:

- Artificial Bacon Bits
- Artificial Mashed Potato Mix
- Batter
- Beans
- Bouillon
- Bread or Bread Crumbs
- Breading
- Cakes, Cookies or Biscuits
- Clean Water
- Colors or Flavors
- Croutons
- Dedicated Fryer
- Fish Sauce
- Fluffing Agent
- Garnishes
- Imitation Crabmeat or Seafood
- Malt
- Malt Vinegar
- Marinades
- Noodles or Pasta
- Oil
- Salad Dressing
- Sauce
- Seasonings
- Sides or Accompaniments
- Soy Sauce
- Stabilizers
- Thickening Agent
- Tortillas or Tortilla Chips
- Wheat Flour
- Wheat Flour Dusting

3

Artificial Bacon Bits are used as substitutes for bacon primarily in North America and may contain gluten/wheat, corn and soy, as well as other ingredients. They are typically offered with baked potatoes and in salads.

- Sample question: *"Is the bacon included in the baked potato real or artificial?"*

Artificial Mashed Potato Mix is often used as a time saving and inexpensive solution for mashed potatoes in North America and may contain gluten/wheat, corn, dairy, peanuts and soy.

- Sample question: *"Are the mashed potatoes included with this dish real or artificial?"*

Batter typically contains gluten/wheat or corn flour combined with eggs and is used in many types of international cuisines.

- Sample question: *"Is the calamari battered with wheat flour?"*

Beans may include wheat flour as an ingredient in many international cuisines.

- Sample question: *"Do the fava beans contain wheat flour?"*

Bouillon is often used as a time saving and inexpensive solution for soup bases and sauces. It often contains gluten/wheat, corn and soy, as well as other ingredients.

- Sample question: *"Is this soup made with fresh vegetable broth?"*

3

Bread or Bread Crumbs typically contain gluten/wheat, corn, dairy, eggs, peanuts, soy and tree nuts, as well as other ingredients, and are used in many types of international cuisines.

- Sample question: *"Are the escargots (snails) topped with bread crumbs?"*

Breading typically contain gluten/wheat, corn, dairy, eggs and soy and is used in many international cuisines.

- Sample question: *"Is the petti di pollo (Italian chicken breast) breaded?"*

Cake, Cookies or Biscuits can contain gluten/wheat, dairy, eggs, peanuts, soy and tree nuts. They are included as ingredients or accompaniments to desserts in many international cuisines.

- Sample question: *"Is there any gluten/wheat in the flourless chocolate torte?"*

Clean Water is a request that may be necessary to eliminate the possibility of cross-contamination from preparing other menu items such as pasta.

- Sample question: *"Is your rice cooked in the same water as your pasta?"*

Colors or Flavors can be made from a variety of ingredients some of which contain gluten/wheat, corn, dairy, eggs, peanuts, soy and tree nuts. These may be included in pre-fabricated frozen desserts, beverages and food coloring.

- Sample question: *"Is the smoked sausage made in the restaurant or do you use pre-packaged sausage that identifies gluten/wheat or its derivatives on the label?"*

Croutons typically contain gluten/wheat, corn, dairy, eggs, peanuts, soy and tree nuts, as well as other ingredients, and are used in salads and soups in many types of international cuisines.

- Sample question: *"Is the salad topped with croutons?"*

3

Dedicated Fryer is a term used for a fryer that only fries one particular food type (e.g. battered items only or French fried potatoes/chips). Dedicated fryers eliminate the possibility of gluten/wheat cross-contamination from frying battered, breaded or gluten/wheat flour dusted foods with non-gluten containing foods.

- Sample question: *"Are your French fried potatoes/ chips fried in the same fryer as your beer battered onion rings?"*

Fish Sauce is a common sauce in Southeast Asian cuisine and may also contain gluten/wheat based upon manufacturing processes outside of Thailand.

- Sample question: *"Is the brand of fish sauce you use in this dish processed in Hong Kong?"*

Fluffing Agent is a term used for adding an ingredient, such as gluten/wheat, to eggs to enhance their appearance and increase their volume.

- Sample question: *"Do you add gluten/wheat to the egg mix for your omelets?"*

Garnishes containing gluten/wheat, peanuts and tree nuts are common in international cuisines.

- Sample question: *"Is this salad garnished with a breadstick?"*

Imitation Crabmeat or Seafood is also known as surimi and is commonly used in Asian cuisines. It is made of fish paste and a number of additives, then molded into a shape, usually resembling crabmeat. In addition to fish, surimi typically contains gluten/wheat and may contain corn, eggs and soy.

3

- Sample question: *"Do you use imitation crabmeat in your seafood bisque?"*

Malt is typically made from barley or corn. Barley contains gluten and is commonly used in commercially produced beverages, confectionery products and frozen desserts.

- Sample question: *"Does the ice cream container identify malt or barley as an ingredient on the label?"*

Malt Vinegar is made by fermenting barley, which contains gluten, and is not distilled. It is a common condiment in French cuisine and also used regularly in the United Kingdom.

- Sample question: *"Can you hold the malt vinegar with my French fried potatoes order?"*

Marinades may have packaged seasonings which contain gluten/wheat as an ingredient.

- Sample question: *"Does the marinade for gai yang (Thai barbequed chicken) contain gluten/wheat?"*

Noodles or Pasta may contain gluten/wheat and eggs as ingredients.

- Sample question: *"Are the noodles in the pad see yu made with gluten/wheat?"*

Oil is used to cook many gluten containing items. Ensure fresh cooking oil is used to eliminate the possibility of cross-contamination from cooking other menu items.

- Sample question: *"Can you use fresh oil to fry my huevos Mexicanos (Mexican eggs)?"*

Salad Dressing that is commercially produced may contain ingredients derived from gluten/wheat, corn, dairy, eggs, fish and soy.

- Sample question: *"Does the ranch dressing identify gluten/wheat or its derivatives as an ingredient on the label?"*

Sauce may contain gluten/wheat as an ingredient, as well as corn, dairy, eggs, peanuts, soy and tree nuts. Commercially produced sauces may contain a number of different gluten/wheat derivatives.

- Sample question: *"Does the peanut sauce contain gluten/wheat?"*

Seasonings that are commercially produced sometimes contain ingredients derived from gluten/wheat, corn, dairy and soy.

- Sample question: *"What type of seasonings do you use to flavor the French fried potatoes?"*

Sides or Accompaniments may contain gluten/wheat, as well as other ingredients and their derivatives such as corn, dairy, eggs, peanuts, soy and tree nuts.

- Sample question: *"Does the fruit compote that comes with the pork chop contain gluten/wheat?"*

Soy Sauce is a common ingredient in Asian and other international cuisines. In addition to being made from soy, most soy sauces also contain gluten/wheat as an ingredient. It is used in marinades or as an ingredient in sauces and soups.

- Sample question: *"Is there soy sauce in the lemon chicken?"*

Stabilizers containing gluten/wheat may be used in commercially produced frozen desserts.

- Sample question: *"Does the sorbet container identify gluten/wheat stabilizers as an ingredient on the label?"*

Thickening Agent is an ingredient, such as gluten/wheat, added to soups or sauces so they have a higher viscosity or thickness.

- Sample question: *"Do you use gluten/wheat to thicken the broth of the egg drop soup?"*

Tortillas or Tortilla Chips may contain gluten/wheat, corn or soy and are common in Central and South American cuisines. They can be made from either corn or wheat flour and lard or vegetable oil containing corn and soy.

- Sample question: *"Can I have corn tortillas with my carnitas (Mexican simmered pork)?"*

Wheat Flour can be used as an ingredient in the most unlikely places. Non-traditional food preparation techniques involving wheat flour are indicated throughout this book.

- Sample question: *"Do you add wheat flour to your hollandaise sauce?"*

Wheat Flour Dusting is a technique used for coating meat or fish with an ingredient, such as gluten/wheat, for texture prior to pan-frying.

- Sample question: *"Do you dust the beef in gluten/wheat prior to pan frying?"*

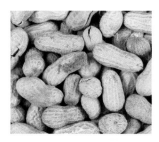

Peanuts

Peanuts are legumes like peas or beans and are used frequently in Asian, Central and South American cuisines. Peanut oil, also known as arachis oil in Europe, is commonly used for frying in Asian, Indian, French and French-influenced cuisines. Other names for peanuts include: beer nuts, cacahouéte, cacahouette, cacahuéte, earth nuts, goober nuts, ground nuts, mandelonas and valencias.

The following potential ingredients and preparation techniques represent areas of concern while managing sensitivities to peanuts and its derivatives:

- Artificial Mashed Potato Mix
- Bread or Bread Crumbs
- Cakes, Cookies or Biscuits
- Colors or Flavors
- Croutons
- Garnishes
- Peanut Oil
- Sauce
- Sides or Accompaniments
- Vegetable Oil

Artificial Mashed Potato Mix is often used as a time saving and inexpensive solution for mashed potatoes in North America and may contain peanuts, corn, dairy, gluten/wheat and soy.

- Sample question: *"Are the mashed potatoes included with this dish real or artificial?"*

Bread or Bread Crumbs may contain peanuts, corn, dairy, eggs, gluten/wheat, soy and tree nuts, as well as other ingredients, and are used in many types of international cuisines.

- Sample question: *"Are there peanuts in this fresh bread?"*

Cakes, Cookies or Biscuits can contain peanuts, dairy, eggs, gluten/wheat, soy and tree nuts. They are included as ingredients or accompaniments to desserts in many international cuisines.

- Sample question: *"Are there any peanuts in the cookie?"*

Colors or Flavors can be made from a variety of ingredients some of which contain peanuts, corn, dairy, eggs, gluten/wheat, soy and tree nuts. These may be included in prefabricated frozen desserts, beverages and food coloring.

- Sample question: *"Do you make your gelato fresh in the restaurant or is it from a container that identifies peanuts or its derivatives as an ingredient on the label?"*

Croutons may contain peanuts, corn, dairy, eggs, gluten/wheat, soy and tree nuts, as well as other ingredients, and are used in salads and soups in many types of international cuisines.

- Sample question: *"Is the salad topped with croutons?"*

Garnishes containing peanuts, gluten/wheat and tree nuts are common in international cuisines.

- Sample question: *"Is the kang dang (Thai red curry) garnished with peanuts?"*

Peanut Oil is commonly used to fry or sauté foods in Asian, Indian, French and French-influenced restaurants.

- Sample question: *"Are the pommes frites (French fried potatoes) fried in peanut oil?"*

Sauce may contain peanuts as an ingredient and is typically found in Asian, Central and South American cuisines. Sauces may also contain corn, dairy, eggs, gluten/wheat, soy and tree nuts. Commercially produced sauces may contain a number of different peanut derivatives.

- Sample question: *"Do you include peanuts in your mole sauce?"*

Sides or Accompaniments may contain peanuts, as well as other ingredients and their derivatives such as corn, dairy, eggs, gluten/wheat, soy and tree nuts.

- Sample question: *"Do you sauté the green beans in peanut oil?"*

Vegetable Oil can be a blend of peanuts, corn, soy and other types of oils.

- Sample question: *"Can I have the mushrooms sautéed in butter rather than vegetable oil?"*

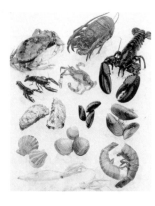

Shellfish

Shellfish are divided into two categories, crustaceans and mollusks. Some crustaceans include copepods, crab, crayfish, lobster, prawns and shrimp. Mollusks include abalone, clam, conch, escargot (snails), limpets, mussels, octopus, oysters, scallops, squid (calamari) and whelks.

The following potential ingredients and preparation techniques represent areas of concern while managing sensitivities to shellfish:

- Calamari
- Crab
- Escargot (Snails)
- Lobster
- Mussels
- Oysters
- Shrimp
- Stocks and Broths

Calamari, the Italian name for squid, may be found in starters, dishes and soups in many international cuisines.

- Sample question: *"Does the salmon bisque contain calamari or any other shellfish?"*

Crab may be found in starters, dishes and soups in many international cuisines.

- Sample question: *"Are the mushrooms stuffed with crab?"*

Escargot (Snails) may be found in starters and dishes in some international cuisines.

- Sample question: *"Are the mushrooms stuffed with escargot (snails)?"*

Lobster may be found in starters, dishes and soups in many international cuisines.

- Sample question: *"Does the risotto special contain lobster or any other shellfish?"*

Mussels may be found in starters, dishes and soups in many international cuisines.

- Sample question: *"Does this paella (Spanish rice dish) contain mussels or any other shellfish?"*

Oysters may be found in starters, dishes and soups in many international cuisines.

- Sample question: *"Does the salmon bisque contain oysters or any other shellfish?"*

Shrimp may be found in starters, dishes and soups in many international cuisines.

- Sample question: *"Do your summer rolls contain shrimp?"*

Stocks and Broths may contain shellfish and fish if they are used in the preparation of seafood dishes.

- Sample question: *"Is your risotto ai funghi (Italian arborio rice and mushroom dish) made with seafood stock?"*

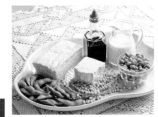

Soy

Soy is a legume like peas or beans and is used frequently in Asian cuisines. In some parts of the world it is referred to as soya or soja. Other names for soy include: edamame, miso, natto, okara, shoyu, tamari, tempeh, tofu (soybean curds) and yuba. Its derivatives are contained in many commercially produced products.

The following potential ingredients and preparation techniques represent areas of concern while managing sensitivities to soy and its derivatives:

- Artificial Bacon Bits
- Artificial Mashed Potato Mix
- Bean Curd
- Bouillon
- Bread or Bread Crumbs
- Breading
- Cakes, Cookies or Biscuits
- Cheese
- Chocolate
- Colors or Flavors
- Croutons
- Imitation Crabmeat or Seafood
- Ketchup
- Masa
- Mayonnaise
- Salad Dressing
- Sauce
- Seasonings
- Sides or Accompaniments
- Soy Sauce
- Tofu
- Tortillas or Tortilla Chips
- Vegetable Oil

Artificial Bacon Bits are used as substitutes for bacon primarily in North America and may contain soy, corn and gluten/wheat, as well as other ingredients. They are typically offered with baked potatoes and in salads.

- Sample question: *"Is the bacon included in this salad real or artificial?"*

Artificial Mashed Potato Mix is often used as a time saving and inexpensive solution for mashed potatoes in North America and may contain soy, corn, dairy, gluten/wheat and peanuts.

- Sample question: *"Are the mashed potatoes included with this dish real or artificial?"*

Bean Curd is made from soy and is similar in consistency to medium-hard cheese. It is often used in Asian cuisines.

- Sample question: *"Is there bean curd in the kaw pad (Thai fried rice)?"*

Bouillon is often used as a time saving and inexpensive solution for soup bases and sauces. It often contains soy, corn and gluten/wheat, as well as other ingredients.

- Sample question: *"Is this bouillabaisse (French seafood stew) made with fresh seafood stock?"*

3

Bread or Bread Crumbs may contain soy, corn, dairy, eggs, gluten/wheat, peanuts and tree nuts, as well as other ingredients, and are used in many types of international cuisines.

- Sample question: *"Do you make your bread with vegetable oil?"*

Breading may contain soy, corn, dairy, eggs and gluten/wheat and is used in many international cuisines.

- Sample question: *"Is the melanzane alla griglia (Italian grilled eggplant) prepared with breading that contains vegetable oil?"*

Cakes, Cookies or Biscuits can contain soy, dairy, eggs, gluten/wheat, peanuts and tree nuts. They are included as ingredients or accompaniments to desserts in many international cuisines.

- Sample question: *"Is there any soy in this wafer?"*

Cheese contains dairy. Pasteurized processed cheese may also contain soy or corn depending upon the manufacturer. It is used as an ingredient in sauces, salads, dishes, sides and desserts.

- Sample question: *"Does the cheese sauce contain pasteurized processed cheese with soy as an ingredient?"*

Chocolate may contain soy if made in the United States and contains dairy if it is identified as milk chocolate or listed on the label. It is used as an ingredient in desserts and some sauces.

- Sample question: *"Can you check to see if the chocolate in the mole sauce contains soy?"*

Colors or Flavors can be made from a variety of ingredients some of which contain soy, corn, dairy, eggs, gluten/wheat, peanuts and tree nuts. These may be included in prefabricated frozen desserts, beverages and food coloring.

- Sample question: *"Do you make your sorbet fresh in the restaurant or is it from a container that identifies soy or its derivatives as an ingredient on the label?"*

Croutons may contain soy, corn, dairy, eggs, gluten/wheat, peanuts and tree nuts, as well as other ingredients, and are used in salads and soups in many types of international cuisines.

- Sample question: *"Is the salad topped with croutons?"*

Imitation Crabmeat or Seafood is also known as surimi and is commonly used in Asian cuisines. It is made of fish paste and a number of additives, then molded into a shape, usually resembling crabmeat. In addition to fish, surimi typically contains gluten/wheat and may contain soy, corn and eggs.

- Sample question: *"Do you use imitation crabmeat in your paella mariscos (Mexican seafood and rice dish)?"*

Ketchup is made from tomatoes, vinegar and many other ingredients which may include soy. It is provided as a condiment and used in some sauces.

- Sample question: *"Do you prepare your cocktail sauce with ketchup that lists soy as an ingredient?"*

Masa is made from corn meal and lard or vegetable oil which may be made with soy and corn. It is used primarily in Central and South American cuisine.

- Sample question: *"Is the masa in your tamales made with vegetable oil containing soy?"*

Mayonnaise contains eggs and is used as an ingredient in sauces, as well as a condiment. Commercially produced mayonnaise may also include soy.

- Sample question: *"Does the mayonnaise you use for the dipping sauce come from a container that identifies soy as an ingredient on the label?"*

Salad Dressing that is commercially produced may contain ingredients derived from soy, corn, dairy, eggs, fish and gluten/wheat. Vinaigrettes made fresh in restaurants with vegetable oil may also include corn and soy. If used in a fresh vinaigrette, olive oil that does not state 100% on the container may be mixed with vegetable oil.

- Sample question: *"Does the Russian salad dressing come from a container that identifies soy or its derivatives as an ingredient on the label?"*

Sauce may contain soy as an ingredient, as well as corn, dairy, eggs, fish, gluten/wheat, peanuts and tree nuts. Commercially produced sauces may contain a number of different soy derivatives.

- Sample question: *"Does the chili sauce contain vegetable oil identifying soy as an ingredient?"*

Seasonings that are commercially produced sometimes contain ingredients derived from soy, corn, dairy and gluten/wheat.

- Sample question: *"What type of seasonings do you use to flavor the hash browns?"*

Sides or Accompaniments may contain soy, as well as other ingredients and their derivatives such as corn, dairy, eggs, gluten/wheat, peanuts, soy and tree nuts.

- Sample question: *"Do you sauté the broccoli rabe in vegetable oil?"*

Soy Sauce is a common ingredient in Asian and other international cuisines. In addition to being made from soy, most soy sauces also contain gluten/wheat as an ingredient. It is used in marinades or as an ingredient in sauces or soups.

- Sample question: *"Does the marinade for your roasted chicken contain soy sauce?"*

Tofu is made from soy and is similar in consistency to soft cheese. It is often used in Asian cuisines.

- Sample question: *"Does the Buddha's Feast include tofu?"*

Tortillas or Tortilla Chips may contain soy, corn or gluten/wheat and are common in Central and South American cuisines. They can be made from either corn or wheat flour and lard or vegetable oil containing corn and soy.

- Sample question: *"Are your tortilla chips made from vegetable oil containing soy?"*

Vegetable Oil can be a blend of soy, corn, peanuts and other types of oils.

- Sample question: *"Can I have the broccoli rabe sautéed in butter rather than vegetable oil?"*

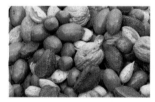

Tree Nuts

Tree nuts are considered "true nuts" and are used in many international cuisines. Various tree nuts from around the world include: almonds (marzipan, amaretti or almondine), beechnuts, Brazil nuts (cream nuts or para nuts), cashews, chestnuts, gevuina nut, gianduja, hazlenuts (filberts), hickory nuts, macadamia nuts (Australian nuts or Queensland nuts), pecans, pine nuts (pignoli, pinon, pinyon, Indian nuts or stone nuts), pistachios, pralines and walnuts (butternuts).

The following potential ingredients and preparation techniques represent areas of concern while managing sensitivities to tree nuts and their derivatives:

- Almonds or Almond Extract
- Bread or Bread Crumbs
- Cakes, Cookies or Biscuits
- Cashews or Cashew Powder
- Colors or Flavors
- Croutons
- Garnishes
- Pistachios
- Sauce
- Sides or Accompaniments
- Walnuts

Almonds or Almond Extract are used in many cuisines and found primarily in breads, desserts and pastries or as an ingredient in vegetable sides. Almond extract typically contains tree nuts and corn.

- Sample question: *"Are there almonds in the haricots verts (French green beans)?"*

Bread or Bread Crumbs may contain tree nuts, corn, dairy, eggs, gluten/wheat, peanuts and soy, as well as other ingredients, and are used in many types of international cuisines.

- Sample question: *"Are the escargots (snails) topped with bread crumbs that contain tree nuts?"*

Cakes, Cookies or Biscuits can contain tree nuts, dairy, eggs, gluten/wheat, peanuts and soy. They are included as ingredients or accompaniments to desserts in many international cuisines.

- Sample question: *"Are there any almonds in this cookie?"*

Cashews or Cashew Powder is often used in Middle Eastern and Indian cuisines, as well as in desserts in many other international cuisines.

- Sample question: *"Are the kabobs made with cashew powder?"*

Colors or Flavors can be made from a variety of ingredients some of which contain tree nuts, corn, dairy, eggs, gluten/wheat, peanuts and soy. These may be included in prefabricated frozen desserts, beverages and food coloring.

- Sample question: *"Do you make your helados (Mexican ice cream, sherbet or sorbet) fresh in the restaurant or is it from a container that identifies tree nuts or their derivatives as an ingredient on the label?"*

Croutons may contain tree nuts, corn, dairy, eggs, gluten/wheat, peanuts and soy, as well as other ingredients, and are used in salads and soups in many types of international cuisines.

- Sample question: *"Is the salad topped with croutons?"*

Garnishes containing tree nuts, gluten/wheat and peanuts are common in international cuisines.

- Sample question: *"Is the kang massaman (Thai tamarind curry) garnished with cashews or any other tree nuts?"*

Pistachios are often used in Middle Eastern and Indian cuisines, as well as in desserts in many other international cuisines.

- Sample question: *"Does the kulfi (Indian ice cream) contain pistachios or any other tree nuts?"*

Sauce may contain tree nuts as an ingredient, as well as corn, dairy, eggs, gluten/wheat, peanuts and soy. Commercially produced sauces may contain a number of different tree nut derivatives.

- Sample question: *"Does the murg korma (Indian chicken in cream curry) contain almonds or any other tree nuts?"*

Sides or Accompaniments may contain tree nuts, as well as other ingredients and their derivatives such as corn, dairy, eggs, gluten/wheat, peanuts and soy.

- Sample question: *"Is there almond oil in the chutney?"*

Walnuts are often used in breads, desserts and salads in many international cuisines.

- Sample question: *"Are walnuts included in the spinach salad?"*

Summary

As you can see, there is more to managing a special diet than simply avoiding the allergens of concern. You will no doubt need, at some time, to return to the previous pages of this chapter to re-familiarize yourself with these potential considerations. As a reminder, if this book indicates that an ingredient may be included in a particular dish, it doesn't necessarily preclude you from ordering it or from serving it to guests with special dietary considerations. You do, however, need to confirm the possibility of its presence.

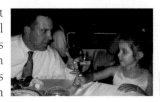

If it is indicated that a dish contains an allergen you are trying to avoid, then it is best to choose another menu option or request a substitution, if applicable. Armed with this knowledge, you will soon realize that there is a whole new world of food options open to you. Ask the right questions, embrace the eating out experience and enjoy your new freedom!

Enjoy Your Meal!

好胃口

Bon Appetit!

Buon Appetitto!

Chalo, sub khana khao!

Buen Provecho!

Gkin Kao!

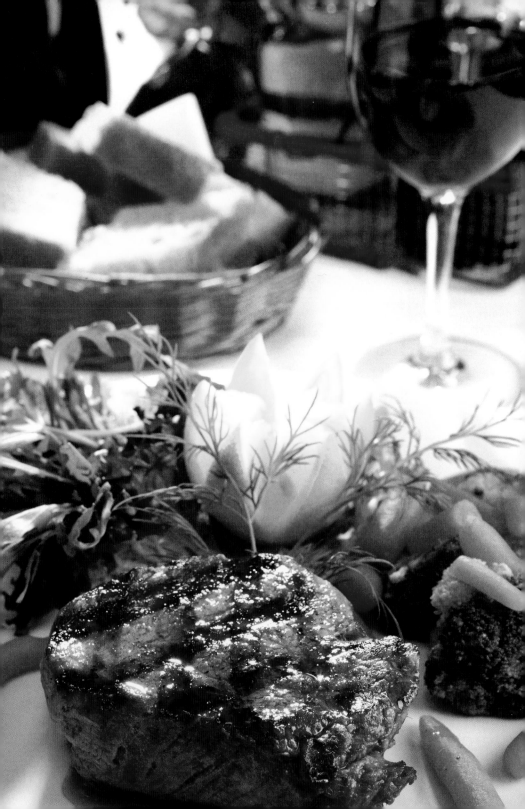

*Of all the contributions this country
has made to dining out, none is so quintessentially
American as the Steak House.*
—John Mariani

4

Chapter 4
Let's Eat American Steak and Seafood Cuisine

Cuisine Overview

The United States of America is a nation of immigrants, whose culture is a unique mixture of international influences and home grown Americana. The US is comprised of 50 states and a number of territories. It is roughly two and a half times the size of Western Europe. It is the world's third largest nation in both population and land mass.

The Steak and Seafood restaurant is the greatest representation of the bountiful harvests of American farmers, fishermen and ranchers. At these establishments, produce, meat and seafood are prepared in a simple culinary fashion that produces a wholesome and satisfying dining experience. This is due to a belief that using good quality ingredients requires few advanced culinary preparation techniques. With this in mind, the American Steak and Seafood restaurant is one of the safer cuisines for those with celiac / coeliac, food allergies or sensitivities.

The range and style of Steak and Seafood houses in America is diverse. Whether you are dining at a single independent restaurant or a large restaurant chain,

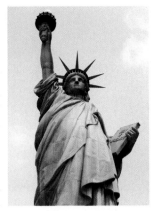
Statue of Liberty

4

each establishment has a unique atmosphere and feeling. There is the classic New York style steakhouse with its career waiters in white coats and bistro aprons or the casual wait staff at the family-oriented theme restaurants. Some restaurants choose the fusion approach of blending other international cuisines with standard steak and seafood dishes, while others give you the feeling of eating at an authentic western saloon. The quality of meat, produce and seafood is in line with the price differential between the finest steak houses and moderately priced restaurant establishments. The finest American Steak and Seafood restaurants are among the most expensive you will find in the United States. Regardless of preference, most steak and seafood restaurants can offer you a wholesome meal.

Traditional Ingredients

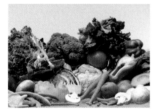
Vegetables

Vegetables play a big part in the American Steak and Seafood restaurant dining experience. Both in salads and in sides, you may see asparagus, artichokes, broccoli, carrots, green beans, hearts of palm, many types of lettuce, olives, onions, potatoes and tomatoes. Herbs include basil, garlic, rosemary and thyme. For seasoning purposes, most restaurants simply use salt and pepper; however, some chefs incorporate exotic seasonings, such as saffron, into their culinary palate.

American Steak and Seafood restaurants carry a variety of beef cuts and follow the scale of quality set forth by the U.S. government. Beef is graded for quality by U.S. Department of Agriculture (USDA) graders according to standards established by the USDA. Grades are based on the amount of marbling (flecks of fat within the cut of meat) and the age of the animal. These quality grades are an indication of palatability characteristics such as tenderness, juiciness and flavor. While there are eight quality grades for beef, the top three grades available to most consumers are prime, choice and select. In addition to beef, you may find lamb, pork and chicken on many Steak and Seafood menus.

Many types of seafood may also be available including Maine lobster, Alaskan king crab, oysters, mussels, salmon and shrimp. Again, the preparation of these dishes is minimal and in most cases involves baking, boiling, grilling, pan frying or steaming. In some establishments, there is a special food service area generally located in the front of the restaurant where raw shellfish is prepared. This "raw bar" is a common menu section that is usually enjoyed as the starter portion of a meal and in some cases can serve as the entire meal all by itself.

Starch dishes available are usually potato-based, such as baked potatoes, French fried potatoes, mashed potatoes, roasted potatoes and hash browns. Rice dishes and pastas are also available. Finally, wine is a popular accoutrement in the American Steak and Seafood dining experience. Most restaurants usually feature a wine list that gives a number of varieties, both white and red, to choose from. In the finer establishments, it is likely that you will have to make a difficult decision on wines from the US and other parts of the world.

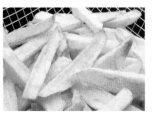
French Fried Potatoes/Chips

Gluten Awareness

Since gluten can be found in some areas of American Steak and Seafood cuisine, we have outlined 30-plus items in our sample menu. It is important to keep in mind that American food is influenced by many international culinary practices. There are seven primary points that you need to consider when dining at an American Steak and Seafood restaurant. To ensure a gluten-free experience, the areas of food preparation that you need to inquire about with your server or chef are listed below.

Sauces	Ensure the *liaison* of the sauce is butter, egg yolks or puréed vegetables—ensure no wheat flour
Flour Dusting	Wheat flour is typically used—request plain
Stocks and Broths	Ensure all are made fresh or from allergen-free mixes and not from bouillon, which may contain gluten
Cooking Oil	Ensure frying oil has not been used to fry battered foods that may contain gluten
Bread, Bread Crumbs & Croutons	Wheat flour is typically used—ensure no bread, bread crumbs or croutons
Marinades	Although uncommon, ensure marinades do not contain soy sauce or wheat flour
Cross-Contamination	Ensure all utensils and cooking surfaces have been cleaned prior to the preparation of your meal

Sauces

Sauces are typically served on the side at American Steak and Seafood restaurants and are often influenced by French cuisine. Of the many different sauces you may encounter, always be sure the *liaison* that binds the sauce together is not wheat flour. Other acceptable *liaisons* include egg yolks, butter and puréed vegetables.

Below is a list of common and typically gluten-free sauces adapted from the French and their ingredients:

4

Hollandaise:	A sauce that contains butter, egg yolks as its liaison and lemon juice
Béarnaise:	A reduction of white wine vinegar, tarragon and shallots that is finished with egg yolks and butter
Reduction:	A mixture that results from rapidly boiling a liquid (like fresh stock, wine or a sauce without wheat flour) and causing evaporation—"reducing" the sauce—which creates a thicker sauce with a more intense flavor than the original liquid

Flour Dusting

Flour dusting is not common in American Steak and Seafood restaurants. If used, most restaurants prefer to dust meat or fish with wheat flour for texture prior to pan-frying, allowing a sauce to be evenly distributed. When meat or fish is grilled over an open flame, flour dusting is not necessary. Ensure that this practice is not used in the preparation of your meal.

Stocks and Broths

Stocks and broths are used frequently in American Steak and Seafood restaurants. They are present in sauces and soups, as well as in marinades for meats and vegetables. Ensure all are made fresh or from allergen-free mixes and not from bouillon, which may contain gluten.

Cooking Oil

Any type of oil such as canola, corn or sunflower may be used in American Steak and Seafood restaurants. Some establishments influenced by French cooking may also use peanut oil. Olive oil may be incorporated from time to time, but is rarely used for frying. Oil is used to fry or sauté foods. When ordering food that is prepared by frying, ensure that there is a dedicated fryer in the kitchen for non-battered menu items. Since battered foods may contain wheat flour, this practice minimizes the potential of gluten cross-contamination from frying.

4

Bread, Bread Crumbs and Croutons

Croutons and bread crumbs are used regularly as an ingredient in starters, soups and salads. Croutons in particular are included with most salads, while bread crumbs are used in some baked vegetable sides. When ordering these dishes, always be sure to request no croutons or bread crumbs. In addition, a basket of bread is usually served, so be certain to request no bread.

Marinades

Marinades are used infrequently in American Steak and Seafood restaurants. If used, ensure that the marinade does not include soy sauce, which contains wheat, or wheat flour.

Cross-Contamination

Cross-contamination occurs in two primary instances and should be considered at any restaurant you choose to dine in. One may occur when your meal is prepared in the same frying oil as foods containing other possible allergens. The second may occur when food particles are transferred from one food to another by using the same knife, cutting board, pots, pans or other utensils without washing the surfaces or tools in between uses. In the case of open flamed grills, the extreme temperature turns most food particles into carbon. Use of a wire brush designed for grill racks typically removes residual contaminants.

To avoid cross-contamination, restaurants need to dedicate fryers for specific foods and wash all materials that may come in contact with food in hot, soapy water prior to preparing items for those with special dietary requirements. It is important to ensure that the restaurant follows these procedures for an allergen-free dining experience.

Other Allergy Considerations

If you have other food allergies or sensitivities, it is important to remain diligent in your approach to dining out. Because American Steak and Seafood restaurants offer a wide variety of foods, there are many common food allergens used on a regular basis.

Know that vegetable oil can always be substituted for any oil and may contain corn, peanuts or soy. It should be noted that unless an olive oil container specifically states 100% olive oil, it may be mixed with vegetable oil. Some restaurants may also use peanut oil for frying. If used, bouillon may contain Hydrolyzed Vegetable Protein (HVP) that can be derived from corn, soy or wheat. We have indicated the potential presence of bouillon, peanut oil and vegetable oil.

From the 30-plus items we have listed in our sample menu, we have identified each common allergen typically included in the dish as an ingredient. We have also indicated other potential allergens that may be present based upon non-traditional culinary practices. The chances of encountering common food allergens in items specific to our sample menu are outlined below.

High likelihood	Dairy, eggs, fish and shellfish
Moderate likelihood	Corn, gluten, peanuts, soy and wheat
Low likelihood	Tree nuts

Dining Considerations

American Steak and Seafood restaurants generally offer a limited number of menu items. They are presented in the English language, unless you are traveling abroad. A few large restaurant chains have locations in Europe, Central and South America and Asia. In those countries, you can expect to see menus translated into the native language.

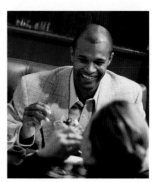

Gentleman enjoying meal

Traditionally, Americans eat two to three meals a day. Breakfast is widely considered the most important meal of the day and usually consists of breads, cereal, coffee, eggs, fruit, juice and meats. Lunch is taken between 11:30 a.m. and 1:30 p.m. and usually lasts about an hour. This meal typically consists of either a large salad, soup and sandwich or a substantial dish. Dinner is eaten anywhere between 5 and 8 p.m. and can range from a single course to a modified course structure inspired by the French *service à la russe,* lasting from one to two hours.

Today, the standard American Steak and Seafood dining experience begins with starters and is followed by soup or salad, main course, and dessert. Since most American Steak and Seafood restaurants serve *à la carte,* it may be necessary to order sides of vegetables and starches with your dishes. The portions of these sides are usually quite large, so be sure to order appropriately and consider sharing them with the table. It is a rare occurrence, indeed, to leave without a full stomach. If you order too much food, you may want to leave with a doggie bag—a very American concept!

Enjoy Your Meal!

4

Sample American Steak and Seafood Menu

Starters
Oysters on the Half Shell
Shrimp Cocktail

Soups
Bisque (Cream Soup)

Salads
Buffalo Mozzarella and Tomato Salad
Chopped Salad
Cobb Salad
Hearts of Palm Salad
Mixed Green Salad

Meat Dishes
Hamburgers
Pork Chops
Lamb Chops
Steaks

Chicken Dishes
Grilled Chicken Breast
Roasted Chicken

Seafood Dishes
Crab
Fish Filet
Lobster

Sample American Steak and Seafood Menu

Sides
Asparagus
Baked Potato
Broccoli
French Fried Potatoes
Green Beans
Hash Browns
Mashed Potatoes
Potatoes Lyonnaise
Spinach

Desserts
Chocolate Mousse
Crème Brulée (Baked Custard)
Flourless Chocolate Torte
Fresh Berries with Whipped Cream
Ice Cream
Sorbet

4

We would like to thank Tim Gannon, Founder and Executive Chef of Outback Steakhouse™ headquartered in Tampa, Florida and Domenica Catelli, Chef from domenica's way in Houston, Texas for their valuable contributions in reviewing the following menu items.

American Steak and Seafood Menu Item Descriptions

Starters
Oysters on the Half Shell
Oysters on the half shell can be served raw with lemon and a cocktail sauce made of tomato sauce, horseradish and lemon juice. They may also be baked or poached

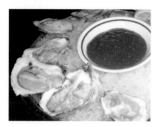

Oysters on the Half Shell served with cocktail sauce

in fresh fish stock and topped with béarnaise or hollandaise sauce.

Gluten-Free Decision Factors:
- Ensure no wheat flour in sauce
- Ensure stocks and broths are not made from bouillon which may contain gluten

Food Allergen Preparation Considerations:
- Contains shellfish from oysters
- May contain corn from bouillon and corn syrup in cocktail sauce
- May contain dairy from béarnaise or hollandaise sauce
- May contain eggs from béarnaise or hollandaise sauce
- May contain fish from fish stock
- May contain soy from bouillon

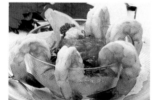

Shrimp Cocktail

Shrimp Cocktail

Shrimp cocktail is a common starter in many international cuisines. Most restaurants prepare and serve this starter in a similar fashion. Large shrimp are steamed or boiled in water or fish stock, shelled and chilled. The shrimp are served with a cocktail sauce (tomato sauce, horseradish and lemon juice), lemon wedges and sometimes an additional mayonnaise-based sauce.

Gluten-Free Decision Factors:
- Ensure stocks and broths are not made from bouillon which may contain gluten

Food Allergen Preparation Considerations:
- Contains shellfish from shrimp
- May contain corn from bouillon and corn syrup in cocktail sauce
- May contain eggs from mayonnaise-based sauce

- May contain fish from fish stock

- May contain soy from bouillon and mayonnaise-based sauce

Soups
Bisque (Cream Soup)
Bisque is a cream soup that usually features seafood, although vegetable bisques are also common. There are hundreds of recipes for this soup, but most call for standard ingredients. The base of the soup is butter, cream, some type of fresh stock or broth and wine. Onions, puréed tomatoes and potatoes are common vegetables and the soup can be seasoned with anything from sea salt to saffron. Vegetarian bisques may also include any type of ground nut. Bisques are usually garnished with parsley and sometimes may contain croutons.

Gluten-Free Decision Factors:
- Ensure no croutons or breadsticks as garnish

- Ensure no wheat flour as thickening agent

- Ensure stocks and broths are not made from bouillon which may contain gluten

- Ensure no imitation crabmeat or seafood which may contain gluten

Food Allergen Preparation Considerations:
- Contains dairy from butter and cream and possibly from croutons

- May contain corn from bouillon, croutons and imitation crabmeat

- May contain eggs from croutons and imitation crabmeat

- May contain fish as an ingredient and from imitation crabmeat and stock if ordered

- May contain peanuts as an ingredient and from croutons

- May contain shellfish as an ingredient and from stock if ordered

- May contain soy from bouillon, croutons and imitation crabmeat

- May contain tree nuts as an ingredient and from croutons

4

Salads
Buffalo Mozzarella and Tomato Salad

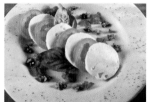

Buffalo Mozzarella and Tomato Salad

Buffalo mozzarella and tomato salad is an Italian classic that has secured a prominent place on American Steak and Seafood restaurant menus. Large slices of buffalo mozzarella are stacked with freshly cut beefsteak tomatoes. Large leafs of basil garnish this dish, which is dressed in olive oil and sometimes balsamic vinegar.

Gluten-Free Decision Factors:
- None

Food Allergen Preparation Considerations:
- Contains dairy from cheese

- May contain corn from vegetable oil

- May contain peanuts from vegetable oil

- May contain soy from vegetable oil

Chopped Salad

Think of a chopped salad as everything that is crunchy in a salad in bite sized pieces. Most chopped salads include bacon, green beans, onions and tomatoes. Some restaurants may include other crunchy vegetables, chopped nuts or add blue cheese for extra flavor. Salad dressings vary from restaurant to restaurant, but balsamic vinaigrette is typically available.

Gluten-Free Decision Factors:
- Ensure bacon bits are real since artificial bacon bits may contain gluten

- Ensure no croutons or breadsticks as garnish

- Ensure salad dressings do not contain gluten

Food Allergen Preparation Considerations:
- May contain corn from artificial bacon bits, cheese, croutons, salad dressing and vegetable oil

- May contain dairy from cheese, croutons and salad dressing

- May contain eggs from croutons and mayonnaise-based dressing

- May contain fish from salad dressing

- May contain peanuts from croutons and vegetable oil

- May contain soy from artificial bacon bits, cheese, croutons, mayonnaise-based dressing and vegetable oil

- May contain tree nuts from croutons

Cobb Salad
This classic salad was invented in the late 1920's by Bob Cobb, manager of Hollywood's famous Brown Derby restaurant. Today, it is considered an American classic. Mixed greens, preferably Boston lettuce, endive and watercress, are topped with avocado, bacon, chicken breast, hard boiled eggs, tomatoes and Roquefort cheese. The traditional dressing is Dijon vinaigrette, consisting of Dijon mustard, olive oil, red wine vinegar, salt and pepper; however, other types of dressing may be available and balsamic vinaigrette can easily be substituted.

Gluten-Free Decision Factors:
- Ensure bacon bits are real since artificial bacon bits may contain gluten

- Ensure no croutons or breadsticks as garnish

- Ensure salad dressings do not contain gluten

Food Allergen Preparation Considerations:

- Contains dairy from cheese and possibly from croutons and salad dressing
- Contains eggs from hard-boiled eggs and possibly from croutons and mayonnaise-based dressing
- May contain corn from artificial bacon bits, cheese, croutons, salad dressing and vegetable oil
- May contain fish from salad dressing
- May contain peanuts from croutons and vegetable oil
- May contain soy from artificial bacon bits, cheese, croutons, mayonnaise-based dressing and vegetable oil
- May contain tree nuts from croutons

Hearts of Palm Salad

Hearts of palm are the center of the sable palmetto, a tough-barked palm tree that grows in Central and South America. They are an important export of Brazil and Costa Rica, ending up on some menus in American Steak and Seafood restaurants. This salad usually includes hearts of palm, hard boiled eggs, olives and tomatoes. It is simply dressed in olive oil and vinegar.

Gluten-Free Decision Factors:

- None

Food Allergen Preparation Considerations:

- May contain corn from vegetable oil
- May contain eggs from hard-boiled eggs
- May contain peanuts from vegetable oil
- May contain soy from vegetable oil

Mixed Green Salad

A mixed green salad may also be presented as the house salad. It is usually a combination of mixed greens, cucumbers, onions and tomatoes. Some restaurants may add bacon bits, croutons, shredded cheese and the type of salad dressing may vary.

Gluten-Free Decision Factors:
- Ensure bacon bits are real since artificial bacon bits may contain gluten

- Ensure no croutons or breadsticks as garnish

- Ensure salad dressings do not contain gluten

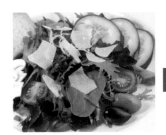
Mixed Green Salad

Food Allergen Preparation Considerations:
- May contain corn from artificial bacon bits, cheese, croutons, salad dressing and vegetable oil

- May contain dairy from cheese, croutons and salad dressing

- May contain eggs from croutons and mayonnaise-based dressing

- May contain fish from salad dressing

- May contain peanuts from croutons and vegetable oil

- May contain soy from artificial bacon bits, cheese, croutons, mayonnaise-based dressing and vegetable oil

- May contain tree nuts from croutons

Meat Dishes
Hamburgers
Considered an American classic, the hamburger's invention has been claimed by numerous individuals in the later part of the 19th century. In actuality, the hamburger was invented by the hoards of Genghis Kahn hundreds of years before the United States was formed. Although there are many styles of hamburgers, most are made with ground meats including beef, chicken and pork. The most common is the beef hamburger, which is made of ground chuck or ground sirloin and either grilled or pan-fried. In upscale establishments you can find Kobe beef burgers, which are made from

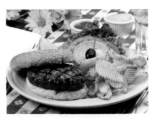
Hamburger with potato chips

a special breed of cattle that is fed a diet of beer and corn. Some restaurants may add bread crumbs to the ground meat prior to cooking. Hamburgers are generally served on a bun with pickles, lettuce, onions and tomatoes, with French fried potatoes on the side. Ketchup, mustard and mayonnaise are usually offered as condiments.

Gluten-Free Decision Factors:
- Ensure no bread crumbs

- Ensure potatoes are not dusted with wheat flour or seasonings that contain gluten

- Ensure oil used for frying is designated for potatoes only and is not used to fry other items that may be battered or dusted with wheat flour

- Ensure no bun—order gluten-free bun if available

Food Allergen Preparation Considerations:
- May contain corn from bread crumbs, bun, corn syrup in ketchup, seasonings and vegetable oil

- May contain dairy from bread crumbs, bun and seasonings

- May contain eggs from bread crumbs, bun and mayonnaise

- May contain peanuts from bread crumbs, bun, peanut oil and vegetable oil

- May contain soy from bread crumbs, bun, ketchup, mayonnaise, seasonings and vegetable oil

- May contain tree nuts from bread crumbs and bun

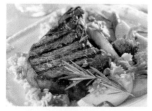
Pork Chops are generally broiled, grilled or roasted.

Pork Chops

Pork chops come from the loin of the animal and there are many variations of the cut. They are generally broiled, grilled or roasted, and may be offered marinated or smoked in some restaurants. Pork chops can also be pan-fried in butter or oil. Accompaniments vary widely from restaurant to restaurant and can include fruit relish, sauerkraut and sauces.

Gluten-Free Decision Factors:
- Ensure pork is not dusted with wheat flour
- Ensure no soy sauce or wheat flour in marinade
- Ensure no wheat flour in sauce

Food Allergen Preparation Considerations:
- May contain corn from vegetable oil
- May contain dairy from butter
- May contain peanuts from vegetable oil
- May contain soy from soy sauce in marinade and vegetable oil

Lamb Chops

The lamb chop, or whole rack of lamb where the chop is separated from, is widely considered the most flavorful cut of lamb. It is taken from the rib and has a good amount of marbling, which provides the rich flavor. The chops are usually browned on both sides in a frying pan with butter or olive oil, then roasted to perfection. They may also be marinated prior to cooking and served with a sauce. If the menu description states that the dish is herb encrusted, bread crumbs may be used. Lamb chops and rack of lamb are usually served with mint jelly on the side for dipping.

Gluten-Free Decision Factors:
- Ensure lamb is not dusted with wheat flour
- Ensure no bread crumbs
- Ensure no soy sauce or wheat flour in marinade
- Ensure no wheat flour in sauce

Food Allergen Preparation Considerations:
- May contain corn from bread crumbs and vegetable oil
- May contain dairy from bread crumbs and butter
- May contain eggs from bread crumbs

- May contain peanuts from bread crumbs and vegetable oil

- May contain soy from bread crumbs, soy sauce in marinade and vegetable oil

- May contain tree nuts from bread crumbs

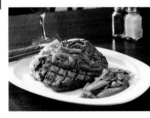

The most popular steak cuts include: filet mignon, New York strip, porterhouse and rib eye.

Steaks

Steaks come in a variety of cuts, the most popular being filet mignon, New York strip, porterhouse and rib eye. Steaks are generally broiled or grilled and seasoned with salt and pepper. They may also be pan-fried in butter or oil. Some restaurants may marinate their steaks or serve them with a sauce, usually a béarnaise, hollandaise or a reduction.

Gluten-Free Decision Factors:

- Ensure beef is not dusted with wheat flour

- Ensure no soy sauce or wheat flour in marinade

- Ensure no wheat flour in sauce

Food Allergen Preparation Considerations:

- May contain corn from vegetable oil

- May contain dairy from butter and béarnaise or hollandaise sauce

- May contain eggs from béarnaise or hollandaise sauce

- May contain peanuts from vegetable oil

- May contain soy from soy sauce in marinade and vegetable oil

Chicken Dishes
Grilled Chicken Breast

Grilled chicken breast is a relatively common menu item in American Steak and Seafood restaurants. In addition to grilled, chicken breasts may also be pan-fried in butter or oil. Occasionally, they may be marinated and come with a sauce. Fortunately, you can usually order a plain grilled chicken breast without any sauce. This dish is typically accompanied by one or two side vegetables, even though many restaurants serve *à la carte*.

Gluten-Free Decision Factors:
- Ensure chicken is not dusted with wheat flour
- Ensure no soy sauce or wheat flour in marinade
- Ensure no wheat flour in sauce

Food Allergen Preparation Considerations:
- May contain corn from vegetable oil
- May contain dairy from butter and milk in marinade
- May contain peanuts from vegetable oil
- May contain soy from soy sauce in marinade and vegetable oil

Roasted Chicken

Chicken is typically roasted on a spit or in a pan with butter or oil. The chicken may be buttered, rubbed with herbs and oil or marinated prior to cooking. A reduction sauce may also be served in some restaurants. The common portion served is half a chicken, complete with breast, wing and thigh on the bone. This dish is typically accompanied by one or two side vegetables, even though many restaurants serve *à la carte*.

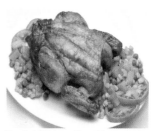
Roasted Chicken with a side vegetable.

Gluten-Free Decision Factors:
- Ensure chicken is not dusted with wheat flour
- Ensure no soy sauce or wheat flour in marinade
- Ensure no wheat flour in sauce

Food Allergen Preparation Considerations:
- May contain corn from vegetable oil
- May contain dairy from butter
- May contain peanuts from vegetable oil

- May contain soy from soy sauce in marinade and vegetable oil

Seafood Dishes
Crab

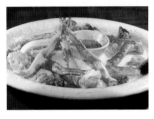

Crab Legs

Alaskan king crab, Maryland blue crab, snow crab and stone crab are the most common varieties of this crustacean offered. Crabs are usually baked or boiled in water or fish stock. The smaller crabs, like Maryland blue crab and stone crab, may be stuffed prior to baking and may contain bread crumbs. Crabs are usually served with drawn butter (melted butter and vegetable oil) and lemon wedges. Unless you are dining at the source of the catch, you may find that your crab has been frozen prior to preparation.

Gluten-Free Decision Factors:
- Ensure no bread crumbs if baked

- Ensure stocks and broths are not made from bouillon which may contain gluten

Food Allergen Preparation Considerations:
- Contains shellfish from crab

- May contain corn from bouillon, bread crumbs and vegetable oil in drawn butter

- May contain dairy from bread crumbs and drawn butter

- May contain eggs from bread crumbs

- May contain fish from fish stock

- May contain peanuts from bread crumbs and vegetable oil

- May contain soy from bouillon, bread crumbs and vegetable oil in drawn butter

- May contain tree nuts from bread crumbs

Fish Filet

Most restaurants offer a fish of the day, which usually revolves around what is in season. Halibut, salmon and sea bass are very common, with many restaurants also offering fresh water fish such as rainbow trout. Fish filets are usually grilled, poached or steamed. They may also be battered or pan-fried with butter or oil and topped with a number of different sauces.

Gluten-Free Decision Factors:
- Ensure no wheat flour in sauce
- Ensure fish is not battered or dusted with wheat flour

Grilled Salmon

4

- Ensure stocks and broths are not made from bouillon which may contain gluten if poached

Food Allergen Preparation Considerations:
- Contains fish as an ingredient
- May contain corn from bouillon and vegetable oil
- May contain dairy from butter
- May contain eggs from batter
- May contain peanuts from vegetable oil
- May contain soy from bouillon and vegetable oil

Lobster
There are two types of lobster typically served at American Steak and Seafood restaurants: Australian and Maine. Australian lobster is known for its large flavorful tail and is usually frozen prior to preparation. Maine lobsters are widely considered to have the sweetest flavor and are typically fresh or live prior to cooking. Lobster tails are usually baked or grilled; whereas, whole Maine lobster is traditionally boiled in water or fish stock. Most lobster is generally served with drawn butter and lemon wedges. Baked Maine Lobster is often halved and topped with bread crumbs and fresh herbs.

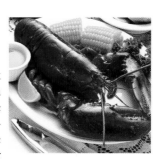
Lobster with butter and lemon

Gluten-Free Decision Factors:
- Ensure no bread crumbs if baked
- Ensure stocks and broths are not made from bouillon which may contain gluten

Food Allergen Preparation Considerations:
- Contains shellfish from lobster

- May contain corn from bouillon, bread crumbs and vegetable oil in drawn butter

- May contain dairy from bread crumbs and drawn butter

- May contain eggs from bread crumbs

- May contain fish from fish stock

- May contain peanuts from bread crumbs and vegetable oil

- May contain soy from bouillon, bread crumbs and vegetable oil in drawn butter

- May contain tree nuts from bread crumbs

Sides
Asparagus
Asparagus is usually prepared in the French style, steamed until they are cooked and still crisp. They are often sautéed in butter or oil, with garlic or onions sometimes added. Some restaurants offer béarnaise or hollandaise sauce on top or on the side for dipping.

Gluten-Free Decision Factors:
- Ensure no wheat flour in sauce

Food Allergen Preparation Considerations:
- May contain corn from vegetable oil

- May contain dairy from butter and béarnaise or hollandaise sauce

- May contain eggs from béarnaise or hollandaise sauce

- May contain peanuts from vegetable oil

- May contain soy from vegetable oil

Baked Potato

A baked potato is typically a safe choice in any restaurant. The accompaniments vary from restaurant to restaurant, but can include bacon bits, butter, cheese, chives and sour cream. Cheese sauce may also be offered. Mix and match what you like or have it plain. Almost all baked potatoes are made to order.

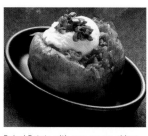

Baked Potato with sour cream, chives and bacon bits

Gluten-Free Decision Factors:
- Ensure bacon bits are real since artificial bacon bits may contain gluten

- Ensure no wheat flour in cheese sauce

Food Allergen Preparation Considerations:
- May contain corn from artificial bacon bits and cheese sauce

- May contain dairy from butter, cheese and sour cream

- May contain soy from artificial bacon bits and cheese sauce

Broccoli

In most cases, broccoli is steamed at American Steak and Seafood restaurants. You may also request it sautéed with butter or olive oil and garlic. In some establishments, the option of cheese sauce may also be available.

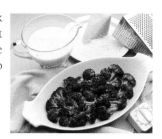

Broccoli with cheese sauce

Gluten-Free Decision Factors:
- Ensure no wheat flour in cheese sauce

Food Allergen Preparation Considerations:
- May contain corn from cheese sauce and vegetable oil

- May contain dairy from butter and cheese sauce

- May contain peanuts from vegetable oil

- May contain soy from cheese sauce and vegetable oil

French Fried Potatoes

French fried potatoes come in many different shapes and sizes. Once cut, the potatoes are fried in oil. Some restaurants may season their fries, while others prefer salting. Ketchup is usually served on the side.

Gluten-Free Decision Factors:

- Ensure potatoes are not dusted with wheat flour or seasonings that contain gluten

- Ensure oil used for frying is designated for potatoes only and is not used to fry other items that may be battered or dusted with wheat flour

Food Allergen Preparation Considerations:

- May contain corn from corn syrup in ketchup, seasonings and vegetable oil

- May contain dairy from seasonings

- May contain peanuts from peanut oil and vegetable oil

- May contain soy from ketchup, seasonings and vegetable oil

Green Beans

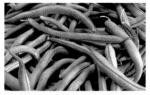

Green Beans

Green beans are usually served in the French style, steamed until they are cooked and still crisp. They are typically served plain or sautéed in butter or oil. Other ingredients such as almonds, garlic and onions may also be included. Green beans may be served with béarnaise or hollandaise sauce on the side.

Gluten-Free Decision Factors:

- Ensure no wheat flour in sauce

Food Allergen Preparation Considerations:

- May contain corn from vegetable oil

- May contain dairy from butter and béarnaise or hollandaise sauce

- May contain eggs from béarnaise or hollandaise sauce

- May contain peanuts from vegetable oil

- May contain soy from vegetable oil

- May contain tree nuts from almonds

4

Hash Browns

Hash browns are a classic side. Julienned potatoes are simply pan fried with butter or vegetable oil, very much like a pancake. They are fried on one side and then carefully flipped over to brown on the other side. Occasionally, they may have sliced onions added to them. Hash browns are usually only seasoned with salt and pepper.

Gluten-Free Decision Factors:
- Ensure no wheat flour or seasonings that contain gluten

Food Allergen Preparation Considerations:
- May contain corn from seasonings and vegetable oil

- May contain dairy from butter and seasonings

- May contain peanuts from vegetable oil

- May contain soy from seasonings and vegetable oil

Mashed Potatoes

Mashed Potatoes are made a variety of ways, most of which include butter and milk to add a creamy texture. The potatoes can be mashed, smashed or whipped with or without the skins left on the spud. Chives and onions are often added to the mix, with garlic mashed potatoes and Parmesan cheese mashed potatoes growing in popularity. Salt and pepper are the standard seasonings used; however, some chefs may add fresh herbs to enhance the flavor.

Gluten-Free Decision Factors:
- Ensure no wheat flour as an ingredient
- Ensure no artificial mashed potato mix which may contain gluten

Food Allergen Preparation Considerations:
- May contain corn from artificial mashed potato mix
- May contain dairy from artificial mashed potato mix, butter, cheese and milk
- May contain peanuts from artificial mashed potato mix
- May contain soy from artificial mashed potato mix

Potatoes Lyonnaise

Potatoes Lyonnaise are a French potato side, very similar to American hash browns. Potatoes are sliced or cubed and then pan fried with sliced onions, butter, salt and pepper. Some restaurants may choose to bake this dish or substitute vegetable oil for butter.

Gluten-Free Decision Factors:
- Ensure no wheat flour as an ingredient

Food Allergen Preparation Considerations:
- May contain corn from vegetable oil
- May contain dairy from butter
- May contain peanuts from vegetable oil
- May contain soy from vegetable oil

Spinach

Spinach is full of vitamins and makes a great side. It is typically steamed or sautéed in olive oil with garlic or onions. Creamed spinach is also usually available; however, most recipes indicate wheat flour as an ingredient.

Gluten-Free Decision Factors:

- Ensure no wheat flour as an ingredient

Food Allergen Preparation Considerations:
- May contain corn from vegetable oil

- May contain dairy from butter and cream

- May contain peanuts from vegetable oil

- May contain soy from vegetable oil

Desserts
Chocolate Mousse

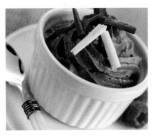
Chocolate Mousse

Chocolate mousse has become a popular dessert and can be found on the menus of many international cuisines. There are a number of variations, but the preparation is typically consistent with the following recipe. Chocolate is melted in a double-boiler with milk and sugar. Whipped eggs are then carefully folded into the chocolate sauce after it has cooled. Next, whipped heavy cream is added to the mixture, which is allowed to sit for a few minutes before the mousse is poured into a container and chilled. Some styles incorporate liqueurs such as coffee, orange and peppermint for a distinctive flavor. Chocolate mousse may be served with whipped cream and a cookie/biscuit.

Gluten-Free Decision Factors:
- Ensure no flavors containing gluten

- Ensure no wheat flour as an ingredient

- Ensure no cookie/biscuit

Food Allergen Preparation Considerations:
- Contains dairy from cream, milk and possibly from chocolate and cookie/biscuit

- Contains eggs as an ingredient and possibly from cookie/biscuit

- May contain corn from colors or flavors in liqueurs

- May contain peanuts from colors or flavors and cookie/biscuit

- May contain soy from chocolate, colors or flavors in liqueurs and cookie/biscuit

- May contain tree nuts from colors or flavors and cookie/biscuit

Crème Brulée (Baked Custard)

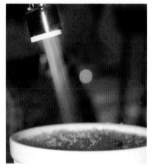

Caramelizing Crème Brulée by hand torch

Crème Brulée is one of the most popular French desserts and is equally popular in American Steak and Seafood restaurants. The custard is made with heavy cream, egg yolks, sugar and vanilla. The whisked ingredients are then baked. After it has cooled, it is topped with brown sugar that is caramelized by placing the custard in a broiler or torched by hand. There are many different types of *Crème Brulée,* some of which may contain different flavors such as almond, chocolate or fresh berries.

Gluten-Free Decision Factors:

- Ensure no wheat flour as an ingredient

- Ensure no cookie/biscuit

Food Allergen Preparation Considerations:

- Contains dairy from cream and possibly from cookie/biscuit

- Contains eggs from egg yolks and possibly from cookie/biscuit

- May contain corn from almond and vanilla extract

- May contain peanuts from cookie/biscuit

- May contain soy from chocolate and cookie/biscuit

- May contain tree nuts from almond extract and cookie/biscuit

Flourless Chocolate Torte

Yes, there is such a thing as flourless chocolate torte...even if some pastry chefs forget the title. Butter, chocolate, eggs and sugar are the standard ingredients and ground nuts may also be added to make up for the lack of flour which would normally hold everything together. Some pastry chefs may use bread crumbs or flour, even though the title suggests they are omitted.

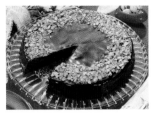

Flourless Chocolate Torte

4

Gluten-Free Decision Factors:
- Ensure no wheat flour as an ingredient or as dusting in pan
- Ensure no bread crumbs

Food Allergen Preparation Considerations:
- Contains dairy from butter, chocolate and possibly from bread crumbs
- Contains eggs as an ingredient and possibly from bread crumbs
- May contain corn from bread crumbs
- May contain peanuts from bread crumbs
- May contain soy from bread crumbs and chocolate
- May contain tree nuts from bread crumbs

Fresh Berries with Whipped Cream

Fresh berries in season usually include blueberries, raspberries and strawberries. Depending on your location, other types such as blackberries, boysenberries and loganberries may be available. They are served chilled and are usually topped with whipped cream.

Gluten-Free Decision Factors:
- Ensure no cookie/biscuit

Food Allergen Preparation Considerations:
- Contains dairy from whipped cream and possibly from cookie/biscuit
- May contain eggs from cookie/biscuit
- May contain peanuts from cookie/biscuit
- May contain soy from cookie/biscuit
- May contain tree nuts from cookie/biscuit

Ice Cream

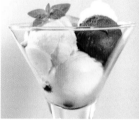

Ice Cream may be pre-fabricated or made by the restaurant.

Ice cream is typically available at American Steak and Seafood restaurants. Some restaurants serve pre-fabricated ice cream, while others choose to make their own. Many ice cream brands are gluten-free and they come in big containers with clear labels. Ask your server to read the ingredients listed on the container and keep your flavor choices simple.

Gluten-Free Decision Factors:
- Ensure no flavors containing gluten
- Ensure no malt and wheat as ingredients
- Ensure no stabilizers which may contain gluten
- Ensure no cookie/biscuit

Food Allergen Preparation Considerations:
- Contains dairy as an ingredient and possibly from chocolate, colors or flavors and cookie/biscuit
- May contain corn from colors or flavors and malt
- May contain eggs from cookie/biscuit
- May contain peanuts from colors or flavors and cookie/biscuit
- May contain soy from chocolate, colors or flavors and cookie/biscuit
- May contain tree nuts from colors or flavors and cookie/biscuit

Sorbet

Sorbet is puréed fruit and sugar that is frozen and served like ice cream. Raspberry, lemon and lime sorbets are the most common, though you may encounter many other fruit flavors or chocolate. Occasionally, sorbet is served with a wafer or another type of cookie/biscuit.

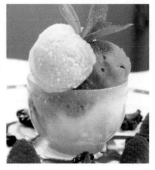

Sorbet

Gluten-Free Decision Factors:

- Ensure no stabilizers which may contain gluten

- Ensure no wheat as an ingredient

- Ensure no cookie/biscuit

Food Allergen Preparation Considerations:

- May contain corn from colors or flavors

- May contain dairy from chocolate, colors or flavors and cookie/biscuit

- May contain eggs from cookie/biscuit

- May contain peanuts from colors or flavors and cookie/biscuit

- May contain soy from chocolate, colors or flavors and cookie/biscuit

- May contain tree nuts from colors or flavors and cookie/biscuit

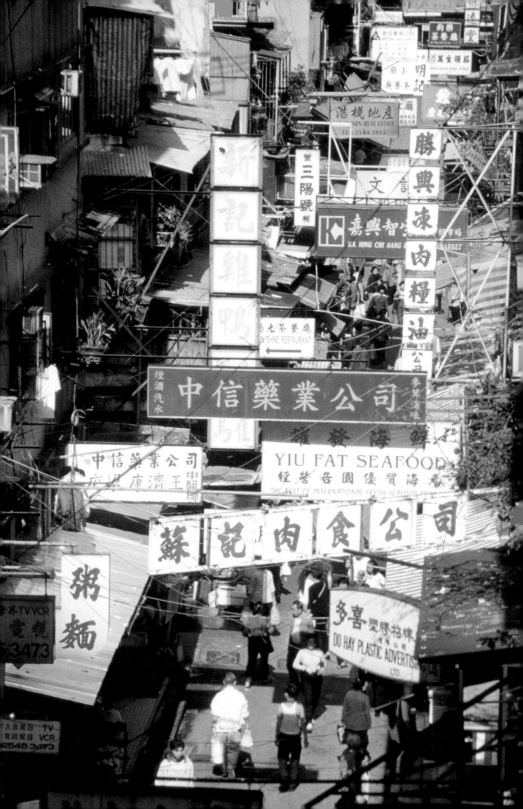

Eating is the utmost important part of life.
—Confucius

5

Chapter 5
Let's Eat Chinese Cuisine

Cuisine Overview

China has the world's largest population with 1.3 billion people and is the third largest country in land mass. As can be expected given these facts, ingredients in Chinese cuisine vary greatly from region to region. All across China, though, food is divided into two categories: *Fan* (starches) and *T'sai* (meat and vegetables).

The Chinese believe that a well-balanced meal can create harmony in one's life and improve mental and physical well being. A traditional Chinese meal consists of many dishes that contain vegetables, meat and starch, which are prepared the way they have been for thousands of years. These dishes feature bite-sized pieces of food, so cutlery is not necessary. In fact, when the Mongols conquered China, they were considered quite barbaric for using knives to cut their meat.

The Chinese technique of preparing food in this fashion grew out of an economic need rather than an aesthetic aspiration, as there were periods of famine and fuel shortage in the nation's history. Stir frying eliminated food waste and reduced the amount of fuel necessary to produce a meal, which ultimately solved two problems at the same time.

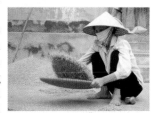
Woman Harvesting Rice

Cooking foods for a short time at a high temperature also allows vegetables to remain crisp, thereby retaining a greater amount of their raw nutritional value. This cooking technique, combined with a balanced approach of including the flavors of bitter, sour, hot, salty and sweet, create a cuisine that is enjoyed by billions of people around the world.

Traditional Ingredients

The vegetables consumed are based upon what is available from region to region and include amaranth, cabbage, carrots, different types of green beans, numerous mushrooms, mustard greens, onions, radishes and turnips. Many spices are incorporated into Chinese cooking, such as cinnamon, ginger, garlic, malva, mint and red pepper. Curry powder also plays an important role in southern Chinese cooking. Soy sauce is the main ingredient used to season dishes, most of which contain wheat.

As far as protein is concerned, the Chinese eat almost everything including: beef, chicken, duck, goose, mutton, pheasant, pork, seafood and venison. Another popular source of protein is tofu, which is derived from soybeans. It is worth mentioning that there are a number of other animal proteins consumed in Asia, such as dog, which you can find in markets and restaurants in China. Luckily, these items are conspicuously missing from restaurant menus in the Western world.

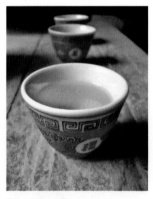
Cha or Chinese Tea

Common forms of starch eaten include buckwheat, maize, millet, *kao-liang* (sorghum), potato, rice, sweet potato and wheat (in breads, dumpling skins and pancakes). The Northern region is cold and not conducive to the cultivation of rice, so breads and pancakes serve as the starch portion of meals there. In the South, rice is abundant and is eaten as either a whole grain or in rice flour that can be used for dumpling dough and noodles.

Tea is the national drink of China and in almost every Chinese dialect is called *cha*. Tea has also played a vital role in Chinese history as it is considered a national treasure, and has even been used as a state currency. There are more than a thousand varieties of tea, with the three main types being oolong, green and black, known as red tea in China.

Tea is to the Chinese what wine is to the French. Most people drink it as part of their daily routine, preserving a nationalistic sense of decorum as part of the Chinese culture.

Gluten Awareness

Since gluten is present in some areas of Chinese cuisine, we have outlined eight items in our sample menu. There are seven primary points that you need to consider when dining at a Chinese restaurant. To ensure a gluten-free experience, the areas of food preparation that you need to inquire about with your server or chef are listed below.

Soy Sauce	Ensure no soy sauce is used. Request gluten-free soy sauce, gluten-free tamari or liquid aminos if available
Flour Dusting	Corn or potato starch is typically used—ensure no wheat flour
Stocks and Broths	Ensure all are made fresh or from allergen-free mixes and not from bouillon, which may contain gluten
Cooking Oil	Ensure frying oil has not been used to fry battered foods that may contain gluten
Noodles and Dumplings	Wheat flour is typically used—ensure no wheat flour
Battering	Request plain-cooked food—ensure no batter
Cross-Contamination	Ensure all utensils and cooking surfaces have been cleaned prior to the preparation of your meal

Soy Sauce

From a gluten perspective, your choices will be extremely limited in traditional Chinese restaurants for a number of reasons, due mostly to the abundant use of soy sauce.

Soy sauce is used in most Chinese dishes and is present in almost every Chinese sauce such as hoi sin, duck sauce and Chinese style barbecue sauce. Soy sauce is made from soybeans, which are considered one of the "seven necessities" of life in China, along with oil, rice, salt, tea, vinegar and firewood. The majority of all soy sauces produced contain wheat. Gluten-free soy sauce, gluten-free tamari or liquid aminos are featured at some restaurants. However, the demand for these products has not necessitated their production and distribution on a global basis as of yet.

Flour Dusting

Flour dusting is common in Chinese cuisine. Most restaurants prefer to dust using corn or potato starch —rather than wheat flour—to texture meats or fish before frying, thereby allowing a sauce to be evenly distributed.

Stocks and Broths

Stocks and broths are used frequently in Chinese cuisines and are present in sauces and soups. Ensure all are made fresh or from allergen-free mixes and not from bouillon, which may contain gluten.

Cooking Oil

Canola oil is typically used in Chinese restaurants; however, other oils such as corn, peanut, sesame or vegetable may be used from time to time. Oil is used to fry or sauté foods. When ordering food that is prepared by frying, ensure that there is a dedicated fryer in the kitchen for non-battered menu items. Since battered foods may contain wheat flour, this practice minimizes the potential of gluten cross-contamination from frying.

Noodles and Dumplings

Wheat flour is used for most dumpling skins, pancakes and noodles, and precludes the majority of *Fan* dishes for those with celiac / coeliac, gluten allergies or sensitivities. Although rice flour based noodles and dumpling skins are used in Southern Chinese cuisine and Asian fusion restaurants, soy sauce is present in most of these dishes.

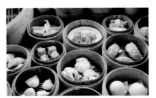

Wheat flour is used for most dumpling skins, pancakes and noodles, and precludes these dishes for those with celiac / coeliac or gluten allergies.

Battering

Battering of meats is common in Chinese cuisine and in some geographic regions, such as the United States, it is especially prevalent. Wheat flour is typically used for batter in Chinese restaurants. Request that your order is cooked plain or steamed.

Cross-Contamination

Cross-contamination occurs in two primary instances and should be considered at any restaurant you choose to dine in. One may occur when your meal is prepared in the same frying oil as foods containing other possible allergens. The second may occur when food particles are transferred from one food to another by using the same knife, cutting board, pots, pans or other utensils without washing the surfaces or tools in between uses. In the case of open flamed grills, the extreme temperature turns most food particles into carbon. Use of a wire brush designed for grill racks typically removes residual contaminants.

To avoid cross-contamination, restaurants need to dedicate fryers for specific foods and wash all materials that may come in contact with food in hot, soapy water prior to preparing items for those with special dietary requirements. It is important to ensure that the restaurant follows these procedures for an allergen-free dining experience.

Other Allergy Considerations

If you have other food allergies or sensitivities, it is important to remain diligent in your approach to dining out. Because Chinese cuisine utilizes a multitude of food products, there are many common food allergens used on a regular basis.

As previously noted, canola oil is typically used in Chinese restaurants; however, corn, peanut and vegetable oil (which may contain corn, peanuts or soy) can also be used. If used, bouillon may contain Hydrolyzed Vegetable Protein (HVP) that can be derived from corn, soy or wheat. We have indicated the potential presence of bouillon and oils.

From the eight menu items we have listed in our sample menu, we have identified each common allergen typically included in the dish as an ingredient. We have also indicated other potential allergens that may be present based upon varied culinary practices. The chances of encountering common food allergens in items specific to our sample menu are outlined on the next page.

High Likelihood   Corn, gluten, soy and wheat

Moderate Likelihood Eggs, fish, peanuts, shellfish and tree nuts

Low Likelihood   Dairy

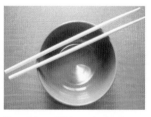
Chopsticks and Chinese rice bowl

Dining Considerations

Menus in Chinese restaurants tend to be presented in the language of the country you are dining in. This is due to the fact that most diners can neither read the Chinese alphabet, nor understand the spoken language.

The names of many dishes serve as a description of the menu item itself, such as lemon chicken. Although, the recipes of these dishes may vary from restaurant to restaurant, the preparation styles remain relatively consistent. There are many dishes that are ubiquitous and can be found in virtually every Chinese restaurant; however, most of these dishes contain soy sauce.

Chopsticks and Chinese-style soup spoons are the only necessary tools needed to enjoy a Chinese meal. Additionally, most Chinese restaurants have adapted Western style cutlery for their guests who prefer to use knives and forks. Whatever utensils you decide to use, they are inconsequential to your enjoyment of Chinese cuisine.

As is the case with most Asian cuisines, Chinese food is designed to be enjoyed family style. Finding a balance between many dishes and sharing them with your table is a very important part of Chinese culture. This grew out of the Chinese idea of incorporating the *ying* and *yang* in every facet of daily life.

Fan (starch) and *Tsai* (meat and vegetable) dishes must be balanced in every meal and the five flavors of bitter, sour, hot, salty and sweet should also be evenly distributed. This creates harmony at the dinner table and is believed to fortify the body and the soul.

好胃口

(This is Chinese for Bon Appetit!)

Sample Chinese Menu

Soups
Egg Drop Soup
Sizzling Rice Soup

Chicken Dishes
Lemon Chicken
Steamed Chicken and Broccoli

Seafood Dishes
Steamed Fish

Vegetarian Dishes
Buddha's Feast

Rice Dishes
Steamed Rice

Desserts
Fresh Tropical Fruits

We would like to thank P.F. Chang's China Bistro® headquartered in Scottsdale, Arizona and Sueson Vess, Founder and President of Special Eats™ in Chicago, Illinois for their valuable contributions in reviewing the following menu items.

Chinese Menu Item Descriptions

Soups
Egg Drop Soup
If it is prepared in the traditional fashion, the base of the soup is fresh chicken stock and is typically thickened with corn or potato starch. Sliced button mushrooms, green onion and spinach are the standard vegetables

and the soup is seasoned with salt and pepper. Tofu may also be added. The ingredients may be sautéed in oil prior to being added to the chicken stock. As its name would suggest, the soup has whisked eggs dropped into the broth, which look like white ribbons. Chinese soups are often garnished with fried noodles or wonton strips.

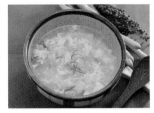
Egg Drop Soup

Gluten-Free Decision Factors:
- Ensure no soy sauce—order gluten-free sauce if available

- Ensure stocks and broths are not made from bouillon which may contain gluten

- Ensure no wheat flour as thickening agent

- Ensure no fried noodles or wonton strips

Food Allergen Preparation Considerations:
- Contains eggs as an ingredient

- May contain corn from bouillon, corn starch and vegetable oil

- May contain peanuts from peanut oil and vegetable oil

- May contain soy from bouillon, soy sauce, tofu and vegetable oil

Sizzling Rice Soup
Sizzling rice soup is a menu item with the final preparation of the dish done table side. The base of the soup is fresh chicken stock or broth that has been thickened with corn starch or potato starch and seasoned with salt and pepper. Strips of chicken and sometimes shrimp are combined with bamboo shoots, eggs, mushrooms and water chestnuts in the broth. Tofu may also be added. At your table, your server adds rice to the soup that has been fried in oil, thus creating the famous "sizzle." Chinese soups are often garnished with fried noodles or wonton strips.

Gluten-Free Decision Factors:
- Ensure no soy sauce—order gluten-free sauce if available
- Ensure clean water is used to cook rice
- Ensure stocks and broths are not made from bouillon which may contain gluten
- Ensure no wheat flour as thickening agent
- Ensure no fried noodles or wonton strips

Food Allergen Preparation Considerations:
- May contain corn from bouillon, corn starch and vegetable oil
- May contain eggs as an ingredient
- May contain peanuts from peanut oil and vegetable oil
- May contain shellfish from shrimp
- May contain soy from bouillon, soy sauce, tofu and vegetable oil

Chicken Dishes

Lemon Chicken

Lemon chicken is a sweet and tangy dish found on most Chinese restaurant menus. Slices of chicken breast are dusted in corn or potato starch and wok fried in oil. Once the chicken is cooked, it is added to a sauce made up of fresh chicken stock, lemons, lemon juice, rice wine vinegar and sugar. Lemon chicken is usually only seasoned with salt and pepper, but some recipes call for ginger. The traditional recipe calls for no vegetables, but many restaurants will add green peppers, mushrooms and onions.

Gluten-Free Decision Factors:
- Ensure no soy sauce—order gluten-free sauce if available
- Ensure chicken is not battered or dusted with wheat flour

- Ensure stocks and broths are not made from bouillon which may contain gluten

- Ensure oil used for frying has not been used to fry other items which may be battered or dusted with wheat flour

Food Allergen Preparation Considerations:
- May contain corn from bouillon, corn starch and vegetable oil

- May contain eggs from batter

- May contain peanuts from peanut oil and vegetable oil

- May contain soy from bouillon, soy sauce and vegetable oil

Steamed Chicken and Broccoli

Chicken and broccoli are common ingredients found in almost every Westernized Chinese restaurant. You must specifically request the dish steamed, as it is typically served in a soy-based sauce. Sliced chicken breast and broccoli are simply steamed and served plain.

Gluten-Free Decision Factors:
- Ensure no soy sauce—order gluten-free sauce if available

Food Allergen Preparation Considerations:
- May contain soy from soy sauce

Seafood Dishes

Steamed Fish

Chinese restaurants generally offer a steamed fish, which can be any fish available. Some restaurants may serve whole steamed fish; however, it is much more common to have a fish filet. The fish is usually accompanied by one of a number of different sauces, most of which contain soy sauce. It may also be served with steamed vegetables, but in many cases you need to order a vegetable dish separately.

Gluten-Free Decision Factors:
- Ensure no soy sauce—order gluten-free sauce if available

Food Allergen Preparation Considerations:
- Contains fish as an ingredient

- May contain soy from soy sauce

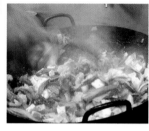

Cooking in a Wok

Vegetarian Dishes
Buddha's Feast

This mixed Asian vegetable dish is either steamed or stir-fried. If it is stir-fried, the dish is tossed in a wok with fresh vegetable or chicken stock and oil. Many restaurants will also add soy sauce to season the dish, so it is typically easier to order the Buddha's Feast steamed. The vegetables of the dish vary, but you can usually expect to see some combination of baby corn, bamboo shoots, bok choy, broccoli, cabbage, Chinese broccoli, carrots, shitake mushrooms and water chestnuts. Garlic and ginger are usually included for flavor and bean curd or tofu may also be included to add extra protein to the dish.

Gluten-Free Decision Factors:
- Ensure no soy sauce—order gluten-free sauce if available

- Ensure stocks and broths are not made from bouillon which may contain gluten

Food Allergen Preparation Considerations:
- May contain corn from baby corn, bouillon and vegetable oil

- May contain peanuts from peanut oil and vegetable oil

- May contain soy from bean curd, bouillon, soy sauce, tofu and vegetable oil

Rice Dishes
Steamed Rice
Plain steamed rice is usually safe to eat. Chinese restaurants typically offer steamed white rice and many now offer steamed brown rice. Since the rice is steamed in a designated rice cooker, the chances of it coming into contact with any foods during cooking are minimal.

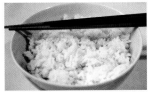
Steamed Rice

Gluten-Free Decision Factors:
- Ensure clean water is used to cook rice

5

Food Allergen Preparation Considerations:
- None

Desserts
Fresh Tropical Fruits
Fresh tropical fruit makes a light choice for dessert. Bite-sized chunks of pineapple, guava, papaya and banana are the most common fruits served.

Gluten-Free Decision Factors:
- Ensure no cookie/biscuit

Food Allergen Preparation Considerations:
- May contain dairy from cookie/biscuit

- May contain eggs from cookie/biscuit

- May contain peanuts from cookie/biscuit

- May contain soy from cookie/biscuit

- May contain tree nuts from cookie/biscuit

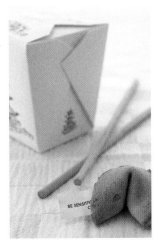
Chinese Take-Out and Fortune Cookie

One final note: Be sure to read your fortune—just don't eat the cookie!

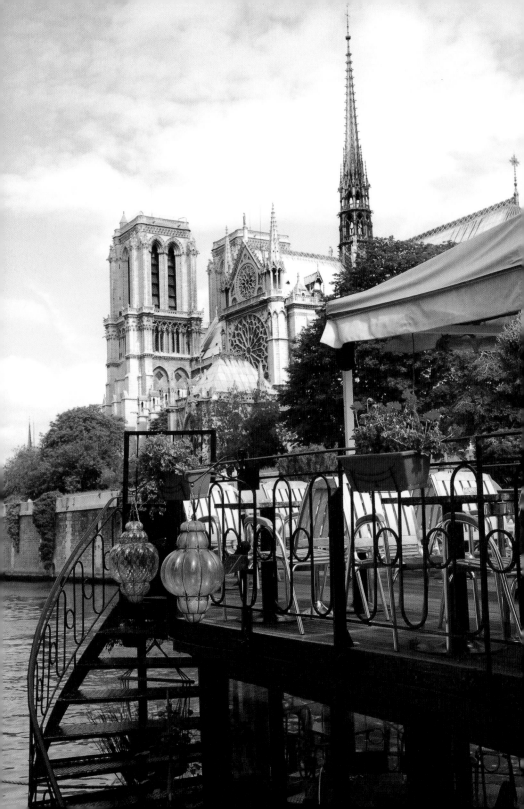

Eating is a serious venture,
if not a patriotic duty, in France.
—Patricia Roberts

Chapter 6

6

Let's Eat French Cuisine

Cuisine Overview

With a population of just over 60 million and a land mass roughly twice the size of Colorado, France is the largest nation in Western Europe. Although its history can be traced back some 30,000 years, most historians agree that the formal history of France began when Clovis, King of the Franks, brought Christianity to the country with his baptism in the 5th century. France is divided into 22 regions, including the island of Corsica and is further represented in territories around the world.

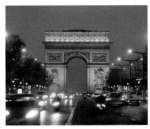

Arc de Triomphe

French cuisine is dynamic to say the least. The food preparation techniques used in France are arguably some of the most sophisticated from a culinary perspective. Chefs must master these techniques, as French food is a passion for millions of people around the world. French cooking is not unified by one school of thought, but rather by regional influences including geography, climate and other international cultures. In the coastal regions of Brittany and Normandy, local culinary specialties revolve around seafood, beef and cheese while cattle is the dominant livestock raised in that area. In the south, Provençal cuisine is influenced by Italy, with its use of olive oil and herbs. The foods of Alsace on the German border feature sweet wines and sausages of a distinctly Germanic flavor. Each region is known for its specific culinary delights, which are assembled on menus around the world under one classification: French!

"Les Champs de Blé" (the fields of wheat) is an important symbol of the French culture. Wheat is a big part of the French gastronomic experience and is present in everything from baguettes to beignets. Be that as it may, there are many French menu items that are traditionally gluten-free.

6

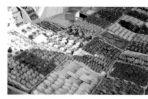

The French are adventurous eaters and vegetables play a huge role in French dining.

Traditional Ingredients

The French are certainly adventurous eaters. Their creative and innovative culinary palate includes everything from saffron to snails. Vegetables play a huge role in French dining along with meat and poultry, but exotic ingredients like frog legs, calf brains and foies gras are just as important. In fact, the most unusual menu items you will encounter in a restaurant are usually quite common to the French.

Asparagus, artichokes, green beans, many types of lettuce, leeks, olives, onions, potatoes and tomatoes are common vegetables. Herbs include basil, fennel, laurel, lavender, marjoram, rosemary, savory, tarragon and thyme.

Beef, chicken, duck, lamb, pork and seafood provide the majority of protein in French food and their desserts are widely considered some of the best in the world. Cheese is a big part of the French diet and plays an important role in their cuisine. There are more varieties of cheese in France than there are days in the year! Brie and Camembert are well known soft cheeses. Chèvre is cheese made from goats' milk that is sweet and creamy when fresh, yet grows to be salty and hard as it ages. Roquefort is one of the more common blue cheeses. When traveling in France, every area you visit will have a local specialty cheese that is prized by its inhabitants.

Like the Italians, the French have been drinking wine for hundreds of years. Wine is to the French what tea is to the English and Chinese. Most people drink it as part of their daily routine, preserving a nationalistic sense of decorum as part of the French culture. Not only do the French drink wine with most meals, but it is used regularly in food preparation. Wines in France are classified by appellation, a term that refers to a viticulture region distinguished by geographical features which produce wines with shared characteristics. The Bordeaux region is held in high regard for its production of some of the world's finest red wine. The wines of Alsace are sweeter and generally revolve around white grape varietals. Champagne is known, of course, for its production of sparkling wines, while wines of Burgundy display a lighter viscosity and subtle flavors.

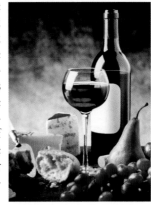

Cheese and Wine

6

Gluten Awareness

Although gluten is present in many areas of French cuisine, we have outlined over 30 items in our sample menu. There are seven primary points that you need to consider when dining at a French restaurant. To ensure a gluten-free experience, the areas of food preparation that you need to inquire about with your server or chef are listed below.

Sauces	Ensure the *liaison* of the sauce is butter, egg yolks or puréed vegetables—ensure no wheat flour
Flour Dusting	Wheat flour is typically used—request plain
Stocks and Broths	Ensure all are made fresh or from allergen-free mixes and not from bouillon, which may contain gluten
Cooking Oil	Ensure frying oil has not been used to fry battered foods that may contain gluten
Bread, Bread Crumbs & Croutons	Wheat flour is typically used—ensure no bread, bread crumbs or croutons
Malt Vinegar	Ensure no malt vinegar as a condiment
Cross-Contamination	Ensure all utensils and cooking surfaces have been cleaned prior to the preparation of your meal

Sauces

Of the many different sauces you may encounter in French cuisine, always be sure the *liaison* that binds the sauce together is not wheat flour. Other acceptable *liaisons* include egg yolks, butter and puréed vegetables. Below is a list of common and typically gluten-free French sauces and their ingredients:

Hollandaise	A sauce that contains butter, egg yolks as its liaison and lemon juice
Béarnaise	A reduction of white wine vinegar, tarragon and shallots that is finished with egg yolks and butter
Reduction	A mixture that results from rapidly boiling a liquid (like fresh stock, wine or a sauce without wheat flour) and causing evaporation— "reducing" the sauce—which creates a thicker sauce with a more intense flavor than the original liquid
Rémoulade	A sauce that contains mayonnaise, mustard, capers, chopped gherkins (French pickles), herbs and anchovies

Other common French sauces include wheat flour as a *liaison* or thickening agent. Below are three common French sauces that you need to avoid:

Roux	A sauce made of flour, fat and butter —a roux can be white, blond, or brown, depending on ingredients and cooking time

Note: Roux is typically not included as part of a menu description. Allergen-free roux mixes are also available.

Béchamel	A white roux with milk
Velouté	A white roux with a light chicken or veal stock added

Flour Dusting
Flour dusting is common in French cuisine. Most restaurants prefer to dust meat or fish with wheat flour for texture prior to pan frying, allowing a sauce to be

evenly distributed. Ensure that this practice is not used in the preparation of your meal.

Stocks and Broths

Stocks and broths are used frequently in French cuisine. They are present in sauces and soups, as well as in marinades for meats and vegetables. Ensure all are made fresh or from allergen-free mixes and not from bouillon, which may contain gluten.

Cooking Oil

The French use mostly peanut, corn and sunflower oil for the purpose of frying. Olive oil can also be used for cooking, but rarely for frying. Outside of France, other oils such as corn or vegetable may be substituted from time to time. Oil is used to fry or sauté foods. When ordering food that is prepared by frying, ensure that there is a dedicated fryer in the kitchen for non-battered menu items. Since battered foods may contain wheat flour, this practice minimizes the potential of gluten cross-contamination from frying.

Bread, Bread Crumbs and Croutons

Croutons and bread crumbs are used regularly as an ingredient in starters, soups and salads. The French generally do not waste any food product, especially old bread. When ordering these dishes, always be sure to request no croutons or bread crumbs. In addition, a basket of bread is usually served, so be certain to request no bread.

Malt Vinegar

Malt vinegar is a common table condiment in French restaurants and is a popular accoutrement for *pommes frites* (French fried potatoes). It is fermented from barley and not distilled; therefore, it contains gluten and must be avoided.

Cross-Contamination

Cross-contamination occurs in two primary instances and should be considered at any restaurant you choose to dine in. One may occur when your meal is prepared in the same frying oil as foods containing other possible allergens. The second may occur when food particles are transferred from one food to another by using the same knife, cutting board, pots, pans or other utensils without washing the surfaces or tools in between uses. In the case of open flamed grills, the extreme temperature turns most food particles into carbon. Use of a wire brush designed for grill racks typically removes residual contaminants.

To avoid cross-contamination, restaurants need to dedicate fryers for specific foods and wash all materials that may come in contact with food in hot, soapy water prior to preparing items for those with special dietary requirements. It is important to ensure that the restaurant follows these procedures for an allergen-free dining experience.

Other Allergy Considerations

If you have other food allergies or sensitivities, it is important to remain diligent in your approach to dining out. Because French cuisine is complex, there are many common food allergens used on a regular basis. While in France, be aware that peanut oil is often used to fry foods. Know that vegetable oil can always be substituted for any oil and may contain corn, peanuts or soy. It should be noted that unless an olive oil container specifically states 100% olive oil, it may be mixed with vegetable oil. If used, bouillon may contain Hydrolyzed Vegetable Protein (HVP) that can be derived from corn, soy or wheat. We have indicated the potential presence of bouillon and non-traditional cooking oils.

From the 30-plus menu items we have listed in our sample menu, we have identified each common allergen typically included in the dish as an ingredient. We have also indicated other potential allergens that may be present based upon non-traditional culinary practices. The chances of encountering common food allergens in items specific to our sample menu are outlined below.

High Likelihood	Dairy, eggs, fish and shellfish
Moderate Likelihood	Corn, gluten, peanuts, soy and wheat
Low Likelihood	Tree nuts

Dining Considerations

French menu items are usually presented in the French language. You often find menu descriptions in the language of the country you are in following the name of the French menu item. While traveling, be sure to familiarize yourself with the common French culinary terms included in this chapter to assist you in your dining experience.

French restaurants serve their cuisine in a style known as *service à la russe,* which is the practice of serving a meal in many courses. Previously, the French dined in a fashion much closer to our modern buffets. Today, the standard French lunch or dinner begins with *hors d'oeuvres* and is followed by soup, main course, salad, cheese and dessert. This multi-course plan was adapted from the Russian culture during the Napoleonic wars in the 19th century and remains the standard for our modern French gastronomic experience.

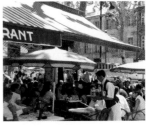

French restaurants serve their cuisine in a style known as *service à la russe,* which is the practice of serving a meal in many courses.

The French generally eat three meals a day. *Le petit déjeuner* is a light breakfast and usually consists of bread, cereals, fruit and coffee. *Le déjeuner* takes place between noon and 2 p.m. and is a larger meal, often consisting of three courses including soup, salad and a main dish. *Le goûter* is a snack sometimes taken in the late afternoon.

The French dinner or *le dîner* is preceded by *l'apéritif,* a national custom that involves setting aside half an hour or so before a meal to share a drink, small starters and conversation with family, friends, neighbors or colleagues. *Le dîner* is a long affair, complete with many courses and lasts two to four hours; thereby allowing ample time to enjoy and savor the meal. It is also a time for the whole family to gather together and talk about their day. Wine is enjoyed throughout the evening, with after dinner drinks such as *calvados, cognac* and *eaux de vie* reserved for the end of the meal.

Bon Appetit!

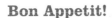

6

Sample French Menu

Starters
Crevette Cocktail (Shrimp Cocktail)
Escargot (Snails)
Foies Gras (Fat Liver)
Les Huîtres (Oysters on the Half Shell)
Steak Tartare (Beef Tartar)
Tartare de Saumon (Salmon Tartar)

Soups
Bisque (Cream Soup)
Vichyssoise (Potato Leek Soup)

Salads
Artichauts à la Vinaigrette (Artichoke Salad)
Asperge à la Vinaigrette (Asparagus Salad)
Mesclun de Salade (Mixed Green Salad)
Salade Niçoise (Nice Style Salad)

Egg Dishes
Les Oeufs (Fried Eggs)
Les Omelettes (Omelets)

Beef Dishes
Filet de Boeuf (Beef Filet)
Fondue Bourguignon (Beef Fondue)
Steak au Poivre (Peppered Steak)
Steak Frites (Steak and French Fried Potatoes)

Chicken Dishes
Poulet Provençal (Roasted Chicken with Herbs)

Seafood Dishes
Bouillabaisse (Seafood Stew)
Moules Frites (Mussels and French Fried Potatoes)
Saumon en Papillote (Baked Salmon)

Sample French Menu

Sides
Gratin Dauphinois (Creamed Potatoes)
Haricots Verts (French Green Beans)
Pommes Frites (French Fried Potatoes)
Ratatouille (Vegetable Stew)

Desserts
Assiette de Fromage (Cheese Plate)
Crème Brulée (Baked Custard)
Fruits à la Crème (Fresh Fruit with Cream)
Mousse au Chocolat (Chocolate Mousse)
Les Sorbets (Sorbet)

6

*We would like to thank Nicolas Bergerault, Founder
and President of L'atelier des Chefs in Paris, France
and Stephane Tremolani, former Executive Chef
de Cuisine at the French Embassy in Rome, Italy
for their valuable contributions in reviewing the
following menu items.*

French Menu Item Descriptions

Starters
Crevette Cocktail (Shrimp Cocktail)
Shrimp cocktail is a common starter across many
international cuisines. *Crevette Cocktail* usually refers
to medium sized shrimp. *Les Gambas,* large shrimp or
prawns, may also be seen on some menus in France.
Most restaurants prepare and serve this starter in
a similar fashion. The shrimp are boiled in water or
fish stock, shelled and chilled. They are traditionally
served with a cocktail sauce (tomato sauce, horseradish and lemon juice), lemon wedges and sometimes an
additional mayonnaise-based sauce.

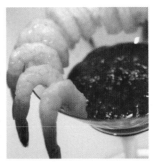

Crevette Cocktail (Shrimp Cocktail)
with cocktail sauce

Gluten-Free Decision Factors:
- Ensure stocks and broths are not made from bouillon which may contain gluten

- Ensure no wheat flour in sauce

Food Allergen Preparation Considerations:
- Contains shellfish from shrimp

- May contain corn from bouillon and corn syrup in cocktail sauce

- May contain eggs from mayonnaise-based sauce

- May contain fish from fish stock

- May contain soy from bouillon and mayonnaise-based sauce

6

Escargot (Snails)

Escargot (Snails)

Escargot is a delicacy that has been enjoyed in Europe since the time of the ancient Romans. The French have carried on this tradition for hundreds of years and have developed many different recipes for the common garden snail. The texture of prepared escargot is very similar to that of a portabella mushroom and the traditional French preparation is very simple. The snails are removed from the shell and salted for a period of usually three days. Next, a purée of butter, garlic, parsley and shallots is placed in the shell. The snails are returned to the shell and topped with the remainder of the purée. They are then baked and garnished with chopped parsley, pepper and salt before serving. Rather than using shells, some recipes call for mushroom caps or a special ceramic dish to hold the ingredients.

Gluten-Free Decision Factors:
- Ensure no bread crumbs

Food Allergen Preparation Considerations:
- Contains dairy from butter and possibly from bread crumbs

- Contains shellfish from escargot (snails)

- May contain corn from bread crumbs
- May contain eggs from bread crumbs
- May contain peanuts from bread crumbs
- May contain soy from bread crumbs
- May contain tree nuts from bread crumbs

Foies Gras (Fat Liver)

Directly translated *foies gras* or *foie gras* means fat liver. Duck (*le canard*) or goose (*l'oie*) liver is predominantly used in French cuisine and is served three different ways: whole, in a pâté or in a mousse. French law requires that any product labeled foies gras must be 80% liver, the other 20% can be other meat from chicken, duck, goose or pork. For whole foies gras, the liver is usually marinated overnight in milk or salt water. After being marinated, the liver is thinly sliced, so that all the nerves can be removed. It is then cooked in a terrine with salt, pepper and cognac. Finally, it is set aside for three to four days before being served. Outside of France, you may encounter foies gras that is roasted or pan seared and then served plain or with various vegetables. Pâté de foies gras differs from mousse de foies gras in the consistency of its texture. Both pâté and mousse may contain dairy, eggs and truffles.

Gluten-Free Decision Factors:

- Ensure no bread

Food Allergen Preparation Considerations:

- May contain corn from bread
- May contain dairy from bread and milk
- May contain eggs as an ingredient and from bread
- May contain peanuts from bread
- May contain soy from bread
- May contain tree nuts from bread

Les Huîtres (Oysters on the Half Shell)

Les Huîtres (Oysters on the Half Shell)

Oysters on the half shell can be served raw with lemon and cocktail sauce. They may also be baked or poached in fresh fish stock and topped with béarnaise or hollandaise sauce.

Gluten-Free Decision Factors:
- Ensure stocks and broths are not made from bouillon which may contain gluten
- Ensure no wheat flour in sauce

Food Allergen Preparation Considerations:
- Contains shellfish from oysters
- May contain corn from bouillon and corn syrup in cocktail sauce
- May contain dairy from béarnaise or hollandaise sauce
- May contain eggs from béarnaise or hollandaise sauce
- May contain fish from fish stock
- May contain soy from bouillon

Steak Tartare (Beef Tartar)

Steak tartare is a traditional starter prepared in French restaurants with many variations. In France, raw ground filet mignon, ground round or ground top sirloin are the common cuts of choice used in this dish. Chopped shallots and capers are served on the side along with lemon, olive oil and white wine vinegar. This allows the guest to pick and choose what ingredients to mix. Outside of France, the dish is usually pre-mixed with the above ingredients and may also include anchovies, garlic and mayonnaise; however, this is uncommon in France. Many recipes also call for a raw egg and white wine. There are a variety of seasonings used including *Herbs de Provence* (marjoram, thyme, summer savory, basil, rosemary, fennel seeds and lavender), mustard powder, pepper and salt. In France, some restaurants may serve Dijon mustard, ketchup (yes, ketchup) and hot pepper sauce on the side.

Gluten-Free Decision Factors:
- Ensure no bread crumbs

Food Allergen Preparation Considerations:
- May contain corn from bread crumbs, corn syrup in ketchup and vegetable oil

- May contain dairy from bread crumbs

- May contain eggs from bread crumbs, mayonnaise and raw egg

- May contain fish from anchovies

- May contain peanuts from bread crumbs and vegetable oil

- May contain soy from mayonnaise and vegetable oil

- May contain tree nuts from bread crumbs

Tartare de Saumon (Salmon Tartar)

There are hundreds of recipes for Salmon Tartar and most are very similar. Raw salmon is either minced or finely cubed. Capers, lemon juice, olive oil, diced scallions and diced shallots are mixed with the salmon and the dish is usually garnished with fresh dill or parsley. In some regions of France, Dijon mustard or mayonnaise may be included.

Gluten-Free Decision Factors:
- None

Food Allergen Preparation Considerations:
- Contains fish from salmon

- May contain corn from vegetable oil

- May contain eggs from mayonnaise

- May contain peanuts from vegetable oil

- May contain soy from mayonnaise and vegetable oil

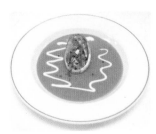

Bisque (Cream Soup) featuring an Oyster

6

Soups
Bisque (Cream Soup)

Bisque is a cream soup that usually features seafood, although vegetable bisques are also common. There are hundreds of recipes for this soup, but most call for standard ingredients. The base of the soup is butter, cream, some type of fresh stock or broth and wine. Onions, puréed tomatoes and potatoes are common vegetables and the soup can be seasoned with anything from sea salt to saffron. Vegetarian bisques may also include any type of ground nut. Bisques are usually garnished with parsley and sometimes may contain croutons.

Gluten-Free Decision Factors:
- Ensure no croutons or breadsticks as garnish
- Ensure no wheat flour as thickening agent
- Ensure stocks and broths are not made from bouillon which may contain gluten
- Ensure no imitation crabmeat or seafood which may contain gluten

Food Allergen Preparation Considerations:
- Contains dairy from butter and cream and possibly from croutons
- May contain corn from bouillon, croutons and imitation crabmeat
- May contain eggs from croutons and imitation crabmeat
- May contain fish as an ingredient and from imitation crabmeat and seafood stock if ordered
- May contain peanuts as an ingredient and from croutons
- May contain shellfish as an ingredient and from seafood stock if ordered
- May contain soy from bouillon, croutons and imitation crabmeat
- May contain tree nuts as an ingredient and from croutons

Vichyssoise (Potato Leek Soup)

Vichyssoise is a chilled vegetable soup. It was created by Chef Louis Diat at New York's Ritz-Carlton Hotel in 1917, but it is a very common menu item in French restaurants. The base of the soup is butter, fresh chicken broth, cream and white wine. Chives, leeks, onions and potatoes are typically included and the soup is seasoned with basil, bay leaf, chervil, pepper, salt and thyme. The soup is usually garnished with chopped chives or parsley.

Gluten-Free Decision Factors:
- Ensure stocks and broths are not made from bouillon which may contain gluten
- Ensure no wheat flour as thickening agent

Food Allergen Preparation Considerations:
- Contains dairy from butter and cream
- May contain corn from bouillon
- May contain soy from bouillon

Salads
Artichauts à la Vinaigrette (Artichoke Salad)

Artichokes with vinaigrette are a popular French salad. There are a number of different recipes that either call for whole artichokes or artichoke hearts, which are steamed first to make the meat of the vegetable tender. Of all the different types of vinaigrettes used to dress the artichokes, most usually contain chives, garlic, olive oil, shallots, wine or sherry vinegar and wine. From time to time, you may encounter vinaigrette made with Dijon mustard.

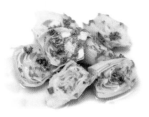

Artichauts à la Vinaigrette (Artichoke Salad)

Gluten-Free Decision Factors:
- None

Food Allergen Preparation Considerations:
- May contain corn from vegetable oil
- May contain peanuts from vegetable oil
- May contain soy from vegetable oil

Asperge à la Vinaigrette (Asparagus Salad)

Asparagus with vinaigrette can be prepared many different ways. After the asparagus has been steamed and chilled, chopped onions, tomatoes, shallots and chives can be added. The vinaigrette will usually contain garlic, olive oil, shallots, tarragon, wine or sherry vinegar and wine. From time to time, you may encounter vinaigrette made with Dijon mustard.

Gluten-Free Decision Factors:
- None

Food Allergen Preparation Considerations:
- May contain corn from vegetable oil

- May contain eggs from egg in vinaigrette

- May contain peanuts from vegetable oil

- May contain soy from vegetable oil

Mesclun de Salade (Mixed Green Salad)

Mesclun is a green salad made from several types of young leaves, typically including arugula, dandelion, radicchio and endive. Some recipes call for fresh berries, carrots, cucumbers, onions, tomatoes and walnuts. When presented as *Mesclun de Salade*, the dish is usually just the greens tossed in varying types of vinaigrette. From time to time, you may encounter vinaigrette made with Dijon mustard.

Gluten-Free Decision Factors:
- Ensure no croutons or breadsticks as garnish

Food Allergen Preparation Considerations:
- May contain corn from croutons and vegetable oil

- May contain dairy from croutons

- May contain eggs from croutons

- May contain peanuts from croutons and vegetable oil

- May contain soy from croutons and vegetable oil

- May contain tree nuts from croutons and walnuts

Salade Niçoise (Nice Style Salad)

Salade Niçoise comes from the south of France and is a favorite at French restaurants. There are many different recipes, but most usually contain anchovies, hard boiled eggs, green beans, mixed greens, potatoes, olives, onions and tomatoes. Seared tuna is a popular ingredient and you may also encounter salmon. The salad is always accompanied by some type of vinaigrette and may contain Dijon mustard.

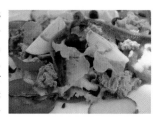
Salade Niçoise (Nice Style Salad)

Gluten-Free Decision Factors
- Ensure no croutons or breadsticks as garnish

Food Allergen Preparation Considerations:
- Contains eggs from hard-boiled eggs and possibly from croutons
- Contains fish from anchovies, salmon and tuna
- May contain corn from croutons and vegetable oil
- May contain dairy from croutons
- May contain peanuts from croutons and vegetable oil
- May contain soy from croutons and vegetable oil
- May contain tree nuts from croutons

Egg Dishes
Les Oeufs (Fried Eggs)

Eggs are usually eaten at *le déjeuner* (lunch) and are typically fried in butter in the north of France or olive oil in the south. *Oeuf dur* means "hard boiled eggs," but their consistency in France can sometimes be between soft and hard boiled. Eggs are often accompanied with *jambon* (ham) or *lardon* (fatty bacon).

Gluten-Free Decision Factors:
- Ensure oil used for frying has not been used to fry other items which may be battered or dusted with wheat flour

Food Allergen Preparation Considerations:
- Contains eggs as an ingredient
- May contain corn from vegetable oil
- May contain dairy from butter
- May contain peanuts from peanut oil and vegetable oil
- May contain soy from vegetable oil

Les Omelettes (Omelets)
Omelets are eaten at *le déjeuner* (lunch) and usually fried in butter in the north of France or olive oil in the south. A variety of omelets are offered including *nature* (plain), *jambon* (ham), *fromage* (cheese), *aux fines herbes* (mixed herbs) and *provençal* (mixed vegetables).

Gluten-Free Decision Factors:
- Ensure oil used for frying has not been used to fry other items which may be battered or dusted with wheat flour
- Ensure no wheat flour as fluffing agent

Food Allergen Preparation Considerations:
- Contains eggs as an ingredient
- May contain corn from vegetable oil
- May contain dairy from butter and cheese
- May contain peanuts from peanut oil and vegetable oil
- May contain soy from vegetable oil

Beef Dishes
Filet de Boeuf (Beef Filet)
Filet de Boeuf, also known as filet mignon, is usually seasoned with salt and pepper and sometimes with other herbs. The beef may be grilled or pan seared in butter or olive oil and accompanied with béarnaise or hollandaise sauce. It should be noted that *Filet de Boeuf*

en Croute, also known as *Filet de Boeuf Wellington,* is wrapped in puff pastry which contains wheat flour.

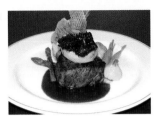

Filet de Boeuf (Beef Filet)

Gluten-Free Decision Factors:
- Ensure no wheat flour in sauce
- Ensure beef is not dusted with wheat flour
- Ensure beef is not breaded

Food Allergen Preparation Considerations:
- May contain corn from breading and vegetable oil
- May contain dairy from breading, butter and sauce
- May contain eggs from breading and sauce
- May contain peanuts from vegetable oil
- May contain soy from breading and vegetable oil

Fondue Bourguignon (Beef Fondue)

Fondue Bourguignon includes raw cubes of beef, usually filet mignon or rump steak, served with a pot of hot vegetable oil. With fondue forks, a diner simply dips the beef into the hot oil until the desired temperature is reached. The dish may be accompanied with a variety of dipping sauces such as béarnaise, hollandaise, mayonnaise and ketchup.

Gluten-Free Decision Factors:
- Ensure no wheat flour in sauce
- Ensure beef is not dusted with wheat flour

Food Allergen Preparation Considerations:
- May contain corn from corn syrup in ketchup and vegetable oil
- May contain dairy from butter and sauce
- May contain eggs from mayonnaise and sauce
- May contain peanuts from peanut oil and vegetable oil
- May contain soy from mayonnaise and vegetable oil

Steak au Poivre (Peppered Steak)

Steak au Poivre is a standard French beef dish. Strip or sirloin steak is salted and pan fried with a little olive oil or butter. The French prefer the cooking temperature to be *bleu* (rare) or *à point* (medium rare). The steak is removed and a reduction of butter, red wine and cracked peppercorn is made in the pan using the fat or jus that remains. Garlic and shallots are sometimes used in the sauce. The dish is usually served with a side of *haricots verts* (French green beans) and carrots.

Gluten-Free Decision Factors:
- Ensure no wheat flour in sauce
- Ensure beef is not dusted with wheat flour

Food Allergen Preparation Considerations:
- Contains dairy from butter
- May contain corn from vegetable oil
- May contain peanuts from vegetable oil
- May contain soy from vegetable oil

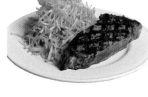
Steak Frites (Steak and French Fried Potatoes)

Steak Frites (Steak and French Fried Potatoes)

Steak Frites can be many cuts of meat including porterhouse, sirloin, rib eye, shell steak or filet mignon. The steak is usually pan fried in butter or oil and seasoned with salt and pepper. Once the steak is done, a reduction can be made with butter, shallots and red wine. The steak is always accompanied by *pommes frites* (French fried potatoes) and may come with herb butter, ketchup, mayonnaise, béarnaise or hollandaise sauce. Malt vinegar is a common table condiment used for *pommes frites* in French restaurants and contains gluten.

Gluten-Free Decision Factors:
- Ensure no wheat flour in sauce
- Ensure beef is not dusted with wheat flour
- Ensure oil used for frying is designated for potatoes only and is not used to fry other items that may be battered or dusted with wheat flour

- Ensure no malt vinegar

Food Allergen Preparation Considerations:
- May contain corn from corn syrup in ketchup and vegetable oil

- May contain dairy from butter and sauce

- May contain eggs from mayonnaise and sauce

- May contain peanuts from peanut oil and vegetable oil

- May contain soy from mayonnaise and vegetable oil

6

Chicken Dishes
Poulet Provençal (Roasted Chicken with Herbs)
Poulet Provençal is a marinated chicken dish that is either roasted in a special rotisserie oven or baked. This dish is a variation of the ubiquitous *Poulet Roti* (roasted chicken) found all over France. The whole chicken is marinated with garlic, *Herbs de Provence* (marjoram, thyme, summer savory, basil, rosemary, fennel seeds and lavender), lemon juice, olive oil, pepper and salt. After it is roasted, the chicken is served with vegetables which may include roasted potatoes with rosemary and salt or *haricots verts* (French green beans).

Gluten-Free Decision Factors:
- Ensure no soy sauce or wheat flour in marinade

Food Allergen Preparation Considerations:

- May contain soy from soy sauce in marinade

Seafood Dishes
Bouillabaisse (Seafood Stew)
More than just a soup or stew, *Bouillabaisse* is a French gastronomic tradition. In a clear fresh fish stock or broth, many types of seafood are combined including clams, crab, any fish, lobster, mussels, oysters, scallops and shrimp. The vegetables usually included are carrots, celery, leeks, onions and potatoes. *Bouillabaisse* is typically seasoned with garlic, pepper, salt

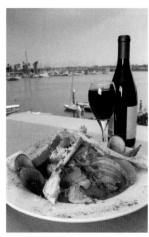

Bouillabaisse (Seafood Stew)

6

and saffron, but may also be seasoned with a *bouquet garni* (cheese cloth bag full of herbs) containing *Herbes de Provence*. Some recipes call for croutons or toasted bread on the side.

Gluten-Free Decision Factors:
- Ensure no bread or croutons
- Ensure no wheat flour as thickening agent
- Ensure stocks or broths are not made from bouillon which may contain gluten

Food Allergen Preparation Considerations:
- Contains fish as an ingredient
- Contains shellfish as an ingredient
- May contain corn from bouillon, bread and croutons
- May contain dairy from bread and croutons
- May contain eggs from bread and croutons
- May contain peanuts from bread and croutons
- May contain soy from bouillon, bread and croutons
- May contain tree nuts from bread and croutons

Moules Frites (Mussels and French Fried Potatoes)
Steamed mussels are served as starters and dishes. The mussels are steamed or boiled in fresh fish stock, then topped with a sauce that contains butter, onions or shallots, white wine and sometimes garlic. They may occasionally be topped with bread crumbs and are typically accompanied with *pommes frites*. *Pommes frites* may come with herb butter, ketchup, mayonnaise, béarnaise or hollandaise sauce. Malt vinegar is a common table condiment used for *pommes frites* in French restaurants and contains gluten.

Gluten-Free Decision Factors:
- Ensure no wheat flour in sauce
- Ensure no bread crumbs

- Ensure stocks and broths are not made from bouillon which may contain gluten

- Ensure potatoes are not dusted with wheat flour

- Ensure oil used for frying is designated for potatoes only and is not used to fry other items that may be battered or dusted with wheat flour

- Ensure no malt vinegar

Food Allergen Preparation Considerations:
- Contains dairy from butter and possibly from béarnaise or hollandaise sauce and bread crumbs

- Contains shellfish from mussels

- May contain corn from bouillon, bread crumbs, corn syrup in ketchup and vegetable oil

- May contain eggs from béarnaise or hollandaise sauce, bread crumbs and mayonnaise

- May contain peanuts from bread crumbs, peanut oil and vegetable oil

- May contain soy from bouillon, bread crumbs and vegetable oil

- May contain tree nuts from bread crumbs

6

Saumon en Papillote (Baked Salmon)

The term *"en Papillote"* refers to the French style of cooking in a parchment paper bag. This is an excellent way to cook any fish, as it allows all the flavors inside to permeate the fish. A filet of salmon is placed in the center of a large piece of parchment paper that has been brushed with butter or olive oil. Blanched vegetables including julienned carrots, leeks and green beans are added to garlic, onions and shallots that are sautéed in butter or olive oil. The dish can be seasoned with various herbs including coriander, fennel, pepper and salt. The parchment paper is then folded in the shape of a bag and baked until brown. Egg whites are sometimes used to seal the parchment paper bag.

Gluten-Free Decision Factors:
- Ensure fish is not dusted with wheat flour

Food Allergen Preparation Considerations:
- Contains fish from salmon

- May contain corn from vegetable oil

- May contain dairy from butter

- May contain eggs from parchment sealing

- May contain peanuts from peanut oil and vegetable oil

- May contain soy from vegetable oil

6

Sides
Gratin Dauphinois (Creamed Potatoes)
A creamed potato casserole, *Gratin Dauphinois* is a common French side. Thinly sliced potatoes are baked in a cream sauce with butter, crème fraîche and milk. It is seasoned with garlic, salt, pepper and possibly nutmeg. Non-traditional recipes call for grated gruyère cheese and bread crumbs.

Gluten-Free Decision Factors:
- Ensure no wheat flour as an ingredient

- Ensure no bread crumbs

Food Allergen Preparation Considerations:
- Contains dairy from butter, crème fraîche, milk and possibly from bread crumbs and cheese

- May contain corn from bread crumbs

- May contain eggs from bread crumbs

- May contain peanuts from bread crumbs

- May contain soy from bread crumbs

- May contain tree nuts from bread crumbs

Haricots Verts (French Green Beans)

The French prepare green beans by steaming them until they are cooked, yet still crisp. *Haricots verts* can be served plain, in butter or olive oil and may contain almonds, garlic and onions. They may also be topped with béarnaise or hollandaise sauce.

Gluten-Free Decision Factors:

- Ensure no wheat flour in sauce

Food Allergen Preparation Considerations:

- May contain corn from vegetable oil

- May contain dairy from butter and sauce

- May contain eggs from sauce

- May contain peanuts from peanut oil and vegetable oil

- May contain soy from vegetable oil

- May contain tree nuts from almonds

6

Pommes Frites (French Fried Potatoes)

Pommes Frites are classic French fried potatoes, although many give credit to the Belgians for creating this dish. The potatoes are typically sliced very thin, fried in peanut or vegetable oil and seasoned with salt. Various dipping sauces may be available such as herb butter, ketchup, mayonnaise, béarnaise or hollandaise sauce and sometimes a butter, garlic and parsley sauce. Malt vinegar is a common table condiment used for *pommes frites* in French restaurants and contains gluten.

Pommes Frites (French Fried Potatoes)

Gluten-Free Decision Factors:

- Ensure potatoes are not dusted with wheat flour prior to frying

- Ensure oil used for frying is designated for potatoes only and is not used to fry other items that may be battered or dusted with wheat flour

- Ensure no malt vinegar

Food Allergen Preparation Considerations:
- May contain corn from corn syrup in ketchup and vegetable oil

- May contain dairy from butter and sauce

- May contain eggs from mayonnaise and sauce

- May contain peanuts from peanut oil and vegetable oil

- May contain soy from mayonnaise and vegetable oil

6

Ratatouille (Vegetable Stew)
Ratatouille is a traditional vegetable dish from the south of France served as a side or meal. It resembles a vegetable stew and includes bell peppers, eggplant, onions, tomatoes and zucchini. The vegetables are cooked in olive oil and white wine, then seasoned with garlic, *Herbs de Provence*, pepper and salt. Although uncommon, some recipes call for grated cheese. *Ratatouille* can be served hot or chilled.

Gluten-Free Decision Factors:
- Ensure no wheat flour as an ingredient

- Ensure stocks and broths are not made from bouillon which may contain gluten

Food Allergen Preparation Considerations:
- May contain corn from bouillon and vegetable oil

- May contain dairy from cheese

- May contain peanuts from vegetable oil

- May contain soy from bouillon and vegetable oil

Desserts
Assiette de Fromage (Cheese Plate)
Typically, cheese is eaten with salad prior to the dessert course in France and listed with dessert items. A variety of different cheeses are offered including brie, camembert and chèvre; however, the types may vary based upon

location and availability. Cheese is usually served with bread or crackers and sometimes sliced fruit.

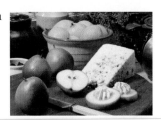

Assiette de Fromage (Cheese Plate) with Fruit

Gluten-Free Decision Factors:
- Ensure no bread or crackers

Food Allergen Preparation Considerations:
- Contains dairy from cheese and possibly from bread
- May contain corn from bread
- May contain eggs as an ingredient and from bread
- May contain peanuts from bread
- May contain soy from bread
- May contain tree nuts from bread

Crème Brulée (Baked Custard)

Crème Brulée is one of the most popular French desserts. The custard is made with heavy cream, egg yolks, sugar and vanilla. The whisked ingredients are then baked. After it has cooled, it is topped with brown sugar that is caramelized by placing the custard in a broiler or torching it by hand. There are many different flavors of crème brulée such as almond, chocolate and fresh berries.

Gluten-Free Decision Factors:
- Ensure no wheat flour as an ingredient
- Ensure no cookie/biscuit

Food Allergen Preparation Considerations:
- Contains dairy from cream and possibly from cookie/biscuit
- Contains eggs from egg yolks and possibly from cookie/biscuit
- May contain corn from almond and vanilla extract
- May contain peanuts from cookie/biscuit
- May contain soy from chocolate and cookie/biscuit

- May contain tree nuts from almond extract and cookie/biscuit

Fruits à la Crème (Fresh Fruit with Cream)

Crème fraîche is a slightly tangy and nutty thick cream that is naturally fermented. The French adore this cream as a dessert with fresh fruit. Mixed berries are usually the fruit of choice, but you can find it with other fruits such as apples and melons. Occasionally, it is served with a cookie/biscuit.

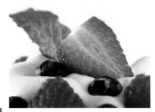

6 Fruits à la Crème (Fresh Fruit with Cream)

Gluten-Free Decision Factors:
- Ensure no cookie/biscuit

Food Allergen Preparation Considerations:
- Contains dairy from cream and possibly from cookie/biscuit
- May contain eggs from cookie/biscuit
- May contain peanuts from cookie/biscuit
- May contain soy from cookie/biscuit
- May contain tree nuts from cookie/biscuit

Mousse au Chocolat (Chocolate Mousse)

Chocolate mousse is a popular dessert and can be found in many international cuisines. Varying slightly, the preparation typically reflects chocolate melted in a double-boiler with milk and sugar. Whipped eggs are then carefully folded into the chocolate sauce after it has cooled. Next, whipped heavy cream is added to the mixture, which is allowed to sit for a few minutes before the mousse is poured into a container and chilled. Some variations incorporate liqueurs such as coffee, orange and peppermint. Chocolate mousse may be served with whipped cream and a cookie/biscuit.

Gluten-Free Decision Factors:
- Ensure no wheat flour as an ingredient
- Ensure no cookie/biscuit

Food Allergen Preparation Considerations:
- Contains dairy from cream, milk and possibly from chocolate and cookie/biscuit

- Contains eggs as an ingredient and possibly from cookie/biscuit

- May contain peanuts from colors or flavors and cookie/biscuit

- May contain soy from cookie/biscuit

- May contain tree nuts from colors or flavors and cookie/biscuit

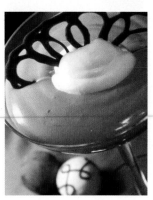

Mousse au Chocolat (Chocolate Mousse)

6

Les Sorbets (Sorbet)

Sorbet is puréed fruit and sugar that is frozen and served like ice cream. If the restaurant uses *service à la russe,* sorbet may be offered in between courses to cleanse your palate. Raspberry, lemon and lime sorbets are the most common. You may also encounter many other fruit flavors or chocolate. Occasionally, sorbet is served with a wafer or another type of cookie/biscuit.

Gluten-Free Decision Factors:
- Ensure no wheat flour as an ingredient

- Ensure no stabilizers which may contain gluten

- Ensure no cookie/biscuit

Food Allergen Preparation Considerations:
- May contain corn from colors or flavors

- May contain dairy from cookie/biscuit

- May contain eggs from cookie/biscuit

- May contain peanuts from colors or flavors and cookie/biscuit

- May contain soy from chocolate, colors or flavors and cookie/biscuit

- May contain tree nuts from colors or flavors and cookie/biscuit

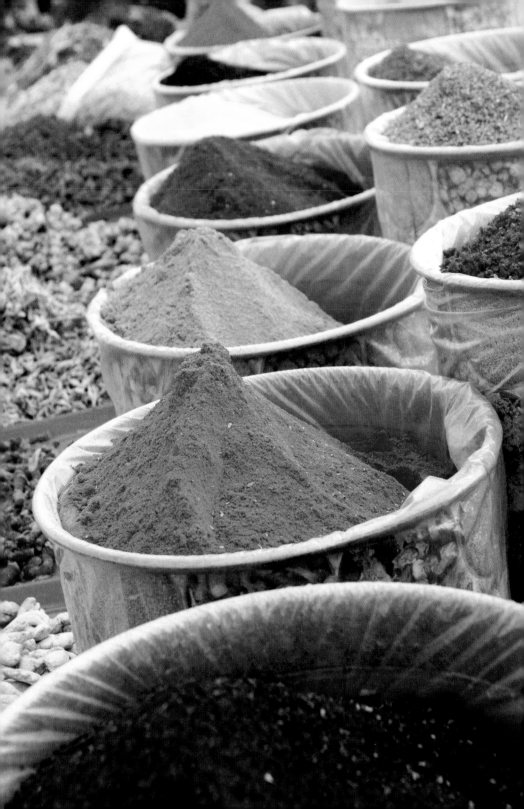

*Far more indispensable than food for the
physical body is spiritual nourishment for the soul.
One can do without food for a considerable time,
but a man of the spirit cannot exist for a single
second without spiritual nourishment.*
—Gandhi

CHAPTER 7
Let's Eat Indian Cuisine

7

Cuisine Overview

With over a billion inhabitants, India is second only
to China in population. The 35 states and territories of
India occupy a landmass roughly the size of Europe.
The cultural identity of India is extraordinarily complex due to the conquest of its lands: From the Aryans,
Mongolians and Persians to the Greeks, Portuguese
and the British. This is further complicated by the fact
that there are 40-plus languages and dialects spoken,
most of which have their own alphabet and script. How
then can one classify the culinary identity of a country
with over a billion people, speaking over 40 languages
and dialects who have been conquered or occupied by
at least 10 different civilizations? One word: *Masala!*

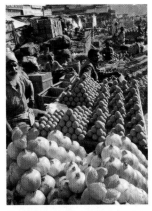

Masala is the Hindi word for spice and
is the single unifying factor of the 16
major schools of Indian cooking.

Masala is the Hindi word for spice and is the
single unifying factor of the 16 major schools of Indian
cooking. Regional cuisines in the North include *Avahd,
Kashmiri, Lucknow, Punjabi, Rajasthan* and *Uttar Pradesh.*
Southern cooking is represented by the *Andhra* or
Hyderabad, Kerala and *Tamil Nadu* cooking styles, while
Bengali is the predominant Eastern Indian cuisine. In
the West, *Goan, Gujarati, Konkani, Maharashtrian* and
Parsi cuisines hold the greatest prominence.

In addition to its conquerors, the original indigenous civilization, the Dravidians, have had a large impact on traditional cuisine. The Dravidians were responsible for the creation and development of the *Ayurveda*, one of the first examples of life sciences in early civilization. The *Ayurveda* was the first documentation of thought that recognized the importance of nutrition and its impact on physical, mental and spiritual health. These early discoveries still remain in practice and are relevant today, serving as the basis for many Indian culinary principles.

Vegetarianism has long been a part of India's culinary history. It is widely believed that the early civilizations of the Indian sub-continent were vegetarian, but this has yet to be confirmed by archeologists. The first documented evidence of vegetarianism in India was in the 6th century BC, through the teachings of both Buddha and Mahavir Jain, the two greatest spiritual influences in Indian culture. The Emperor Ashoka, further popularized the virtue of vegetarianism during his rule in the 2nd century BC. Today, vegetarian dishes hold a prominent place in the Indian gastronomic experience.

Familiarity with Indian cuisine varies greatly depending upon your geographic location. In the United Kingdom, for example, there are over 9,000 Indian restaurants and the cuisine itself has become as common as Mexican food in California. Indian neighborhoods can be found in cities all over the world; this is where you will find the most authentic cuisine outside the Indian sub-continent.

Traditional Ingredients

Legumes, such as lentils, are often used as ingredients (left). Chili peppers are a common Indian spice (right).

Like many cuisines in Asia, Indian culinary ingredients are directly related to the availability of products in each region. Since the country is so large, there is a cornucopia of food products used in the many schools of Indian cooking. Dairy products, legumes, spices and vegetables are regularly consumed at most Indian meals. Breads, crepes and pancakes made from chickpea, lentil, potato, rice and wheat flours are also a daily staple of their diet.

Since the number of vegetarians in India is substantial, there is obviously an extensive variety of vegetables used regularly. Cabbage, carrots, cauliflower, corn, onions, potatoes, pumpkin, shallots, spinach, tomatoes and turnips are common vegetables found across Indian cuisine. Legumes such as black gram, chick peas and lentils are often used as ingredients, as well as ground into flours for bread. Nuts play a big part, with almonds, cashews, peanuts, pistachios and walnuts frequently incorporated into dishes. In addition, Indian cuisine utilizes many different types of fruit such as coconut, mango and raisins as ingredients in their dishes and in chutney, the famous spiced fruit spread.

Masala (spice) is used in the majority of dishes. Although the exact spices for a specific dish vary from chef to chef, their choices for what spices to include are standard across Indian cuisine. These common Indian herbs and spices include bay leaves, black pepper, cardamom, chili pepper, cinnamon, cloves, coriander, cumin, fennel, fenugreek, garlic, ginger, mustard seed and turmeric.

Because the cow is sacred to Hindus, dairy products are prevalent far more often than beef in Indian cooking; although, you may find beef in non-Hindu Indian restaurants. *Ghee* (clarified butter) is traditionally used to cook food, in addition to peanut, seed and other vegetable oils. Yogurt is often included in curry dishes, with buttermilk, cream and milk incorporated from time to time. *Paneer,* a soft Indian cheese, is used in vegetarian dishes and desserts.

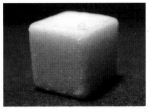

Paneer, a soft Indian cheese, is used in vegetarian dishes and desserts.

Sources of protein in Indian restaurants are directly reflective of each restaurant owner's religious beliefs. Generally speaking, most Indian restaurants offer chicken, fish and lamb dishes, with *paneer* (Indian cheese), lentils and yogurt serving as the major sources of protein for vegetarians. A Hindu restaurant would never serve beef; whereas, one would expect to find it in a Muslim restaurant, where you would not find pork or shellfish. In fact, it is rare to see pork on a typical Indian menu.

The Indian culture is known for its consumption of non-alcoholic specialty beverages. Tea is considered a national treasure, with the orange pekoe blend being the most common. Because of India's geographic location, thousands of tea varieties are available including red, green and black. *Masala Chai* is a popular Indian beverage enjoyed around the world that is made with black tea, cardamom, hot milk and sugar. Another non-alcoholic specialty beverage is *Lassi*. It is made with yogurt and salt or sugar, which can be requested plain or with a variety of natural flavors such as mint, mango or strawberry.

Gluten Awareness

Although gluten is present in some areas of Indian cuisine, we have outlined 25-plus items in our sample menu. There are six primary points that you need to consider when dining at an Indian restaurant. To ensure a gluten-free experience, the areas of food preparation that you need to inquire about with your server or chef are listed below.

Sauces	Ensure sauces do not contain wheat flour
Stocks and Broths	Ensure all are made fresh or from allergen-free mixes and not from bouillon, which may contain gluten
Cooking Oil	Ensure frying oil has not been used to fry battered foods that may contain gluten
Bread and Dosas	Wheat flour is typically used—ensure no wheat flour
Marinades	Although uncommon, ensure marinades do not contain wheat flour or soy sauce
Cross-Contamination	Ensure all utensils and cooking surfaces have been cleaned prior to the preparation of your meal

Sauces

Culinary practices vary in Indian restaurants. Although it is uncommon, some sauces may have wheat flour added to them as a thickening agent. Many standard Indian condiments such chutney, Indian pickles or *raita* resemble sauces. Chutneys are spicy fruit or vegetable spreads and are very common in Indian restaurants. Indian pickles are made with fruit or vegetables in oil with aromatic spices and differ from western pickles in that they resemble relish. They almost never contain vinegar and are not made from cucumbers. *Raita* is a yogurt dipping sauce.

Although ingredients will vary widely from restaurant to restaurant, below is a list of common and typically gluten-free condiments and their ingredients.

Coconut Chutney	Coconut, chili pepper, vegetable oil, yogurt, Indian herbs and spices
Mango Chutney	Mango, ginger, onions, raisins, Indian herbs and spices
Mint Chutney	Mint, chili pepper, lemon juice, onions, salt, sugar, oil, Indian herbs and spices
Tamarind Chutney	Tamarind pulp, sugar, oil, water, Indian herbs and spices
Tomato Chutney	Tomato, chili pepper, cilantro, garlic, salt, sugar, tamarind juice, Indian herbs and spices
Indian Pickles	Any type of fruit or vegetable with Indian herbs and spices in oil
Raita	A yogurt sauce with Indian herbs and spices, which may also contain sliced onions and tomatoes

Stocks and Broths

Stocks and broths are used frequently in Indian cuisine and are present in sauces and soups. Ensure all are made fresh or from allergen-free mixes and not from bouillon, which may contain gluten.

Cooking Oil

Indians sometimes use *ghee* (clarified butter) to fry foods because of its perceived health benefits and high smoking point. The flavor is rather strong, so many chefs prefer to use other types of oils including: canola, coconut, corn, mustard seed, olive, peanut, sesame and sunflower. Outside of India, vegetable oil may be substituted from time to time. Oil is used to fry or sauté foods. When ordering food that is prepared by frying, ensure that there is a dedicated fryer in the kitchen for non-battered menu items. Since battered foods may contain wheat flour, this practice minimizes the potential of gluten cross-contamination from frying.

Bread and Dosas

Dosas, a South Indian version of the crepe or pancake, are usually stuffed with a filling and served with chutneys. In some cases, they resemble a pizza, with the ingredients placed on the top of the crepe or pancake. *Dosas* are often made with black gram, lentil, potato or rice flour. If ordered, ensure that *dosas* do not contain wheat flour.

With the exception of many *dosas,* most breads and pancakes are made with wheat flour in Indian restaurants. At left is a list of common breads and pancakes made with wheat flour that should be avoided.

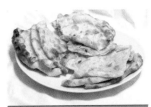

Common bread and pancakes with wheat flour that should be avoided:	
Bhatura	Poori
Chappati	Puri
Kulcha	Rava Dosa
Naan	Roti
Paratha	

Marinades

Marinades are used frequently in Indian restaurants and differ from most cuisines in that they are typically citrus or yogurt based. Although uncommon, other types of marinades may be used in restaurants that incorporate non-traditional culinary practices. If this is the case, ensure that the marinade does not include soy sauce, which contains wheat, or wheat flour.

Cross-Contamination

Cross-contamination occurs in two primary instances and should be considered at any restaurant you choose to dine in. One may occur when your meal is prepared in the same frying oil as foods containing other possible allergens. The second may occur when food particles are transferred from one food to another by using the same knife, cutting board, pots, pans or other utensils without washing the surfaces or tools in between uses. In the case of open flamed grills, the extreme temperature turns most food particles into carbon. Use of a wire brush designed for grill racks typically removes residual contaminants. To avoid cross-contamination, restaurants need to dedicate fryers for specific foods and wash all materials that may come in contact with food in hot, soapy water prior to preparing items for those with special dietary requirements. It is important to ensure that the restaurant follows these procedures for an allergen-free dining experience.

Other Allergy Considerations

If you have other food allergies or sensitivities, it is important to remain diligent in your approach to dining out. Because Indian cuisine is complex, there are many common food allergens used on a regular basis. While in India, be aware that *ghee* (clarified butter) is often used to fry foods. Know that vegetable oil can always be substituted for any oil and may contain corn, peanuts or soy. Peanuts and tree nuts are frequently used both as an ingredient and in cooking oils. If used, bouillon may contain Hydrolyzed Vegetable Protein (HVP) that can be derived from corn, soy or wheat. We have indicated the potential presence of bouillon and cooking oils.

7

From the 25-plus items we have listed in our sample menu, we have identified each common allergen typically included in the dish as an ingredient. We have also indicated other potential allergens that may be present based upon non-traditional culinary practices. The chances of encountering common food allergens in items specific to our sample menu are outlined below.

High likelihood	Corn, dairy, fish, peanuts and soy
Moderate likelihood	Gluten, shellfish, tree nuts and wheat
Low likelihood	Eggs

In addition, your sensitivity to spice levels can be an important concern. Indian food is often extremely spicy due to the use of chili peppers and powders. *Tandoor* dishes tend to be far less spicy than curries. In most cases, you can order dishes mild. Keep in mind that mild to an Indian chef may still be quite spicy. If you are especially sensitive, it is important to discuss these concerns with your server or chef.

Dining Considerations

Menus in Indian restaurants tend to be presented in the language of the country you are dining in. This is due to the fact that most people neither read the Indian language alphabets, nor understand the 40-

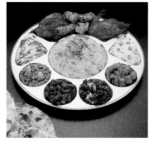

Indian Meal Tray

plus languages and dialects spoken in India. Since Indian languages have different alphabets than the English language, menus may have the name of a dish spelled phonetically in English. With this in mind, you will soon realize that there are many different ways to phonetically spell an Indian dish. Kabobs, whether it is spelled kababs, kebobs or kebabs, is the same skewered meat dish.

Depending on where you are dining, it may be acceptable to eat with your hands; however, most restaurants offer Western cutlery for your convenience. As is the case with most Asian cuisines, Indian food is designed to be enjoyed "family style." Finding a balance between many dishes and sharing them with your table is a very important part of the Indian culture.

Dining schedules in India vary according to religious practices. The customary eating schedule for many Hindus includes a light meal in the morning, a heavier meal in the afternoon and another light meal in the evening. For Muslims, the dining schedule is similar; however, during the month of Ramadan, fasting is observed during daylight hours.

Chalo, sub khana khao!
(Bon Appetit in Hindi.
It literally means
"Come, let's start eating!")

Sample Indian Menu

Starters
Aloo Tikki (Potato Patty)
Kabobs (Skewered Meat)
Pakoras (Vegetable Fritters)
Papadam (Spicy Crackers)

Sample Indian Menu

Soups
Curried Coconut Soup
Mulligatawny (Chicken and Vegetable Soup)
Sambar (Lentil and Vegetable Stew)

Salads
Kachumber (Chopped Salad)

Curry Dishes
Channa Masala (Chickpeas in Tomato Curry)
Gosht Vindaloo (Spicy Lamb Curry)
Jhinga Masala (Shrimp in Coconut Curry)
Malai Kofta (Vegetarian Croquettes in Mild Curry)
Murg Korma (Chicken in Cream Curry)
Murg Tikki Masala (Chicken in Tomato Curry)
Rogan Josh (Mild Lamb Curry)
Saag Paneer (Indian Cheese and Spinach Curry)

Tandoor Specialties
Boti Kabob (Skewered Lamb)
Murg Tandoori (Tandoori Barbeque Chicken)
Murg Tikka (Yogurt Marinated Chicken)
Seekh Kabob (Skewered Minced Lamb)

Dosas (South Indian Specialties)
Masala Dosa (Spicy Vegetable Filled Crepe)
Sada Dosa (Lentil and Rice Crepe)
Uthappam (Lentil and Rice Pancake)

Desserts
Kheer (Rice Pudding)
Kulfi (Indian Ice Cream)
Rasmalai (Cheese Balls in Sweet Cream)

7

We would like to thank Samir Majmudar, owner of Rani Indian Bistro in Brookline, Massachusettes and Tariq Zaman, owner of The Spice Company in Moseley, United Kingdom for their valuable contributions in reviewing the following menu items.

Indian Menu Item Descriptions

Starters
Aloo Tikki (Potato Patty)
Aloo Tikki is a popular North Indian starter. The preparation involves combining slightly mashed potatoes with vegetable flour, usually chickpea (*besan*), corn (*makai*) or water chestnut (*singara*). Some chefs may also add yogurt curd. The potato mixture is seasoned with spices, which vary from kitchen to kitchen and usually include chili powder, cumin, salt and pepper. The resulting mixture is then formed into balls or patties and pan fried in *ghee* (clarified butter) or oil. *Aloo Tikki* is typically garnished with coriander leaves (cilantro), chopped green chili peppers, onions, tomatoes and some type of chutney on the side for dipping.

Gluten-Free Decision Factors:
- Ensure no wheat flour—chickpea, corn or water chestnut flour is typically used

- Ensure no wheat flour in chutney

Food Allergen Preparation Considerations:
- May contain corn from corn flour and vegetable oil

- May contain dairy from butter and yogurt curd

- May contain peanuts from peanut oil and vegetable oil

- May contain soy from vegetable oil

Kabobs (Skewered Meat)

Indian *Kabobs* are usually offered with chicken or lamb; however, fish, shrimp and vegetarian *Kabobs* are available in some restaurants. In most cases, the ingredients are marinated in a yogurt sauce with Indian spices, which usually include chili powder, cumin, coriander, garlic, ginger and turmeric. The marinade may also include lime juice or vegetable oil. The meat is then skewered and grilled over an open flame or baked in a tandoori oven. *Kabobs* may be served with some type of chutney or *raita* (a yogurt sauce) on the side for dipping.

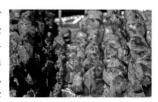
Kabobs (Skewered Meat)

Gluten-Free Decision Factors:

- Ensure no wheat flour in chutney

- Ensure no soy sauce or wheat flour in marinade

Food Allergen Preparation Considerations:

- Contains dairy from yogurt sauce

- May contain corn from vegetable oil

- May contain fish if ordered

- May contain peanuts from peanut oil and vegetable oil

- May contain shellfish if ordered

- May contain soy from soy sauce in marinade and vegetable oil

Pakoras (Vegetable Fritters)

Pakoras are popular hot starters eaten in India, enjoyed especially during the rainy season. A thick batter is made with chickpea flour *(besan)*, chili powder, cumin, salt and pepper. Chopped cabbage, cauliflower, chili pepper, coriander leaves, mint leaves, onions, potatoes and spinach are added. The resulting mixture is then formed into balls or patties and pan fried in *ghee* or oil. *Pakoras* are usually garnished with coriander or mint leaves and served with some type of chutney on the side for dipping.

Gluten-Free Decision Factors:
- Ensure no wheat flour—chickpea, corn or water chestnut flour is typically used
- Ensure no wheat flour in chutney

Food Allergen Preparation Considerations:
- May contain corn from corn flour and vegetable oil
- May contain dairy from butter
- May contain peanuts from peanut oil and vegetable oil
- May contain soy from vegetable oil

Papadam (Spicy Crackers)

Papadam are crackers made out of lentil (*urad daal*) or chickpea (*besan*) flour and are eaten very much like tortilla chips in Mexico. The dough is lentil or chickpea flour with salt, water and may include other Indian spices. They come in many flavors, including black or red pepper, garlic or plain and can be pan fried in *ghee* or oil or baked. *Papadam* are then served with dipping sauces which usually include *raita* and some type of chutney.

Papadam (Spicy Crackers)

Gluten-Free Decision Factors:
- Ensure no wheat flour—chickpea, corn or water chestnut flour is typically used
- Ensure no wheat flour in chutney

Food Allergen Preparation Considerations:
- May contain corn from corn flour and vegetable oil
- May contain dairy from butter and yogurt sauce
- May contain peanuts from peanut oil and vegetable oil
- May contain soy from vegetable oil

Soups
Curried Coconut Soup

Curried coconut soup is very common in Indian restaurants and can be served chilled or hot. The base of the soup consists of coconut milk, milk, water and sometimes egg yolks or *ghee*. In most cases, the soup is seasoned with a curry powder consisting of cardamom, chili powder, cloves and cumin. It may also contain various spices such as nutmeg or fennel. Although ingredients vary, almonds, coconut flakes, onions and pistachios are typically included. The soup is usually garnished with toasted coconut flakes.

Gluten-Free Decision Factors:
- Ensure no wheat flour as thickening agent

Food Allergen Preparation Considerations:
- Contains dairy from milk and possibly from butter

- May contain eggs from egg yolks

- May contain tree nuts from almonds and pistachios

Mulligatawny (Chicken and Vegetable Soup)

Mulligatawny is the most common version of spicy chicken soup found in Indian restaurants. There are hundreds of variations, but most follow a basic recipe. Fresh chicken stock is the base of the soup, with standard ingredients including carrots, celery, chicken, chili peppers, lentils, lemon juice, onions, potatoes, tomatoes and rice. Some chefs include coconut milk and milk. The ingredients of the soup are sautéed in *ghee* or oil with various types of Indian spices and then added to the fresh chicken stock. *Mulligatawny* can be garnished with cream or coconut cream, chopped coriander leaves or parsley and toasted almonds or pistachios.

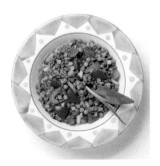
Mulligatawny (Chicken and Vegetable Soup)

Gluten-Free Decision Factors:
- Ensure stocks and broths are not made from bouillon which may contain gluten

- Ensure no wheat flour as thickening agent

Food Allergen Preparation Considerations:
- May contain corn from bouillon and vegetable oil

- May contain dairy from butter, cream and milk

- May contain peanuts from peanut oil and vegetable oil

- May contain soy from bouillon and vegetable oil

- May contain tree nuts from almonds and pistachios

7

Sambar (Lentil and Vegetable Stew)
Sambar is a South Indian vegetable stew. The base of the stew is a fresh vegetarian stock made with water, tamarind juice or paste and *sambar* powder (ground black pepper, chili powder, coconut, coriander, cumin, fenugreek seed, lentils, mustard seed and tumeric). Many types of chopped vegetables, which usually include onions, potatoes, shallots, tomatoes and turnips, are sautéed in *ghee* or oil. The vegetables are then added to the fresh stock with lentils or rice. It is served as a stew or a side dish with *dosas* (South Indian crepes or pancakes).

Gluten-Free Decision Factors:
- Ensure stocks and broths are not made from bouillon which may contain gluten

- Ensure no wheat flour as thickening agent

- Ensure no wheat flour in *dosas*

Food Allergen Preparation Considerations:
- May contain corn from bouillon, corn flour in *dosas* and vegetable oil

- May contain dairy from butter

- May contain peanuts from peanut oil and vegetable oil

- May contain soy from bouillon and vegetable oil

Salads
Kachumber (Chopped Salad)
Kachumber is an Indian chopped salad which is common with every meal. A salad in an Indian restaurant serves only as an accompaniment rather than a course in itself. This salad usually consists of chopped carrots, chili peppers, cucumbers, onions, radishes and tomatoes. It is seasoned with chopped coriander leaves, cumin, red chili powder and salt. These ingredients are then tossed in a bowl with lemon juice and sometimes oil.

Gluten-Free Decision Factors:
- None

Food Allergen Preparation Considerations:
- May contain corn from vegetable oil

- May contain peanuts from peanut oil and vegetable oil

- May contain soy from vegetable oil

Curry Dishes
Channa Masala (Chickpeas in Tomato Curry)
Channa Masala is usually a vegetarian dish, however fresh chicken stock is used from time to time. Chopped chili, garlic, ginger and onions are sautéed in *ghee* or oil. Chopped or crushed tomatoes are then added with water or occasionally chicken stock. Boiled and drained chickpeas are then added with *garam masala* powder (a spice mixture which varies, but typically includes black pepper, cloves, coriander, cumin and red chili powder). The dish is usually garnished with chopped coriander leaves.

Gluten-Free Decision Factors:
- Ensure stocks and broths are not made from bouillon which may contain gluten

- Ensure no wheat flour in sauce

Food Allergen Preparation Considerations:
- May contain corn from bouillon and vegetable oil
- May contain dairy from butter
- May contain peanuts from peanut oil and vegetable oil
- May contain soy from bouillon and vegetable oil

Gosht Vindaloo (Spicy Lamb Curry)

Gosht Vindaloo is a spicy lamb curry dish. Cubed lamb is marinated in a paste made of black pepper, cinnamon, cloves, coriander, cumin, garlic, ginger, red chili powder, turmeric and cider or wine vinegar for a period of up to 24 hours. Chopped onions and potatoes are sautéed in *ghee* or oil. The lamb and the marinade are then added with diced chili peppers and crushed tomatoes and all the ingredients are simmered for about a half an hour. The dish is usually served with basmati rice and garnished with chopped coriander leaves or bay leaves.

Gluten-Free Decision Factors:
- Ensure no wheat flour in sauce
- Ensure no soy sauce or wheat flour in marinade

Food Allergen Preparation Considerations:
- May contain corn from vegetable oil
- May contain dairy from butter
- May contain peanuts from peanut oil and vegetable oil
- May contain soy from soy sauce in marinade and vegetable oil

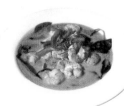

Jhinga Masala
(Shrimp in Coconut Curry)

Jhinga Masala (Shrimp in Coconut Curry)

Jhinga Masala is one of the most common shrimp dishes found in Indian restaurants. The base of the curry is typically coconut milk; however, this ingredient may be omitted in some restaurants. *Garam masala* powder, garlic, ginger and tamarind are sautéed in *ghee* or oil. Chopped onions, crushed tomatoes and shrimp are then added and the entire mixture is brought to a boil. Once the shrimp is cooked, coconut milk and salt are added. Sometimes lemon or tamarind juice may also be used. The dish is usually served with basmati rice and garnished with chopped coriander leaves or bay leaves.

Gluten-Free Decision Factors:
- Ensure no wheat flour in sauce

Food Allergen Preparation Considerations:
- Contains shellfish from shrimp

- May contain corn from vegetable oil

- May contain dairy from butter

- May contain peanuts from peanut oil and vegetable oil

- May contain soy from vegetable oil

7

Malai Kofta (Vegetarian Croquettes in Mild Curry)

Malai Kofta is a traditional vegetarian dish that may be traced back to the Muslim Moghul Empire which once controlled most of the Indian subcontinent. The croquettes are made with mashed potatoes or rice, cashews, chopped green chili, coriander, *paneer* and raisins. They are dusted with corn, lentil (*urad daal*) or chickpea (*besan*) flour and pan fried in *ghee* or oil. The croquettes are then added to a mild curry sauce made with *garam masala* powder, cream or yogurt, garlic, ginger, onions, *paneer*, puréed tomatoes and *ghee* or oil. The dish is usually served with basmati rice and garnished with chopped coconut.

Gluten-Free Decision Factors:
- Ensure no wheat flour—chickpea, corn or lentil flour is typically used

- Ensure croquettes are not dusted with wheat flour

- Ensure no wheat flour in sauce

Food Allergen Preparation Considerations:
- Contains dairy from cheese, cream, yogurt and possibly from butter
- Contains tree nuts from cashews
- May contain corn from vegetable oil
- May contain peanuts from peanut oil and vegetable oil
- May contain soy from vegetable oil

Murg Korma (Chicken in Cream Curry)

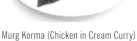

Murg Korma (Chicken in Cream Curry)

Murg Korma is a popular curry dish made in Indian restaurants all over the world. Garlic and onions are sautéed in *ghee* or oil with cardamom, cloves, coriander, ginger and salt. Yogurt is then stirred in, along with other spices such as *garam masala* powder and often almonds. Cubed boneless chicken is added and the dish is simmered for about twenty minutes. Milk or cream is then added a few minutes prior to serving. The dish is usually served with basmati rice and garnished with chopped coriander leaves (cilantro).

Gluten-Free Decision Factors:
- Ensure no wheat flour in sauce

Food Allergen Preparation Considerations:
- Contains dairy from cream, yogurt and possibly from butter
- May contain corn from vegetable oil
- May contain peanuts from peanut oil and vegetable oil
- May contain soy from vegetable oil
- May contain tree nuts from almonds

Murg Tikka Masala (Chicken in Tomato Curry)

Murg Tikka Masala may be the most popular dish found in Indian restaurants across the globe. In fact, it is estimated that over 23 million portions are sold annually in restaurants in the United Kingdom alone. Although recipes for this dish vary widely, the basic preparation of the dish remains consistent. Cubed boneless chicken is marinated in yogurt, lemon juice, cumin, cinnamon, red chili powder, black pepper, ginger and salt for a period of up to 24 hours. It is then grilled over an open flame or baked in a tandoori oven. To prepare the tomato curry sauce, onions are sautéed in *ghee* or oil. Tomato purée and crushed tomatoes are added along with garlic paste, ginger paste and *garam masala* powder. Occasionally, almonds or cashews may be included. To give the dish a red color, red food coloring may also be added. The chicken is then added to the tomato curry and finished with cream. The dish is usually served with basmati rice and garnished with sliced almonds, chopped coriander leaves (cilantro) or shaved coconut.

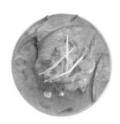

Murg Tikka Masala (Chicken in Tomato Curry)

Gluten-Free Decision Factors:
- Ensure no wheat flour in sauce
- Ensure no soy sauce or wheat flour in marinade

Food Allergen Preparation Considerations:
- Contains dairy from cream, yogurt and possibly from butter
- May contain corn from food coloring and vegetable oil
- May contain peanuts from peanut oil and vegetable oil
- May contain soy from food coloring, soy sauce in marinade and vegetable oil
- May contain tree nuts from almonds and cashews

Rogan Josh (Mild Lamb Curry)
Rogan Josh is a popular lamb dish that is typically less spicy than *Gosht Vindaloo*. Cubed lamb is marinated in a paste made of cardamom, cinnamon, coriander, cumin, red chili powder, turmeric and yogurt for a period of up to 24 hours. Puréed garlic, ginger, onions

and tomatoes are then mixed with *garam masala* powder. This mixture is brought to a boil with a touch of *ghee* or oil. The lamb and the marinade are then added and all the ingredients are simmered for about a half an hour or until the curry is reduced to a thick sauce. The dish is usually served with basmati rice and garnished with chopped coriander leaves (cilantro).

Gluten-Free Decision Factors:
- Ensure no wheat flour in sauce
- Ensure no soy sauce or wheat flour in marinade

Food Allergen Preparation Considerations:
- Contains dairy from yogurt and possibly from butter
- May contain corn from vegetable oil
- May contain peanuts from peanut oil and vegetable oil
- May contain soy from soy sauce in marinade and vegetable oil

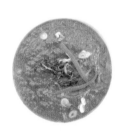
Saag Paneer (Indian Cheese and Spinach Curry)

Saag Paneer (Indian Cheese and Spinach Curry)
Saag Paneer is a common Indian vegetarian dish. A paste is made of garlic, onions and ginger, then sautéed in a pan with *ghee* or oil. Buttermilk or cream, chili powder, *garam masala* powder, spinach and yogurt are added and simmered for 20 to 30 minutes. *Paneer* is added and all the ingredients are cooked for approximately five minutes. The dish is usually served with basmati rice.

Gluten-Free Decision Factors:
- Ensure no wheat flour in sauce

Food Allergen Preparation Considerations:
- Contains dairy from buttermilk, cream, cheese, yogurt and possibly from butter
- May contain corn from vegetable oil

- May contain peanuts from peanut oil and vegetable oil

- May contain soy from vegetable oil

Tandoor Specialties
Boti Kabob (Skewered Lamb)
Boti Kabobs are a direct influence of the Muslim culture on traditional Indian culinary practices. Cubed lamb is marinated in yogurt with cardamoms, cinnamon, coriander seeds, garlic, lemon juice and red chili powder for a period of up to 24 hours. The lamb is then skewered and grilled over an open flame or baked in a tandoori oven. While cooking, the *Kabobs* are continually basted with the marinade which has had vegetable oil added to it. The dish is usually served with basmati rice, a variety of grilled vegetables and garnished with cucumber, lemon wedges, lettuce and sliced onions.

7

Gluten-Free Decision Factors:
- Ensure no soy sauce or wheat flour in marinade

Food Allergen Preparation Considerations:
- Contains dairy from yogurt

- May contain corn from vegetable oil

- May contain peanuts from peanut oil and vegetable oil

- May contain soy from soy sauce in marinade and vegetable oil

Murg Tandoori (Tandoori Barbeque Chicken)
Murg Tandoori is the typical Indian version of barbequed chicken. Quartered chicken or boneless cubed chicken is marinated in yogurt, chili powder, garlic, ginger, *garam masala* powder, lemon juice and mustard oil for a period of up to 24 hours. The chicken is then skewered and grilled over an open flame or baked in a tandoori oven. While cooking, the chicken is continually basted with the marinade which has

had *ghee* or oil added to it. The dish is usually served with basmati rice and garnished with lemon wedges and sliced onions.

Gluten-Free Decision Factors:
- Ensure no soy sauce or wheat flour in marinade

Food Allergen Preparation Considerations:
- Contains dairy from yogurt and possibly from butter

- May contain corn from vegetable oil

- May contain peanuts from peanut oil and vegetable oil

- May contain soy from soy sauce in marinade and vegetable oil

Murg Tikka (Yogurt Marinated Chicken)

Murg Tikka is prepared exactly the same way as *Murg Tikka Masala,* except it is served without the tomato curry sauce. Cubed boneless chicken is marinated in yogurt, lemon juice, cumin, cinnamon, black pepper, ginger, red chili powder and salt for a period of up to 24 hours and grilled over an open flame or baked in a tandoori oven. To give the chicken a red color, red food coloring or tomato sauce may also be added. While cooking, the chicken is continually basted with *ghee* or oil. The dish is usually served with basmati rice and garnished with lemon wedges and sliced onions.

Gluten-Free Decision Factors:
- Ensure no soy sauce or wheat flour in marinade

Food Allergen Preparation Considerations:
- Contains dairy from yogurt and possibly from butter

- May contain corn from food coloring and vegetable oil

- May contain peanuts from peanut oil and vegetable oil

- May contain soy from food coloring, soy sauce in marinade and vegetable oil

Seekh Kabob (Skewered Minced Lamb)

Like *Boti Kabobs, Seekh Kabobs* are a direct influence of the Muslim culture on traditional Indian culinary practices. They are similar to sausage, without the sausage casings or skins. Lamb is ground or minced with cashew powder, chickpea flour (*besan*), caraway seeds, coriander, eggs, fenugreek, garlic paste, ginger paste, *garam masala* powder, green chili pepper, nutmeg powder, onions, papaya pulp and tomato paste or red food coloring. The mixture is then formed around skewers and grilled over an open flame or baked in a tandoori oven. The dish is usually served with basmati rice and dipping sauces, usually *raita* and some type of chutney. It is typically garnished with lemon wedges and sliced onions.

Gluten-Free Decision Factors:

- Ensure no wheat flour in chutney

Food Allergen Preparation Considerations:

- Contains eggs as an ingredient

- Contains tree nuts from cashew powder

- May contain corn from food coloring

- May contain dairy from yogurt sauce

- May contain soy from food coloring

Dosas (South Indian Specialties)

Masala Dosa (Spicy Vegetable Filled Crepe)

Masala Dosas are a spicy version of this South Indian specialty. A fermented dough is made with a combination of chickpea (*besan*), lentil (*dal*) or rice flour and salt. A vegetable filling is prepared by sautéing sliced chili peppers, onions, peas and sometimes garlic in *ghee* or oil. Cooked cubed potatoes are then added with Indian spices, usually *garam masala* powder. Once fermented, the batter is placed on a griddle which has been lightly brushed with *ghee* or oil to make a thin crepe or pancake. The vegetable filling is then placed in the center and the crepe is wrapped around it like a small burrito. *Dosas* are usually served with common Indian condiments such as chutney, Indian pickles, *raita* and *sambar.*

Gluten-Free Decision Factors:
- Ensure no wheat flour—chickpea, lentil or rice flour are typically used

- Ensure no wheat flour in chutney and *sambar*

- Ensure stocks and broths are not made from bouillon which may contain gluten—if *sambar* is served

Food Allergen Preparation Considerations:
- May contain corn from bouillon and vegetable oil

- May contain dairy from butter and yogurt sauce

- May contain peanuts from peanut oil and vegetable oil

- May contain soy from bouillon and vegetable oil

Sada Dosa (Lentil and Rice Crepe)
Sada Dosas are the perfect substitute for bread when available in Indian restaurants. A fermented dough is made using a combination of lentil (*dal*) and rice flour with salt. Once fermented, the batter is placed on a griddle which has been lightly brushed with *ghee* or oil to make a thin crepe or pancake. *Dosas* are usually served with common Indian condiments such as chutney, Indian pickles, *raita* and *sambar.*

Gluten-Free Decision Factors:
- Ensure no wheat flour—lentil and rice flour are typically used

- Ensure no wheat flour in chutney and *sambar*

- Ensure stocks and broths are not made from bouillon which may contain gluten—if *sambar* is served

Food Allergen Preparation Considerations:
- May contain corn from bouillon and vegetable oil

- May contain dairy from butter and yogurt sauce

- May contain peanuts from peanut oil and vegetable oil

- May contain soy from bouillon and vegetable oil

Uthappam (Lentil and Rice Pancake)
Uthappam is an Indian version of the Italian favorite: pizza. A fermented dough is made using a combination of lentil (*dal*) and rice flour with salt. Once fermented, chopped onions, tomatoes, green chili, cashews and coriander (cilantro) are added to the batter. The resulting mixture is then placed on a griddle which has been lightly brushed with *ghee* or oil to make a pancake. *Uthappam* is usually served with common Indian condiments such as chutney, pickles, *raita* and *sambar*.

Gluten-Free Decision Factors:
- Ensure no wheat flour—lentil and rice flour are typically used

- Ensure no wheat flour in chutney and *sambar*

- Ensure stocks and broths are not made from bouillon which may contain gluten—if *sambar* is served

Food Allergen Preparation Considerations:
- Contains tree nuts from cashews

- May contain corn from bouillon and vegetable oil

- May contain dairy from butter and yogurt sauce

- May contain peanuts from peanut oil and vegetable oil

- May contain soy from bouillon and vegetable oil

Desserts
Kheer (Rice Pudding)

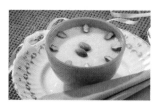

Kheer (Rice Pudding)

Kheer is one of the more popular Indian desserts. Milk is brought to a boil with basmati rice, cardamom and sugar. Once the liquid is reduced in half, sliced nuts are added such as almonds, cashews or pistachios and the mixture is allowed to cool. Saffron and raisins may also be added from time to time. *Kheer* is usually topped with sliced tree nuts.

Gluten-Free Decision Factors:
- Ensure no wheat flour as an ingredient

Food Allergen Preparation Considerations:
- Contains dairy from milk

- Contains tree nuts from almonds, cashews and pistachios

Kulfi (Indian Ice Cream)

Kulfi is an Indian ice cream made with a mixture of sweet condensed milk, cream and ground cardamom. For different flavors, fresh fruit purée, ground nuts and occasionally, a touch of saffron may be added. The mixture is then poured into molds and frozen for 12 hours. *Kulfi* can be garnished with rose water or ground nuts.

Gluten-Free Decision Factors:
- Ensure no wheat flour as an ingredient

Food Allergen Preparation Considerations:
- Contains dairy from cream and milk

- May contain tree nuts as an ingredient

Rasmalai (Cheese Balls in Sweet Cream)

Rasmalai is a common Indian dessert. *Paneer* and powdered sugar are mixed together and shaped into flat balls similar to a biscuit. They are then cooked in a light syrup made of sugar and water until they have a spongy consistency. In another pan, cardamom, cream, saffron, sugar and vanilla are brought a boil. The cheese balls are then added to the sweet cream and allowed to cool. *Rasmalai* is garnished with sliced tree nuts such as almonds, cashews or pistachios.

Gluten-Free Decision Factors:

- None

Food Allergen Preparation Considerations:

- Contains dairy from cheese and cream

- Contains tree nuts from almonds, cashews and pistachios

- May contain corn from vanilla extract

7

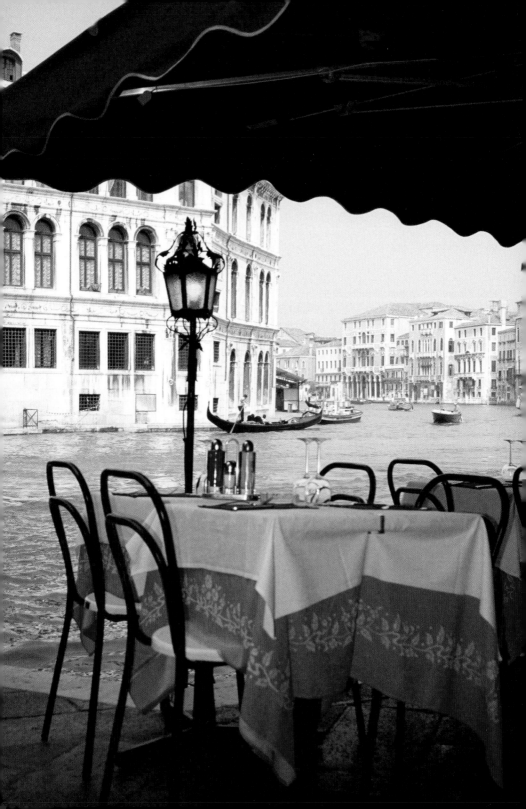

*One of the very nicest things about life
is the way we must regularly stop whatever it is we
are doing and devote our attention to eating.*
—Luciano Pavarotti

Chapter 8
Let's Eat Italian Cuisine

8

Cuisine Overview

Italy has a population of over 58 million and is slightly larger than the United Kingdom or the state of California. There are 20 different regions or states, each of which has developed its own culinary practices. For classification purposes, these regions can be divided into three categories of cuisine: Northern, Central and Southern. Climate and environment have been the greatest influences to culinary practices in these regions and their respective diets have remained virtually unchanged for centuries.

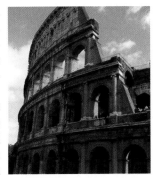
Roman Colosseum

What one eats really depends on where one is located in Italy. Northern Italian cuisine is famous for polenta and risotto, as well as popular cheeses and pesto sauce. Pasta, red wine and carbonara sauce are indicative of Central Italian cuisine. Southern Italian cuisine is known for seafood dishes, pizza and dark rich olive oil.

The foods of Italy are perhaps the most common ethnic cuisine found around the world. Restaurants, regardless of location, generally offer dishes that represent a number of the regional specialties found in Italy. Although some staples of the Italian diet contain gluten, there are numerous gluten-free dishes available at restaurants.

Traditional Ingredients

The Italian diet is rich in carbohydrates and vegetables; yet surprisingly limited in its use of meats. Vegetables, bread, pasta, cheese and olive oil are the hallmarks of Italian cuisine. The use of these traditional ingredients, in a variety of styles represented by the three major regions of Italy, is the essence of their national cuisine.

Italy is known for its bounty of bright vegetables. Artichokes, asparagus, cauliflower, eggplant, legumes, olives, peppers, porcini mushrooms, spinach, tomatoes and zucchini are abundant. Fresh herbs such as bay leaves, basil, garlic, mint, oregano, parsley, pepper, rosemary, sage, salt and thyme are regularly used, with olive oil prominently positioned in most kitchens.

Cheeses are a big part of the Italian diet and there are wide variety of choices. *Asiago, bel paese, fontina, crescienza, gorgonzola, mascarpone, pecorino sardo, provolone, ricotta, robiola* and *taleggio* are Italian table cheeses. *Mozzarella* and *provatura* are cooking cheeses, whereas, *parmigiano reggiano* and *pecorino romano* are cheeses that are usually grated and used to top dishes.

Although meats are used in limited quantities, most meals include protein of some kind. Prosciutto (cured ham) and salami are usually eaten during the starter portion of the meal. Chicken, fish, beef and lamb are typically featured in dishes and shellfish may be available with every course.

Like the French, Italians have been drinking wine for hundreds of years. Most Italians drink wine as part of their daily routine. Not only do they drink wine with most meals, but it is used regularly in food preparation. Each individual state or region produces its own style of wine. Italians produce twice as much red wine annually as they do white, most prominently in the Northern and Central regions of Tuscano, Piemonte and Veneto. These red wines include *Barolo, Barbaresco, Brunello di Montalcino, Chianti* and *Vallpolicella.* White wines, which are produced all over Italy, include *Asti Spumanti, Marsala, Pinot Grigio* and *Soave.*

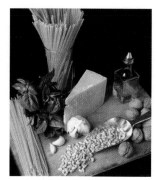

Although some staples of the Italian diet contain gluten, there are numerous gluten-free dishes available at restaurants.

8

Gluten Awareness

Although gluten is present in many areas of Italian cuisine, we have outlined 25-plus items in our sample menu. There are seven primary points that you need to consider when dining at an Italian restaurant. To ensure a gluten-free experience, the areas of food preparation that you need to inquire about with your server or chef are listed below

Sauces	Ensure sauces do not contain wheat flour
Flour Dusting	Wheat flour is typically used—request plain
Stocks and Broths	Ensure all are made fresh or from allergen-free mixes and not from bouillon, which may contain gluten
Cooking Oil	Ensure frying oil has not been used to fry battered foods that may contain gluten
Pasta	Wheat flour is typically used—request gluten-free pasta or substitute polenta, if available
Battering, Bread & Breading	Wheat flour is typically used—request plain-cooked food. Ensure no batter, bread or breading
Cross-Contamination	Ensure all utensils and cooking surfaces have been cleaned prior to the preparation of your meal

8

Sauces

Of the many different sauces you may encounter in Italian cuisine, always be sure the sauce is not thickened with wheat flour or made from a roux. Below is a list of common and typically gluten-free Italian sauces and their ingredients:

Alfredo	A white sauce made of butter, cream and Parmesan cheese
Bolognese	A meat sauce made with pancetta, ground meat, tomatoes, onions and garlic
Carbonara	A white sauce made with butter, eggs, pancetta, pecorino and Parmesan cheese
Marinara	A red sauce made with basil, garlic, olive oil, onions, oregano, tomatoes and possibly Parmesan cheese

Pesto	A garlic and olive oil sauce made with basil, pine nuts, Parmesan cheese and possibly cashews
Piccata	A lemon and caper sauce made with white wine and butter
Pomodoro	Means tomato in Italian and can be any type of tomato sauce

Some Italian sauces include bread crumbs or wheat flour. Below are three common Italian sauces that you need to avoid:

Agliata	A garlic sauce made with bread crumbs, olive oil and vinegar
Pesto Ericino	A Sicilian pesto sauce made with almonds, basil, bread crumbs, garlic, olive oil and tomatoes
Roux	A sauce made with flour, fat and butter.

Note: Roux is typically not included as part of a menu description. Allergen-free roux mixes are also available.

Flour Dusting

Flour dusting is common in Italian cuisine. Most restaurants prefer to dust using wheat flour to texture meats or fish prior to pan frying, thereby allowing a sauce to be evenly distributed. Ensure that this practice is not used in the preparation of your meal.

Stocks and Broths

Stocks and broths are used frequently in Italian cuisine. They are used in sauces and soups, as well as in marinades for meats and vegetables. Ensure all are made fresh or from allergen-free mixes and not from bouillon, which may contain gluten.

Cooking Oil

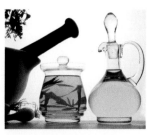

Olive oil is typically used in Italian restaurants. Outside of Italy, other oils such as corn or vegetable may be substituted from time to time.

Olive oil is typically used in Italian restaurants, but rarely used for frying. Outside of Italy, other oils such as corn or vegetable may be substituted from time to time. Oil is used to fry or sauté foods. When ordering food that is prepared by frying, ensure that there is a dedicated fryer in the kitchen for non-battered menu items. Since battered foods may contain wheat flour, this practice minimizes the potential of gluten cross-contamination from frying.

Pasta
There are over 400 different types of pasta produced in Italy, the vast majority of which are made from wheat flour. Depending upon your geographic location, gluten-free pasta may be available at restaurants. In Italy, for example, there are thousands of restaurants that offer gluten-free alternatives to wheat flour pasta. Polenta may also be available as a gluten-free alternative to wheat flour pasta.

Battering, Bread & Breading
Battering is used for frying foods like calamari and breading is used for meat cutlets. Wheat flour is typically used for battering and breading in Italian restaurants. Bread crumbs are used regularly as an ingredient in appetizers, soups and entrées. When ordering these dishes, request that your order is plain-cooked to ensure no battering, breading or bread crumbs. In addition, a basket of bread is usually served with most meals, so be certain to request no bread.

Cross-Contamination
Cross-contamination occurs in two primary instances and should be considered at any restaurant you choose to dine in. One may occur when your meal is prepared in the same frying oil as foods containing other possible allergens. The second may occur when food particles are transferred from one food to another by using the same knife, cutting board, pots, pans or other utensils without washing the surfaces or tools in between uses. In the case of open flamed grills, the extreme temperature turns most food particles into carbon. Use of a wire brush designed for grill racks typically removes residual contaminants.

To avoid cross-contamination, restaurants need to dedicate fryers for specific foods and wash all materials that may come in contact with food in hot, soapy water prior to preparing items for those with special dietary requirements. It is important to ensure that the restaurant follows these procedures for an allergen-free dining experience.

Other Allergy Considerations

If you have other food allergies or sensitivities, it is important to remain diligent in your approach to dining out. Because Italian cuisine is complex, there are many common food allergens used on a regular basis.

Know that vegetable oil can always be substituted for any oil and may contain corn, peanut or soy. It should be noted that unless an olive oil container specifically states 100% olive oil, it may be mixed with vegetable oil. If used, bouillon may contain Hydrolyzed Vegetable Protein (HVP) that can be derived from corn, soy or wheat. We have indicated the potential presence of bouillon and non-traditional cooking oils.

From the 25-plus items we have listed in our sample menu, we have identified each common allergen typically included in the dish as an ingredient. We have also indicated other potential allergens that may be present based upon non-traditional culinary practices. The chances of encountering common food allergens in our sample menu are outlined below.

High likelihood Dairy, eggs, fish, gluten, shellfish and wheat

Moderate likelihood Corn and soy

Low likelihood Peanuts and tree nuts

Dining Considerations

Italian menu items are usually presented in the Italian language. You may often find menu descriptions in the language of the country you are in following the name of the Italian menu item. While traveling, be sure to familiarize yourself with the common Italian culinary terms included in this chapter to assist you in your dining experience.

Italians generally eat two meals a day. In the morning, they usually drink coffee with warm milk and may have a *biscotti* or sweet biscuit. The first big meal of the day happens between 1 p.m. and 3 p.m. and is called *pranzo*. This is usually the largest meal of the day and consists of four to five courses.

The evening meal or *cena* is usually a quick affair when eaten at home with the family, beginning at 8 p.m. and ending before nine. As a special meal, *cena* can be enjoyed later than many people are used to, sometimes beginning at 9 or 10 p.m. It is a lighter meal than the afternoon *pranzo*. When dining out or entertaining guests in the home, Italians like to eat slowly and savor their food. Most meals typically last between two to three hours. Wine and conversation are a must at an Italian table, so it is best to relax and enjoy the experience.

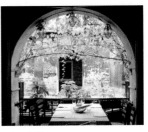
Italian Café

There are generally four courses to an Italian meal:

- *Antipasto* (soups, salads or starters)

- *Primo* (pasta)

- *Secondo* (dishes)

- *Dolce* (desserts)

Occasionally, an additional vegetable course may be added after the *secondo* and is called the *contorno*. Wine is served continually throughout the meal, with sweet dessert wines enjoyed at the end of the meal.

Buon Appetito!

Sample Italian Menu

Starters
Calamari alla Griglia (Grilled Calamari)
Carpaccio di Manzo (Beef Carpaccio)
Carpaccio di Salmone (Salmon Carpaccio)
Cocktail di Gamberi (Shrimp Cocktail)
Cozze al Vapore (Steamed Mussels)
Prosciutto e Melone (Cured Ham and Melon)

Soups
Gazpaccio

Salads
Insalata Caprese (Mozzarella Tomato Salad)
Insalata Mista (Mixed Green Salad)

Italian Specialties
Risotto ai Frutti di Mare (Arborio Rice and Seafood Dish)
Risotto ai Funghi (Arborio Rice and Mushroom Dish)
Risotto ai Quattro Formaggi (Arborio Rice and Cheese Dish)
Risotto al Pollo (Arborio Rice and Chicken Dish)

Meat Dishes
Costatella D'Agnello (Rack of Lamb)
Fileto di Manzo (Filet Mignon)
Medalione di Manzo (Beef Tenderloin Medallions)
Vitello (Veal)

Chicken Dishes
Petti di Pollo (Chicken Breast)
Pollo Arrosto Rosmarino (Rosemary Roasted Chicken)

Seafood Dishes
Salmone alla Griglia (Grilled Salmon)
Scampi (Prawns)

8

Sample Italian Menu

Sides
Broccoli Rabe (Broccoli Florets)
Funghi all' Aglio e Olio (Mushrooms in Garlic and Olive Oil)
Melanzane alla Griglia (Grilled Eggplant)
Polenta (Boiled Corn Meal)

Desserts
Gelato (Italian Ice Cream or Sherbet)
Granita (Italian Ice)
Zabaglione (Italian Custard)

8

We would like to thank Arber Murici of Lumi in New York, New York and Stephane Tremolani, former Executive Chef de Cuisine of the French Embassy in Rome, Italy for their valuable contributions in reviewing the following menu items.

Italian Menu Item Descriptions

Starters
Calamari alla Griglia (Grilled Calamari)
Many Italian restaurants offer grilled calamari; however, it is more commonly fried. Slices of calamari are marinated in lemon juice or olive oil then cooked on a grill over an open flame. Lemon wedges and marinara sauce for dipping are usually served on the side.

Gluten-Free Decision Factors:
- Ensure no wheat flour in sauce

- Ensure calamari is not battered

- Ensure calamari is not dusted with wheat flour
- Ensure no bread crumbs

Food Allergen Preparation Considerations:
- Contains shellfish from calamari
- May contain corn from batter, bread crumbs, dipping sauce and vegetable oil
- May contain dairy from bread crumbs and dipping sauce
- May contain eggs from batter, bread crumbs and dipping sauce
- May contain peanuts from bread crumbs, dipping sauce and vegetable oil
- May contain soy from bread crumbs and vegetable oil
- May contain tree nuts from bread crumbs and dipping sauce

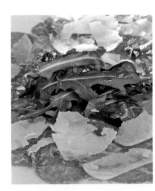
Carpaccio di Manzo (Beef Carpaccio)

Carpaccio di Manzo (Beef Carpaccio)
Beef Carpaccio is thinly sliced rare beef lightly dressed with olive oil and sometimes balsamic vinegar. Shaved *parmigiano reggiano,* capers and dried herbs top the beef. This dish is generally garnished with fresh basil.

Gluten-Free Decision Factors:
- Ensure no gluten containing garnish

Food Allergen Preparation Considerations:
- Contains dairy from cheese
- May contain corn from vegetable oil
- May contain peanuts from vegetable oil
- May contain soy from vegetable oil

Carpaccio di Salmone (Salmon Carpaccio)
Like Beef Carpaccio, Salmon Carpaccio is thinly sliced raw salmon marinated in olive oil and lemon. There

are many different recipes for this dish; however, they are all similar. In some variations, balsamic vinegar, shallots, fresh dill and capers can be present. You may encounter a version of *Carpaccio di Salmone* at a restaurant that includes fava beans. The preparation of the fava beans most likely contains wheat flour.

Gluten-Free Decision Factors:
- Ensure no wheat flour in fava beans

Food Allergen Preparation Considerations:
- Contains fish from salmon

- May contain corn from vegetable oil

- May contain peanuts from vegetable oil

- May contain soy from vegetable oil

8

Cocktail di Gamberi (Shrimp Cocktail)
Shrimp cocktail is a common starter in many international cuisines. Most restaurants prepare and serve this starter in a similar fashion. Large shrimp are boiled in water or fish stock, shelled and chilled. The shrimp are served with a cocktail sauce (tomato sauce, horseradish and lemon juice) and lemon wedges. Italians prefer a mayonnaise-based cocktail sauce made with ketchup, a dash of pepper sauce and a touch of liquor such as whiskey or cognac.

Gluten-Free Decision Factors:
- Ensure stocks and broths are not made from bouillon which may contain gluten

Food Allergen Preparation Considerations:
- Contains shellfish from shrimp

- May contain corn from bouillon and corn syrup in cocktail sauce

- May contain eggs from mayonnaise-based sauce

- May contain fish from fish stock

- May contain soy from bouillon and mayonnaise-based sauce

Cozze al Vapore (Steamed Mussels)

Steamed mussels are a very popular starter in Italian restaurants. They are served both as a starter or as a main course, which is usually accompanied with pasta. The mussels are steamed or boiled in fish stock, then topped with a sauce that contains butter, onions or shallots, white wine and sometimes garlic. Occasionally, the mussels may be topped with bread crumbs.

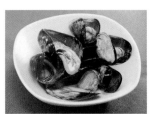
Cozze al Vapore (Steamed Mussels)

Gluten-Free Decision Factors:
- Ensure no bread crumbs
- Ensure no wheat flour pasta—order gluten-free pasta or polenta if available
- Ensure stocks and broths are not made from bouillon which may contain gluten

Food Allergen Preparation Considerations:
- Contains dairy from butter and possibly from bread crumbs
- Contains shellfish from mussels
- May contain corn from bouillon and bread crumbs
- May contain eggs from bread crumbs and pasta
- May contain peanuts from bread crumbs
- May contain soy from bouillon and bread crumbs
- May contain tree nuts from bread crumbs

Prosciutto e Melone (Cured Ham and Melon)

Prosciutto e Melone is a common dish found in many Italian restaurants. It is fresh cantaloupe or honey dew wrapped with *prosciutto di parma,* an Italian cured ham. Sometimes the dish contains aged hard cheese such as *parmigiano reggiano.*

Gluten-Free Decision Factors:
- None

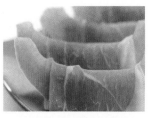
Prosciutto e Melone (Cured Ham and Melon)

Food Allergen Preparation Considerations:
- May contain dairy from cheese and prosciutto

Soups
Gazpaccio
This chilled soup usually consists of puréed tomatoes, onions, peppers and garlic, but may contain any fresh vegetable. It is seasoned with salt and pepper and may also contain other fresh Italian herbs. The popularity of gazpaccio has allowed this soup to be adapted into many regional cuisines in Europe. Although it is uncommon in Italy, restaurants outside the country may add wheat flour and croutons.

Gluten-Free Decision Factors:
- Ensure no croutons
- Ensure no wheat flour as thickening agent

Food Allergen Preparation Considerations:
- May contain corn as an ingredient and from croutons
- May contain dairy from croutons
- May contain eggs from croutons
- May contain peanuts from croutons
- May contain soy from croutons
- May contain tree nuts from croutons

8

Salads
Insalata Caprese (Mozzarella Tomato Salad)
Buffalo mozzarella and tomato salad is an Italian classic. Large slices of buffalo mozzarella are stacked with freshly sliced tomatoes. It is usually seasoned with salt and pepper and other dried herbs on occasion. Large leafs of basil garnish this dish, which is lightly dressed in olive oil and sometimes balsamic vinegar.

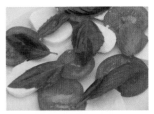

Insalata Caprese (Mozzarella Tomato Salad)

Gluten-Free Decision Factors:
- None

Food Allergen Preparation Considerations:
- Contains dairy from cheese

- May contain corn from vegetable oil

- May contain peanuts from vegetable oil

- May contain soy from vegetable oil

Insalata Mista (Mixed Green Salad)

A mixed green salad in Italy is usually a combination of mixed greens, cucumbers, onions and tomatoes. Some Italian restaurants may add anchovies or croutons and the type of salad dressings may vary.

Gluten-Free Decision Factors:
- Ensure no croutons or breadsticks as garnish

Food Allergen Preparation Considerations:
- May contain corn from vegetable oil

- May contain eggs from croutons

- May contain fish from anchovies

- May contain peanuts from vegetable oil

- May contain soy from vegetable oil

Italian Specialties
Risotto ai Frutti di Mare (Arborio Rice and Seafood Dish)

Risotto is a Northern Italian dish with seafood being one of the common varieties. The preparation techniques of *risotto* dishes are usually similar, but the ingredients vary depending on the type of *risotto* that you order. In *Risotto ai Frutti di Mare,* arborio rice is boiled in fresh stock, usually chicken, fish or shrimp. In a separate pan, white wine is simmered with garlic, olive oil, onions or shallots, salt and pepper. Mushrooms such as porcini or portabella are often added. Mixed seafood (usually calamari, clams, fish, oysters, mussels, scallops and shrimp) is then cooked in the wine until its temperature is somewhere between rare and medium rare. The seafood is then added to the rice, which has had fresh stock continually added to it as the moisture evaporates. As the moisture continues to evaporate, butter, *parmigiano reggiano* and *romano* cheese are added. The dish is usually garnished with parsley.

Gluten-Free Decision Factors:
- Ensure stocks and broths are not made from bouillon which may contain gluten

- Ensure clean water is used to cook rice

Food Allergen Preparation Considerations:
- Contains dairy from butter and cheese

- Contains fish as an ingredient

- Contains shellfish as ingredient

- May contain corn from bouillon and vegetable oil

- May contain peanuts from vegetable oil

- May contain soy from bouillon and vegetable oil

8

Risotto ai Funghi (Arborio Rice and Mushroom Dish)

In *Risotto ai Funghi,* arborio rice is boiled in fresh stock, usually chicken or mushroom. In a separate pan, white wine is simmered with garlic, olive oil, onions or shallots, salt and pepper. Mushrooms such as cremini, porcini and portabella are added. Some recipes may even call for *tartufi,* which are black or white truffles. The mushrooms are then added to the rice, which has had fresh stock continually added to it as the moisture evaporates. As the moisture continues to evaporate, butter, *parmigiano reggiano* and *romano* cheese are added. The dish is usually garnished with parsley.

Gluten-Free Decision Factors:
- Ensure stocks and broths are not made from bouillon which may contain gluten

- Ensure clean water is used to cook rice

Food Allergen Preparation Considerations:
- Contains dairy from butter and cheese

- May contain corn from bouillon and vegetable oil

- May contain peanuts from vegetable oil

- May contain soy from bouillon and vegetable oil

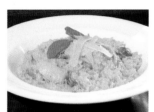

Risotto ai Quattro Formaggi (Arborio Rice and Cheese Dish)

Risotto ai Quattro Formaggi (Arborio Rice and Cheese Dish)

In *Risotto ai Quattro Formaggi,* arborio rice is boiled in fresh stock, usually chicken or vegetable. In a separate pan, white wine is simmered with garlic, olive oil, onions or shallots, salt and pepper. This is then added to the rice, which has had fresh stock continually added to it as the moisture evaporates. As the moisture continues to evaporate, butter, *fontina, parmigiano reggiano, pecorino* and *romano* cheese are added. The dish is usually garnished with parsley.

Gluten-Free Decision Factors:
- Ensure stocks and broths are not made from bouillon which may contain gluten
- Ensure clean water is used to cook rice

Food Allergen Preparation Considerations:
- Contains dairy from butter and cheese
- May contain corn from bouillon and vegetable oil
- May contain peanuts from vegetable oil
- May contain soy from bouillon and vegetable oil

Risotto al Pollo (Arborio Rice and Chicken Dish)

In *Risotto al Pollo,* arborio rice is boiled in fresh chicken stock. In a separate pan, white wine is simmered with garlic, olive oil, onions or shallots, salt and pepper. Slices of chicken are then added, sometimes with aromatic herbs such as anise, fennel or rosemary. The chicken is then added to the rice, which has had fresh stock continually added to it as the moisture evaporates. As the moisture continues to evaporate, butter, *parmigiano reggiano* and *romano* cheese are added. The dish is usually garnished with parsley.

Gluten-Free Decision Factors:
- Ensure stocks and broths are not made from bouillon which may contain gluten
- Ensure clean water is used to cook rice

Food Allergen Preparation Considerations:
- Contains dairy from butter and cheese

- May contain corn from bouillon and vegetable oil

- May contain peanuts from vegetable oil

- May contain soy from bouillon and vegetable oil

Meat Dishes
Costatella D'Agnello (Rack of Lamb)

Costatella (rack) or *costoletta* (chop) are widely considered the most flavorful cut of lamb. They are taken from the rib and have a good amount of marbling, which provides the rich flavor. Italians traditionally roast lamb with olive oil, rosemary, salt, pepper and plenty of garlic. If the menu description states that the dish is herb encrusted, bread crumbs are usually used. The dish is typically served with a side vegetable or pasta.

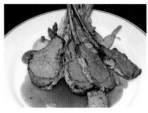

Costoletta D'Agnello (Lamb Chops)

Gluten-Free Decision Factors:
- Ensure lamb is not dusted with wheat flour

- Ensure no wheat flour pasta—order gluten-free pasta or polenta if available

- Ensure no bread crumbs

Food Allergen Preparation Considerations:
- May contain corn from bread crumbs and vegetable oil

- May contain dairy from bread crumbs

- May contain eggs from bread crumbs and pasta

- May contain peanuts from bread crumbs and vegetable oil

- May contain soy from bread crumbs and vegetable oil

- May contain tree nuts from bread crumbs

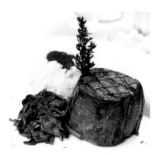

Fileto di Manzo (Filet Mignon)

Fileto di Manzo (Filet Mignon)

Fileto di Manzo is the classic dish known to most as filet mignon. It is usually seasoned with salt and pepper and may sometimes be seasoned with other Italian herbs. The beef may be pan seared in butter or olive oil; it can also be grilled over an open flame. The dish is typically served with a side vegetable or pasta.

Gluten-Free Decision Factors:
- Ensure beef is not dusted with wheat flour
- Ensure no wheat flour pasta—order gluten-free pasta or polenta if available

Food Allergen Preparation Considerations:
- May contain corn from vegetable oil
- May contain dairy from butter
- May contain eggs from pasta
- May contain peanuts from vegetable oil
- May contain soy from vegetable oil

Medalione di Manzo (Beef Tenderloin Medallions)

Slices of beef tenderloin are pan seared in butter or olive oil, or they can be grilled over an open flame. The medallions are usually seasoned with salt and pepper and may also be seasoned with other Italian herbs. It is common for the medallions to be served in *marinara* or *pomodoro* sauce. The dish is typically served with a side vegetable or pasta.

Gluten-Free Decision Factors:
- Ensure no wheat flour in sauce
- Ensure beef is not dusted with wheat flour
- Ensure no wheat flour pasta—order gluten-free pasta or polenta if available

Other Potential Allergens
- May contain corn from vegetable oil
- May contain dairy from butter and sauce
- May contain eggs from pasta
- May contain peanuts from vegetable oil
- May contain soy from vegetable oil
- May contain tree nuts from sauce

Vitello (Veal)

Veal is a very popular type of meat served in Italian restaurants. It is meat from a young calf, usually eight months in age, and considered more tender and flavorful than regular beef. The most common cuts of veal you may encounter are *scallopine* (cutlet), *costatella* (rack of rib) and *costoletta* (chop). Veal can be prepared a number of different ways and is usually grilled, pan seared or roasted. When offered as *scallopine,* it is typically served in a sauce like *parmigiana* (a tomato sauce with *parmigiano reggiano* cheese) or *piccata* (a lemon and caper sauce made with white wine and butter). In the case of *parmigiana* or *piccata,* the veal may be breaded or flour dusted. If the menu description states that the veal is herb encrusted, bread crumbs are typically used. Veal is usually served with a side vegetable or pasta in restaurants outside of Italy. However, pasta with veal in Italy is uncommon.

Gluten-Free Decision Factors:
- Ensure no wheat flour in sauce
- Ensure no breading
- Ensure veal is not dusted with wheat flour
- Ensure no bread crumbs
- Ensure no wheat flour pasta—order gluten-free pasta or polenta if available

Food Allergen Preparation Considerations:
- May contain corn from bread crumbs, breading and vegetable oil

- May contain dairy from bread crumbs, breading, butter, cheese and sauce

- May contain eggs from bread crumbs, breading and pasta

- May contain peanuts from bread crumbs and vegetable oil

- May contain soy from bread crumbs, breading and vegetable oil

- May contain tree nuts from bread crumbs and sauce

8

Chicken Dishes
Petti di Pollo (Chicken Breast)
Grilled chicken breast is a relatively common menu item in Italian restaurants. Chicken breasts can be prepared many different ways and usually come topped with a sauce. Some chicken breast dishes with sauces include; *all' anice* (a cream sauce with anise and fennel), *al limone* (*piccata* style in a lemon and caper sauce made with white wine and butter) and *parmigiana*. In the case of *al limone* or *parmigiana*, the chicken may be breaded or flour dusted. If the menu description states that the chicken is herb encrusted, bread crumbs are typically used. Chicken breast dishes are usually accompanied by a side vegetable or pasta.

Gluten-Free Decision Factors:
- Ensure no wheat flour in sauce

- Ensure no breading

- Ensure chicken is not dusted with wheat flour

- Ensure no bread crumbs

- Ensure no wheat flour pasta—order gluten-free pasta or polenta if available

Food Allergen Preparation Considerations:
- May contain corn from bread crumbs, breading and vegetable oil

- May contain dairy from bread crumbs, breading, butter, cheese, cream and sauce

- May contain eggs from bread crumbs, breading and pasta

- May contain peanuts from bread crumbs and vegetable oil

- May contain soy from bread crumbs, breading and vegetable oil

- May contain tree nuts from bread crumbs and sauce

Pollo Arrosto Rosmarino (Rosemary Roasted Chicken)
Italian restaurants serve many different styles of roasted chicken, with rosemary being the most commonly used herb. A whole chicken is rubbed with olive oil, fresh rosemary, salt, pepper and possibly anise, fennel, garlic, oregano and thyme. It is then roasted in an oven or over an open flame. Half a roasted chicken is the common portion. If the menu description states that the chicken is herb encrusted, bread crumbs are typically used. The dish is usually served with a side vegetable or pasta.

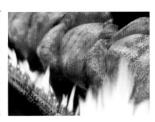
Pollo Arrosto Rosmarino (Rosemary Roasted Chicken)

Gluten-Free Decision Factors:
- Ensure no bread crumbs

- Ensure no wheat flour pasta—order gluten-free pasta or polenta if available

Food Allergen Preparation Considerations:
- May contain corn from bread crumbs and vegetable oil

- May contain dairy from bread crumbs

- May contain eggs from bread crumbs and pasta

- May contain peanuts from bread crumbs and vegetable oil

- May contain soy from bread crumbs and vegetable oil

- May contain tree nuts from bread crumbs

Seafood Dishes
Salmone alla Griglia (Grilled Salmon)
Grilled salmon is popular in many Italian restaurants. Salmon filets are grilled and seasoned with fresh lemon juice and herbs, usually dill or rosemary. Once cooked, the filet may be served *al limone* or with lemon wedges and typically a side vegetable or pasta.

8

Gluten-Free Decision Factors:
- Ensure no wheat flour in sauce

- Ensure no wheat flour pasta—order gluten-free pasta or polenta if available

Food Allergen Preparation Considerations:
- Contains fish from salmon

- May contain corn from vegetable oil

- May contain dairy from butter and sauce

- May contain eggs from pasta

- May contain peanuts from vegetable oil

- May contain soy from vegetable oil

- May contain tree nuts from sauce

Scampi (Prawns)
Scampi are prawns with extremely large ones called *mazzancolle*. In most cases, they are sautéed in butter or olive oil with white wine, garlic, salt, pepper and topped with minced basil or parsley. Cream and lemon juice are other ingredients used occasionally. *Fra diavolo* (sautéed in a spicy tomato sauce) and *al forno* (baked in tomato sauce and topped with cheese)

are other common variations. If baked, although rare, bread crumbs may be present. Scampi is often served with pasta as a side.

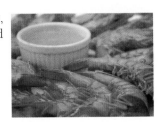

Scampi simply means prawns; extremely large ones called mazzancolle are very popular in Rome.

Gluten-Free Decision Factors:
- Ensure no wheat flour in sauce
- Ensure no bread crumbs
- Ensure no wheat flour pasta—order gluten-free pasta or polenta if available

Food Allergen Preparation Considerations:
- Contains shellfish from shrimp
- May contain corn from bread crumbs and vegetable oil
- May contain dairy from bread crumbs, butter, cheese, cream and sauce
- May contain eggs from bread crumbs and pasta
- May contain peanuts from bread crumbs and vegetable oil
- May contain soy from bread crumbs and vegetable oil
- May contain tree nuts from bread crumbs and sauce

Sides
Broccoli Rabe (Broccoli Florets)

Broccoli Rabe is a slightly bitter tasting relative of broccoli. Also called *brocoletti di rape, rape* and *rapini*, it resembles the leafy flower of regular broccoli. Many restaurants may substitute *broccoli rabe* with regular broccoli. The Italian preference is to boil *broccoli rabe* for a few minutes to take out the bitterness, then sauté it in olive oil with garlic, salt and chili peppers. In Northern Italian restaurants, butter and various Italian herbs may be added and is usually garnished with chopped parsley and sometimes lemon wedges.

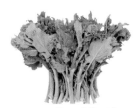

Broccoli Rabe (Broccoli Florets)

Gluten-Free Decision Factors:
- None

Food Allergen Preparation Considerations:
- May contain corn from vegetable oil
- May contain dairy from butter
- May contain peanuts from vegetable oil
- May contain soy from vegetable oil

Funghi all' Aglio e Olio (Mushrooms in Garlic and Olive Oil)

A very popular Italian side, mushrooms, such as cremini, porcini and portabella, are sautéed in olive oil, garlic, salt and pepper. In Northern Italian restaurants, butter may be added along with various Italian herbs and bread crumbs. The dish is usually garnished with chopped parsley.

Gluten-Free Decision Factors:
- Ensure no wheat flour as an ingredient
- Ensure no bread crumbs

Food Allergen Preparation Considerations:
- May contain corn from bread crumbs and vegetable oil
- May contain dairy from bread crumbs and butter
- May contain eggs from bread crumbs
- May contain peanuts from bread crumbs and vegetable oil
- May contain soy from bread crumbs and vegetable oil
- May contain tree nuts from bread crumbs

Melanzane alla Griglia (Grilled Eggplant)

Many Italian restaurants feature grilled eggplant. Slices of eggplant are marinated in garlic, olive oil, salt and pepper, then scored and grilled over an open flame. In some cases, the eggplant may be dusted with wheat flour or coated with bread crumbs. Grilled eggplant is usually garnished with chopped parsley.

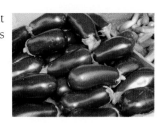
Melanzane (Eggplant)

Gluten-Free Decision Factors:
- Ensure eggplant is not dusted with wheat flour
- Ensure no bread crumbs

Food Allergen Preparation Considerations:
- May contain corn from bread crumbs and vegetable oil
- May contain dairy from bread crumbs
- May contain eggs from bread crumbs
- May contain peanuts from bread crumbs and vegetable oil
- May contain soy from bread crumbs and vegetable oil
- May contain tree nuts from bread crumbs

Polenta (Boiled Corn Meal)

Polenta has been a starch staple in Northern Italy for hundreds of years. The standard preparation involves boiling corn meal in water with salt. Once boiled out, the corn meal is malleable and can be formed into different shapes. *Polenta* may be topped with butter and various Italian cheeses or cut into sticks or wedges and fried crisp in oil. Grilling is another popular preparation style. *Polenta* is a great substitute for pasta when available and can be topped with any type of Italian sauce.

Gluten-Free Decision Factors:
- Ensure no wheat flour in sauce
- Ensure oil used for frying is designated for polenta only and is not used to fry other items that may be battered or dusted with wheat flour

Food Allergen Preparation Considerations:
- Contains corn from corn meal and possibly from vegetable oil

- May contain dairy from butter, cheese and sauce

- May contain peanuts from vegetable oil

- May contain soy from vegetable oil

- May contain tree nuts from sauce

Desserts
Gelato (Italian Ice Cream or Sherbet)

Gelato is somewhere between ice cream and sherbet and includes many flavors such as chocolate, custard, fruits and nuts. Some restaurants make it fresh while others may purchase it pre-made. Puréed fruit or other natural flavors and sugar are mixed with heavy whipping cream and frozen, either in a freezer or an ice cream machine. As with ice cream, ask your server to read the ingredients listed on the container if available and keep your flavor choices simple. Gelato may be served with a cookie/biscuit.

Gluten-Free Decision Factors:
- Ensure no stabilizers which may contain gluten

- Ensure no cookie/biscuit

Food Allergen Preparation Considerations:
- Contains dairy as an ingredient and possibly from cookie/biscuit

- May contain corn from colors or flavors

- May contain eggs from colors or flavors and cookie/biscuit

- May contain peanuts from colors or flavors and cookie/biscuit

- May contain soy from colors or flavors and cookie/biscuit

- May contain tree nuts from colors or flavors and cookie/biscuit

Granita (Italian Ice)

It was known as *Ghiaccio Italiano* (Italian ice) in the immigrant neighborhoods of New York City, as well as other US east coast cities for part of the 20th century. *Granita* is shaved ice with fruit syrup poured over the top, rather like a snow cone. What separates it from the standard snow cone is that the syrups are made fresh. Fruit is puréed and boiled with sugar and sometimes wine or liquor added to flavor the syrup.

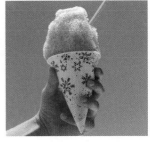
Granita (Italian Ice)

Gluten-Free Decision Factors:
- Ensure no malt or stabilizers which may contain gluten

Food Allergen Preparation Considerations:
- May contain corn from colors or flavors
- May contain soy from colors or flavors

8

Zabaglione (Italian Custard)

Unlike most custards, *zabaglione* is usually free of dairy products. It is made by whipping egg yolks and sugar together while cooking in a double boiler. Sweet *Marsala* wine and sometimes cookie/biscuit crumbs are added toward the end. When finished, it resembles a thick whipped cream with a yellow tint. *Zabaglione* is served warm or chilled, by itself or over fresh fruit, and possibly on top of cake.

Gluten-Free Decision Factors:
- Ensure no cake or cookie/biscuit crumbs

Food Allergen Preparation Considerations:
- Contains eggs from egg yolks and possibly from cake and cookie/biscuit crumbs
- May contain dairy from cake and cookie/biscuit crumbs
- May contain peanuts from cake and cookie/biscuit crumbs
- May contain soy from cookie/biscuit crumbs
- May contain tree nuts from cake and cookie/biscuit crumbs

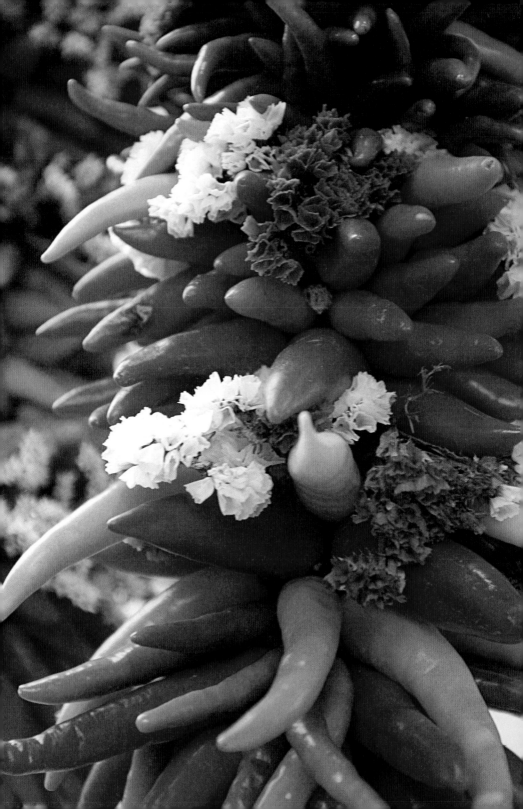

Conversation is food for the soul.
—Mexican proverb

Chapter 9
Let's Eat Mexican Cuisine

Cuisine Overview

9

With a landmass almost four times the size of Spain or three times the size of Texas, Mexico consists of 31 states, each of which has its own culinary traditions. The cultural identity of Mexico comes from a mixture of three distinct groups of people: The native Indians, the descendants of Spanish settlers and a mixture of the two groups known as Mestizos. Mexican food, like its history, is reflective of these three distinctive cultural influences.

Each region of Mexico is known for certain culinary specialties. The central plains, called the *Altiplano,* are credited with *antojos* (snacks) or *antojitos* (little snacks), which include foods such as tacos, tamales and enchiladas. The coastal state of Veracruz is known for its seafood dishes, whereas Puebla is famous for its complex mole sauce. Sauces in Yucatan are fruit-based and not as spicy as the chili fortified sauces you encounter in Sonora or Chihuahua. Restaurants in Mexico City serve bread with every meal, which is reminiscent of the French who ruled for a brief time. The state of Oaxaca is famous for its strong coffee and *mezcal,* a cousin of tequila made from the *agave* plant.

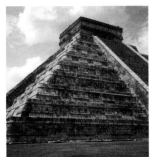
Chit'zen Itza

Mexican cuisine is based on fresh, seasonal produce. Chefs love to create dishes full of color and texture and typically present their plates in a simple fashion. Common culinary practices vary from state to state within Mexico. As you encounter restaurants outside the borders of Mexico, both authentic and derivative styles of Mexican cuisine maintain similar ingredients, while potentially incorporating different methods of preparation.

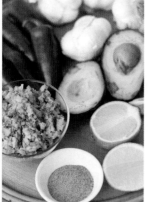

Traditional Mexican Ingredients

Traditional Ingredients

The traditional Mexican diet is rich in fresh vegetables, which are generally used only when in season. Various meats and seafood are balanced with vegetables. Cornmeal is the most common starch. Beans and rice are staples of every meal. The spices used in Mexican cooking are common to many cuisines, and yet, there are a number of seasonings that are unique to Mexican food. Desserts can range from simple tropical fruits to elaborate custards and cakes.

Called *verduras* in Spanish, vegetables are a part of the majority of Mexican meals, either as a side or in salads, soups and sauces. Onions, potatoes and tomatoes are common, with exotic fruits and vegetables such as avocado, *chayote* (gourd), *huitlacoche* (black mushrooms), jicama, prickly pear cactus and squash often featured. The most important spice used in Mexican cooking is also a vegetable in its fresh form: the chili pepper, spelled *chile* in Mexico.

Chile peppers are used as a dry spice as well as a fresh ingredient. There are many types, with the most common being ancho, habeñero, jalepeño, New Mexican green, New Mexican red, poblano and serrano. These peppers range from mild, like the poblano, to the extremely hot habeñero. Other herbs and spices that flavor Mexican cuisine are anise, cilantro, cinnamon, clove, cumin, garlic, marjoram, Mexican oregano and thyme. *Azafran* (Mexican saffron) and the pungent *epazote* (wormseed) are popular indigenous spices. Contrary to popular belief, most Mexican cuisine is rather mild, yet there are certain regional specialties that are extraordinarily spicy.

Queso (cheese) is eaten on a daily basis in Mexico. There are many different types of Mexican cheese and they come in a variety of textures. The most common are queso añejo (a soft cheese), queso blanco (a fresh, white cheese) and queso Chihuahua (a semi-soft cheese). Most Mexican cheese is made from cow or goat's milk; however, some cheeses like queso fresco are a combination of the two.

Prior to the arrival of the Spanish, the Aztec and Mayan Indians survived on wild game and fowl such as rabbit, boar, venison, quail, turkey and pigeons. Today, wild game and fowl specialties are considered a delicacy. The Spanish introduced domesticated live-stock, which is the predominate meat currently served in Mexican restaurants. Beef, chicken and pork are most common and can be prepared every imaginable way in a Mexican kitchen including:

- Baked (*al horno*)
- Broiled (*asado*)
- Grilled (*a la parilla*)
- Fried (*frito*)
- Steamed (*al vapor*)

Salt water fish and shellfish are naturally popular in coastal areas, but you can also find fresh water fish on some menus.

Beer and tequila are the most popular alcoholic beverages in Mexico, with the popularity of wine gradually gaining prominence. There is also a unique type of Mexican non-alcoholic beverage called *aguas frescas*. They are frappe-type drinks made with fresh fruit and puréed rice, melon seed or hibiscus flower. *Café de olla* is a popular form of Mexican coffee that is spiced with clove and cinnamon and is very high in caffeine.

Gluten Awareness

Although gluten is present in some areas of Mexican cuisine, we have outlined 30-plus items in our sample menu. There are six primary points that you need to consider when dining at a Mexican restaurant. To ensure a gluten-free experience, the areas of food preparation that you need to inquire about with your server or chef are listed below.

Sauces	Ensure sauces do not contain wheat flour
Stocks and Broths	Ensure all are made fresh or from allergen-free mixes and not from bouillon, which may contain gluten
Cooking Oil	Ensure frying oil has not been used to fry battered foods that may contain gluten
Tortillas	Corn tortillas are typically used—ensure no wheat flour
Marinades	Although uncommon, ensure marinades do not contain soy sauce or wheat flour
Cross-Contamination	Ensure all utensils and cooking surfaces have been cleaned prior to the preparation of your meal

Sauces

Culinary practices vary in Mexican restaurants. Although it is uncommon, some sauces may have wheat flour added to them as a thickening agent. Tex-Mex and New Mexican style cuisines tend to add flour to sauces more frequently. Always be sure to confirm that flour is not added to any sauce. Below is a list of common Mexican sauces and their ingredients:

Green Chile	Green chile, garlic, onions with a cream or milk base
Red Chile	Puréed red chile, garlic, onions and water
Mole	Over 30 ingredients and spices, including chile, cinnamon, cardamom, garlic, chopped nuts, sesame seeds and chocolate
Pico de Gallo	A fresh salsa consisting of tomatoes, onions, garlic, jalapenos and cilantro
Salsa Picante	Puréed tomatoes, chile, garlic, onions and cilantro
Salsa Ranchero	A milder version of salsa picante with more tomato sauce

9

Stocks and Broths

Stocks and broths are used frequently in Mexican cuisines. They are present in sauces and soups, as well as in marinades for meats and vegetables. Ensure all are made fresh or from allergen-free mixes and not from bouillon, which may contain gluten.

Cooking Oil

Corn oil is typically used in Mexican restaurants; however, other vegetable oils may be used from time to time. Oil is used to fry or sauté foods. When ordering food that is prepared by frying, ensure that there is a dedicated fryer in the kitchen for non-battered menu items. Since battered foods may contain wheat flour, this practice minimizes the potential of gluten cross-contamination from frying.

Tortillas

There are more than 160 different varieties of tortillas and nearly every Mexican meal will include at least one of them. Corn tortillas are the most common. The popularity of wheat flour tortillas has grown considerably during the last century in Northern Mexico and the United States. Cornmeal or wheat flour is combined with lard (animal fat) or vegetable oil/shortening to produce a thick dough. The dough is then made into thin circles and pre-cooked on a flat iron or griddle. Cross-contamination may occur during this process, as the cooking area and utensils might be used for both corn and flour tortillas. It is also important to ensure that a restaurant has a separate designated fryer for tortilla chips to avoid cross-contamination, as some establishments use only one. They may be served at room temperature, steamed, pan-fried or deep fried. Many restaurants make their own, while others prefer to purchase pre-made tortillas. Most dishes that use wheat flour tortillas can be easily modified by the substitution of corn tortillas.

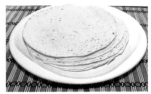

Nearly every Mexican meal will include tortillas.

Marinades

Marinades are used frequently in Mexican restaurants. In most cases they are citrus based; however, some restaurants may incorporate non-traditional ingredients in their marinades. If this is the case, ensure that the marinade does not include soy sauce, which contains wheat or wheat flour.

Cross-Contamination

Cross-contamination occurs in two primary instances and should be considered at any restaurant you choose to dine in. One may occur when your meal is prepared in the same frying oil as foods containing other possible allergens. The second may occur when food particles are transferred from one food to another by using the same knife, cutting board, pots, pans or other utensils without washing the surfaces or tools in between uses. In the case of open flamed grills, the extreme temperature turns most food particles into carbon. Use of a wire brush designed for grill racks typically removes residual contaminants.

To avoid cross-contamination, restaurants need to dedicate fryers for specific foods and wash all materials that may come in contact with food in hot, soapy water prior to preparing items for those with special dietary requirements. It is important to ensure that the restaurant follows these procedures for an allergen-free dining experience.

Other Allergy Considerations

If you have other food allergies or sensitivities, it is important to remain diligent in your approach to dining out. Because Mexican cuisine is complex, there are many common food allergens used on a regular basis. While in Mexico, be aware that corn oil is typically used to fry foods. Know that vegetable oil can always be substituted for any oil and may contain corn, peanuts or soy. If used, bouillon may contain Hydrolyzed Vegetable Protein (HVP) that can be derived from corn, soy or wheat. We have indicated the potential presence of bouillon and vegetable oil.

From the 30-plus items we have listed in our sample menu, we have identified each common allergen typically included in the dish as an ingredient. We have also indicated other potential allergens that may be present based upon non-traditional culinary practices. The chances of encountering common food allergens in items specific to our sample menu are outlined on the next page.

High likelihood   Corn, dairy, eggs, fish and shellfish

Moderate likelihood Gluten, soy and wheat

Low likelihood   Peanuts and tree nuts

Dining Considerations

Mexican menu items are usually presented in Spanish. You may often find menu descriptions in the language of the country you are in following the name of the Mexican menu item. While traveling, be sure to familiarize yourself with the common Mexican culinary terms included in this chapter to assist you in your dining experience.

Native Mexicans generally eat four meals a day. The first meal of the day, *desayuno,* is taken early in the morning and consists of coffee, juice, fruit and hot cereal. At around 11 a.m., *almuerzo* is served and usually consists of eggs, beans and rice. *Comida* takes place between 2 p.m. and 5 p.m. and serves as the largest meal of the day. *Antojos* (snacks) or *antojitos* (little snacks) are featured in a *plato fuerte* (main dish) with rice and beans at this meal, along with *sopas* (soups). This usually tides over the appetite until 8 p.m. when *cena* is served, which is a light meal similar in size to *desayuno.* A more substantial evening meal, called *merienda,* is sometimes eaten in the evening depending upon how extensive the *comida* of the day was.

Like the Italians and French, Mexicans like to eat slowly and savor their food. The afternoon and evening meals are usually served in a modified course structure inspired by the French *service à la russe* and can last about two to three hours. This casual dining style means that the check, or *la cuenta*, is typically delivered when asked for. This relaxed style of service can often be confused with poor service. If you have time constraints, it is best to let your server know in advance so that they may expedite your meal appropriately.

Buen Provecho!

Sample Mexican Menu

Starters
Ceviche (Raw Fish Salad)
Chile con Queso (Chili Cheese Dip)
Guacamole (Avocado Dip)
Queso Fundido (Cheese Dip)
Tortillas y Salsa (Chips and Salsa)

Soups
Posole (Chili Corn Soup)
Sopa Azteca (Lime Chicken Soup)

Salads
Ensalada (House Salad)
Taco Salad

Egg Dishes
Huevos Mexicanos (Mexican Eggs)
Huevos Rancheros (Ranch Style Eggs)

Antojos (Mexican Specialties)
Enchiladas
Enfrijoladas
Tacos
Tamales (Stuffed Corn Meal)
Tostadas Compuestas (Filled Corn Tortillas)

Meat Dishes
Arracheras (Flank or Skirt Steak)
Bistek (Steak)
Carne Asada (Broiled Beef)
Carnitas (Simmered Pork)
Machaca (Shredded Beef)

Sample Mexican Menu

Chicken and Turkey Dishes
Mole
Pechuga de Pollo (Chicken Breast)
Pollo Asado (Broiled Chicken)

Seafood Dishes
Langosta (Lobster)
Paella Mariscos (Seafood and Rice)

Sides
Arroz (Rice)
Frijoles (Beans)

Desserts
Arroz con Leche (Rice Pudding)
Flan (Custard)
Helados (Ice Cream, Sherbet or Sorbet)

9

We would like to thank Freddie Sanchez, owner and chef of Adobo Grill in Chicago, Illinois and the Crawley Family of El Sombrero Patio Cafe in Las Cruces, New Mexico for their valuable contributions in reviewing the following menu items.

Mexican Menu Item Descriptions

Starters
Ceviche (Raw Fish Salad)
Ceviche is a popular starter enjoyed worldwide, specifically in Latin America and Spain. In most cases, it is raw white fish with chopped jalepeños, cilantro and onions tossed in lime juice with salt. Ceviche may also include other *mariscos* (seafood) such as calamari, crab,

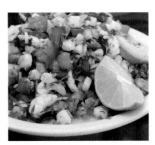
Ceviche (Raw Fish Salad)

lobster, octopus or shrimp; however, these ingredients are usually cooked. The dish may be served with corn tortilla chips.

Gluten-Free Decision Factors:
- Ensure corn tortilla chips—no wheat flour
- Ensure oil used for frying is designated for corn tortilla chips only and is not used to fry other items that may be battered or dusted with wheat flour

Food Allergen Preparation Considerations:
- Contains fish as an ingredient
- May contain corn from tortilla chips and vegetable oil
- May contain peanuts from vegetable oil
- May contain shellfish as an ingredient
- May contain soy from tortilla chips and vegetable oil

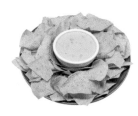

Chile con Queso (Chili Cheese Dip)

Chile con Queso (Chili Cheese Dip)

Traditional *Chile con Queso* is a blend of butter, cheese and chopped chile pepper. Any type of cheese or chile pepper can be used. It is usually served with corn tortilla chips or plain hot tortillas.

Gluten-Free Decision Factors:
- Ensure corn tortillas or chips—no wheat flour
- Ensure oil used for frying is designated for corn tortilla chips only and is not used to fry other items that may be battered or dusted with wheat flour
- Ensure no wheat flour in sauce

Food Allergen Preparation Considerations:
- Contains dairy from butter and cheese
- May contain corn from cheese, tortilla chips and vegetable oil
- May contain peanuts from vegetable oil

- May contain soy from cheese, tortilla chips and vegetable oil

Guacamole (Avocado Dip)

Guacamole is crushed avocado with garlic, lime juice, onions and tomatoes. Other ingredients may include diced chile pepper and cilantro. It is usually served with corn tortilla chips or plain hot tortillas.

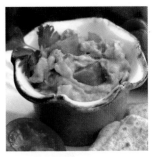

Guacamole is crushed avocado

Gluten-Free Decision Factors:

- Ensure corn tortillas or chips—no wheat flour

- Ensure oil used for frying is designated for corn tortilla chips only and is not used to fry other items that may be battered or dusted with wheat flour

Food Allergen Preparation Considerations:

- May contain corn from tortilla chips and vegetable oil

- May contain peanuts from vegetable oil

- May contain soy from tortilla chips and vegetable oil

Queso Fundido (Cheese Dip)

Queso Fundido is another variety of Mexican cheese dip. Cheese is melted together with butter and served in a hot ceramic dish. It may include sliced vegetables such as bell peppers, onions and tomatoes. Sometimes *chorizo* (Mexican pork sausage) may be added. It is usually served with corn tortilla chips or plain hot tortillas.

Gluten-Free Decision Factors:

- Ensure corn tortillas or chips—no wheat flour

- Ensure oil used for frying is designated for corn tortilla chips only and is not used to fry other items that may be battered or dusted with wheat flour

- Ensure no wheat flour in sauce

Food Allergen Preparation Considerations:
- Contains dairy from butter and cheese

- May contain corn from cheese, tortilla chips and vegetable oil

- May contain peanuts from vegetable oil

- May contain soy from cheese, tortilla chips and vegetable oil

Tortillas y Salsa (Chips and Salsa)

Any Mexican meal would be incomplete without a bowl of chips and salsa. Tortilla chips are accompanied by any type of fresh salsa.

Gluten-Free Decision Factors:
- Ensure corn tortilla chips—no wheat flour

- Ensure oil used for frying is designated for corn tortilla chips only and is not used to fry other items that may be battered or dusted with wheat flour

- Ensure no wheat flour in salsa

Food Allergen Preparation Considerations:
- May contain corn from salsa, tortilla chips and vegetable oil

- May contain peanuts from vegetable oil

- May contain soy from tortilla chips and vegetable oil

Tortillas y Salsa (Chips and Salsa)

Soups
Posole (Chili Corn Soup)

Posole is a traditional, spicy Mexican soup. Although there are many recipes, most follow these guidelines: chunks of pork are simmered in fresh chicken stock with garlic, hominy, onions, chile peppers and tomato. With the exception of hominy, the other ingredients will likely be sautéed in oil prior to being added to the soup. It can be seasoned with *azafran* (Mexican saffron), chile powder, cilantro, Mexican oregano or any other Mexican herbs and spices. Both *Posole* and

Menudo (a similar soup that features tripe) are considered excellent hangover remedies in Mexico.

Gluten-Free Decision Factors:
- Ensure stocks and broths are not made from bouillon which may contain gluten

- Ensure no wheat flour as thickening agent

Food Allergen Preparation Considerations:
- Contains corn from hominy and possibly from bouillon and vegetable oil

- May contain peanuts from vegetable oil

- May contain soy from bouillon and vegetable oil

Sopa Azteca (Lime Chicken Soup)

Sopa Azteca may also be called tortilla soup on some restaurant menus. There are many variations of this soup, but most are similar in preparation. Garlic, onions, sliced chicken and tomatoes are simmered in fresh chicken stock and lime juice. The soup is often topped with crunchy corn tortilla strips and grated cheese. Some recipes call for a greater variety of vegetables and may also include cream.

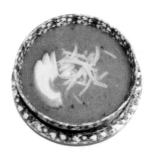

Sopa Azteca (Lime Chicken Soup)

Gluten-Free Decision Factors:
- Ensure stocks and broths are not made from bouillon which may contain gluten

- Ensure no wheat flour as thickening agent

- Ensure corn tortilla chips—no wheat flour

- Ensure oil used for frying is designated for corn tortilla chips only and is not used to fry other items that may be battered or dusted with wheat flour

Food Allergen Preparation Considerations:
- Contains dairy from cheese and possibly from cream

- May contain corn from bouillon, cheese, tortilla chips and vegetable oil

- May contain peanuts from vegetable oil
- May contain soy from bouillon, cheese, tortilla chips and vegetable oil

Salads
Ensalada (House Salad)
An *Ensalada* will usually be included with a *plato fuerte* or main dish. This salad usually consists of lettuce, onions and tomatoes. Salad dressings are uncommon; usually a wine vinegar and oil are available if needed.

Gluten-Free Decision Factors:
- Ensure no wheat tortilla chips as garnish

Food Allergen Preparation Considerations:
- May contain corn from vegetable oil
- May contain peanuts from vegetable oil
- May contain soy from vegetable oil

Taco Salad

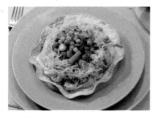
Taco Salad

Taco salads are found on restaurant menus outside of Mexico. They can be served in a corn tortilla bowl, flour tortilla bowl or on a plate, topped with tortilla chips. The dish contains mixed greens, beans, grated cheese, onions and tomatoes. Your options usually include sliced marinated chicken, ground beef or steak. The salad is typically topped with fresh salsa and sour cream since salad dressings are uncommon.

Gluten-Free Decision Factors:
- Ensure no soy sauce or wheat flour in marinade
- Ensure no wheat flour in salsa
- Ensure no wheat flour in beans
- Ensure corn tortilla bowl and chips—no wheat flour
- Ensure oil used for frying is designated for corn tortilla bowl and chips only and is not used to fry

other items that may be battered or dusted with wheat flour

Food Allergen Preparation Considerations:
- Contains dairy from cheese and sour cream
- May contain corn from cheese, salsa, tortillas and vegetable oil
- May contain peanuts from vegetable oil
- May contain soy from cheese, soy sauce in marinade, tortillas and vegetable oil

Egg Dishes
Huevos Mexicanos (Mexican Eggs)
Huevos Mexicanos are scrambled eggs with chopped chile, onions and tomatoes. Eggs are usually cooked with vegetable oil or occasionally butter. They are often served with steamed tortillas and beans, which may be topped with cheese. Salsa picante (puréed tomatoes, chile, garlic, onions and cilantro) or pico de gallo (a fresh salsa consisting of tomatoes, onions, garlic, jalapenos and cilantro) may be offered on the side.

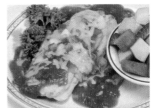
Huevos Mexicanos (Mexican Eggs)

Gluten-Free Decision Factors:
- Ensure no wheat flour in salsa
- Ensure no wheat flour in beans
- Ensure corn tortillas—no wheat flour
- Ensure oil used for frying is designated for corn tortillas only and is not used to fry other items which may be battered or dusted with wheat flour

Food Allergen Preparation Considerations:
- Contains eggs as an ingredient
- May contain corn from cheese, salsa, tortillas and vegetable oil
- May contain dairy from butter and cheese
- May contain peanuts from vegetable oil
- May contain soy from cheese, tortillas and vegetable oil

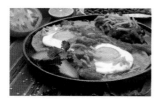
Huevos Rancheros (Ranch Style Eggs)

Huevos Rancheros (Ranch Style Eggs)

Huevos Rancheros consist of eggs fried in vegetable oil or occasionally butter. They are usually sunny side up, on top of a corn tortilla that has been lightly fried in vegetable oil. The eggs are topped with chile con carne (meat simmered in red or green chile) and cheese. Chopped lettuce, onions, tomatoes, beans and pico de gallo may also accompany the dish.

Gluten-Free Decision Factors:

- Ensure no wheat flour in salsa or sauce

- Ensure no wheat flour in beans

- Ensure corn tortillas—no wheat flour

- Ensure oil used for frying is designated for corn tortillas only and is not used to fry other items that may be battered or dusted with wheat flour

Food Allergen Preparation Considerations:

- Contains dairy from cheese and possibly from butter

- Contains eggs as an ingredient

- May contain corn from cheese, salsa, tortillas and vegetable oil

- May contain peanuts from vegetable oil

- May contain soy from cheese, tortillas and vegetable oil

Antojos (Mexican Specialties)
Enchiladas

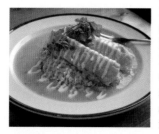
Enchiladas with green chile sauce

Enchiladas are prepared two different ways: rolled and stuffed with ingredients or stacked like pancakes and layered with ingredients. When rolled, the tortillas are lightly fried in vegetable oil, stuffed with the ingredients of your choice and then topped with mole, red chile sauce or green chile sauce and cheese. When stacked, after the tortillas have been lightly fried, they are dipped in red or green chile. They are then layered with the desired ingredients. Standard *enchilada* ingredients include cheese and onions, served plain or with your choice of beef, chicken or pork. There are also hundreds of recipes, including any number of ingredients. Stacked *enchiladas* are often topped with a fried egg.

Gluten-Free Decision Factors:
- Ensure no wheat flour in sauce

- Ensure corn tortillas—no wheat flour

- Ensure oil used for frying is designated for corn tortillas only and is not used to fry other items that may be battered or dusted with wheat flour

Food Allergen Preparation Considerations:
- Contains dairy from cheese and possibly from cream

- May contain corn from cheese, tortillas and vegetable oil

- May contain eggs as an ingredient

- May contain peanuts from mole sauce and vegetable oil

- May contain soy from cheese, mole sauce, tortillas and vegetable oil

- May contain tree nuts from mole sauce

Enfrijoladas

Enfrijoladas are like enchiladas, but feature beans as a major ingredient. Tortillas are lightly fried in oil then dipped in a crushed or puréed bean sauce with garlic. They can be rolled or stacked with cheese and onions and are typically topped with salsa and sour cream. Sometimes beef or chicken may be offered as fillings. Stacked *enfrijoladas* are often topped with a fried egg.

Gluten-Free Decision Factors:
- Ensure no wheat flour in salsa or sauce

- Ensure corn tortillas—no wheat flour

- Ensure oil used for frying is designated for corn tortillas only and is not used to fry other items that may be battered or dusted with wheat flour

Food Allergen Preparation Considerations:
- Contains dairy from cheese and sour cream

- May contain corn from cheese, salsa, tortillas and vegetable oil

- May contain eggs as an ingredient

- May contain peanuts from vegetable oil

- May contain soy from cheese, tortillas and vegetable oil

Tacos

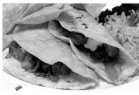
Tacos al Carbon

Tacos are the Mexican version of a sandwich. They come in fried or steamed corn tortillas or in soft wheat flour tortillas. In most cases, they are folded; however, you may come across fried rolled tacos called *Flautas* or *Taquitos*. Ingredients vary widely depending on where you are and what type you decide to order. Some varieties include *al carbon* (grilled beef), *al dorado* (rolled and fried with shredded chicken or beef), *al pastor* (shaved marinated pork), *carnitas* (pork simmered with orange rind), *camarones* (shrimp), *machaca* (shredded beef), *pescado* (fish) and *pollo* (chicken). In addition to shredded lettuce and cheese, other garnishes may include sliced cucumbers, radishes, red and green salsas, sour cream, lime wedges and guacamole.

Gluten-Free Decision Factors:
- Ensure no wheat flour in salsa

- Ensure corn tortillas—no wheat flour

- Ensure oil used for frying is designated for corn tortillas only and is not used to fry other items that may be battered or dusted with wheat flour

Food Allergen Preparation Considerations:
- Contains dairy from cheese and sour cream

- May contain corn from cheese, salsa, tortillas and vegetable oil

- May contain fish if ordered

- May contain peanuts from vegetable oil

- May contain shellfish if ordered

- May contain soy from cheese, tortillas and vegetable oil

Tamales (Stuffed Corn Meal)

Tamales are made of *masa* (corn meal and vegetable oil or lard), which is stuffed with various ingredients, wrapped in a corn husk and steamed. There are a number of different types of tamale ingredients, the most common being shredded beef, chicken or pork that is simmered in red chile sauce.

Gluten-Free Decision Factors:
- Ensure no wheat flour in sauce

Tamales (Stuffed Corn Meal)

Food Allergen Preparation Considerations:
- Contains corn from *masa* and possibly from vegetable oil

- May contain peanuts from vegetable oil

- May contain soy from *masa* and vegetable oil

Tostadas Compuestas (Filled Corn Tortillas)

Tostadas Compuestas are crisp fried corn tortillas, either flat or shaped in a bowl, which are topped or filled with various ingredients. The most common are red or green chile con carne, shredded cheese, lettuce and tomatoes. Some recipes may also call for beans, sliced marinated beef or chicken, pico de gallo and sour cream.

Gluten-Free Decision Factors:
- Ensure no wheat flour in salsa

- Ensure no wheat flour in beans

- Ensure no soy sauce or wheat flour in marinade

- Ensure corn tortillas—no wheat flour

- Ensure oil used for frying is designated for corn tortillas only and is not used to fry other items that may be battered or dusted with wheat flour

Food Allergen Preparation Considerations:
- Contains dairy from cheese and possibly sour cream

- May contain corn from cheese, salsa, tortillas and vegetable oil

- May contain peanuts from vegetable oil

- May contain soy from cheese, soy sauce in marinade, tortillas and vegetable oil

Meat Dishes
Arracheras (Flank or Skirt Steak)

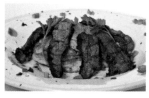

Sliced Arracheras (Flank or Skirt Steak)

Arracheras are thin cuts of meat and are used for making fajitas. The only real difference between the two is that fajitas are sliced into thinner strips. Flank or skirt steak is marinated in lime juice, garlic, salt, pepper and sometimes diced chile peppers. The beef is cooked over an open flame to temperature and served with steamed tortillas, shredded lettuce, tomatoes, beans and rice. The beans may be topped with cheese and salsa picante or pico de gallo.

Gluten-Free Decision Factors:
- Ensure no wheat flour in salsa

- Ensure no wheat flour in beans

- Ensure no soy sauce or wheat flour in marinade

- Ensure corn tortillas—no wheat flour

Food Allergen Preparation Considerations:
- May contain corn from cheese, salsa, tortillas and vegetable oil in beans

- May contain dairy from cheese

- May contain peanuts from vegetable oil in beans

- May contain soy from cheese, soy sauce in marinade, tortillas and vegetable oil in beans

Bistek (Steak)

Steaks come in a variety of cuts, the most popular being filet, New York strip, porterhouse and rib eye depending upon location and availability. Steaks are generally seasoned with salt and pepper and broiled or grilled. They may also be marinated in fresh lime juice, garlic and diced chile peppers. Beans (which may be topped with cheese) and rice are common sides. You may also encounter *papas fritas* (fried potatoes). Occasionally a menu will offer *Bistek Ranchero*, in which case the beef is smothered in salsa ranchero.

Gluten-Free Decision Factors:

- Ensure no wheat flour in salsa

- Ensure no wheat flour in beans

- Ensure no soy sauce or wheat flour in marinade

- Ensure oil used for frying is designated for potatoes only and is not used to fry other items that may be battered or dusted with wheat flour

Food Allergen Preparation Considerations:

- May contain corn from cheese, salsa and vegetable oil in beans and fried potatoes

- May contain dairy from cheese

- May contain peanuts from vegetable oil in beans

- May contain soy from cheese, soy sauce in marinade and vegetable oil in beans and fried potatoes

Carne Asada (Broiled Beef)

Carne Asada is marinated broiled beef and can be any of the smaller cuts of beef not considered bistek. These types include everything from butt steak to tri-tip. Mexican restaurants generally season *Carne Asada* with a marinade of lime juice, garlic, Mexican oregano, salt, pepper and sometimes diced chile peppers. The dish is usually served with steamed tortillas, shredded lettuce, tomatoes, rice and beans, which may be topped with cheese. Salsa picante or pico de gallo may be offered on the side.

9

Gluten-Free Decision Factors:
- Ensure no wheat flour in salsa
- Ensure no wheat flour in beans
- Ensure no soy sauce or wheat flour in marinade
- Ensure corn tortillas—no wheat flour

Food Allergen Preparation Considerations:
- May contain corn from cheese, salsa, tortillas and vegetable oil in beans
- May contain dairy from cheese
- May contain peanuts from vegetable oil
- May contain soy from cheese, soy sauce in marinade, tortillas and vegetable oil in beans

Carnitas (Simmered Pork)

Carnitas are a popular delicacy all over Mexico. Pork is slowly roasted and simmered in its own juices with orange rinds and any number of Mexican spices. In fact, purveyors of *Carnitas* in Mexico closely guard the specific spices they use; however, these secret recipes typically consist of dried Mexican chile powders and herbs such as cumin, *epazote* (wormseed), garlic, Mexican oregano, salt and pepper. The dish is usually served with steamed tortillas, shredded lettuce, tomatoes, rice and beans, which may be topped with cheese. Salsa picante or pico de gallo may be offered on the side.

Gluten-Free Decision Factors:
- Ensure no wheat flour in salsa
- Ensure no wheat flour in beans
- Ensure corn tortillas—no wheat flour

Food Allergen Preparation Considerations:
- May contain corn from cheese, salsa, tortillas and vegetable oil in beans
- May contain dairy from cheese

- May contain peanuts from vegetable oil in beans

- May contain soy from cheese, tortillas and vegetable oil in beans

Machaca (Shredded Beef)

Machaca is a Northern Mexican specialty. Beef shoulder or chuck roast is simmered for hours in water, oil and spices (usually chile powder, cumin, garlic, salt and pepper). Once all the fat has been cooked out of the beef, it is pulled apart or shredded. The dish is usually served with steamed tortillas, shredded lettuce, tomatoes, rice and beans, which may be topped with cheese. Salsa picante or pico de gallo may be offered on the side.

Gluten-Free Decision Factors:

- Ensure no wheat flour in salsa

- Ensure no wheat flour in beans

- Ensure corn tortillas—no wheat flour

Food Allergen Preparation Considerations:

- May contain corn from cheese, salsa, tortillas and vegetable oil

- May contain dairy from cheese

- May contain peanuts from vegetable oil

- May contain soy from cheese, tortillas and vegetable oil

Chicken and Turkey Dishes

Mole

Mole is a specialty from the states of Puebla and Oaxaca. It is a thick brown sauce, usually served over chicken or turkey. Although there are hundreds, if not thousands, of recipes for *Mole*, the sauce is typically made from a lengthy list of ingredients that include unsweetened chocolate, chile peppers, cinnamon, cloves, coriander, cumin, garlic, peanuts, sesame seeds and tree nuts. The dish is usually served with steamed tortillas, shredded lettuce, tomatoes, rice and beans, which may be topped with cheese. Salsa picante or pico de gallo may be offered on the side.

Gluten-Free Decision Factors:
- Ensure no wheat flour in sauce
- Ensure no wheat flour in beans
- Ensure corn tortillas—no wheat flour

Food Allergen Preparation Considerations:
- May contain corn from cheese, tortillas and vegetable oil in beans
- May contain dairy from cheese
- May contain peanuts from sauce and vegetable oil in beans
- May contain soy from cheese, mole sauce, tortillas and vegetable oil in beans
- May contain tree nuts from sauce

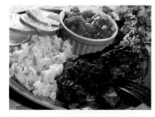
Penchuga de Pollo (Chicken Breast)

Pechuga de Pollo (Chicken Breast)

Chicken breasts are usually marinated in lime juice, garlic, Mexican oregano, salt, pepper and sometimes diced chile peppers. They are cooked *asado* (broiled) or *a la parilla* (grilled). The dish is usually served with steamed tortillas, shredded lettuce, tomatoes, rice and beans, which may be topped with cheese. Salsa picante or pico de gallo may be offered on the side.

Gluten-Free Decision Factors:
- Ensure no wheat flour in salsa
- Ensure no wheat flour in beans
- Ensure no soy sauce or wheat flour in marinade
- Ensure corn tortillas—no wheat flour

Food Allergen Preparation Considerations:
- May contain corn from cheese, salsa, tortillas and vegetable oil in beans

- May contain dairy from cheese

- May contain peanuts from vegetable oil in beans

- May contain soy from cheese, soy sauce in marinade, tortillas and vegetable oil in beans

Pollo Asado (Broiled Chicken)

Pollo Asado is a whole chicken, usually marinated in lime juice, garlic, Mexican oregano, salt, pepper and sometimes diced chile peppers. It is then broiled or charbroiled so that the skin is very crispy. The standard serving is half of a chicken on the bone. The dish is usually served with steamed tortillas, shredded lettuce, tomatoes, rice and beans, which may be topped with cheese. Salsa picante or pico de gallo may be offered on the side.

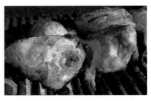
Pollo Asado (Broiled Chicken)

Gluten-Free Decision Factors:

- Ensure no wheat flour in salsa

- Ensure no wheat flour in beans

- Ensure no soy sauce or wheat flour in marinade

- Ensure corn tortillas—no wheat flour

Food Allergen Preparation Considerations:

- May contain corn from cheese, salsa, tortillas and vegetable oil in beans

- May contain dairy from cheese

- May contain peanuts from vegetable oil in beans

- May contain soy from cheese, soy sauce in marinade, tortillas and vegetable oil in beans

Seafood Dishes

Langosta (Lobster)

Mexican restaurants generally offer the clawless spiny lobsters available in the Caribbean or off the coast of the Baja peninsula. Whole lobster or just the tails may be featured on the menu. Lobster tails are usually broiled or grilled, whereas whole lobsters are traditionally boiled in water, fish stock or seafood stock. Most lobster is served with drawn butter (melted butter and vegetable oil), lime wedges and steamed tortillas. Salsa picante or pico de gallo may be offered on the side.

Gluten-Free Decision Factors:
- Ensure no wheat flour in salsa
- Ensure stocks and broths are not made from bouillon which may contain gluten
- Ensure corn tortillas—no wheat flour

Food Allergen Preparation Considerations:
- Contains shellfish from lobster and possibly from seafood stock
- May contain corn from bouillon, salsa, tortillas and vegetable oil in drawn butter
- May contain dairy from drawn butter
- May contain fish from seafood stock
- May contain peanuts from vegetable oil in drawn butter
- May contain soy from bouillon, tortillas and vegetable oil in drawn butter

Paella Mariscos (Seafood and Rice)

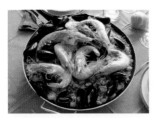
Paella Mariscos (Seafood and Rice)

Paella is a popular Spanish rice dish that is enjoyed all over the Latin world including Mexican restaurants. Rice is boiled in fresh chicken or fish stock. Clams, calamari, fish, mussels, scallops and shrimp that have been sautéed in vegetable oil, herbs and spices are then added. These herbs and spices usually include *azafran* (Mexican saffron), chile powder, garlic, salt and pepper. The dish usually includes bell peppers, sliced chile peppers, onions and tomatoes.

Gluten-Free Decision Factors:
- Ensure stocks and broths are not made from bouillon which may contain gluten

Food Allergen Preparation Considerations:
- Contains fish as an ingredient

- Contains shellfish as an ingredient

- May contain corn from bouillon and vegetable oil

- May contain peanuts from vegetable oil

- May contain soy from bouillon and vegetable oil

Sides
Arroz (Rice)
Most rice served in Mexican restaurants is similar in preparation and may be referred to as Spanish rice. After the rice has been boiled, usually in water or fresh chicken stock, crushed tomatoes or tomato sauce and sliced onions are added. Sometimes the tomatoes and onions may be sautéed in vegetable oil prior to being added. The rice is seasoned with salt and may also be seasoned with *azafran*.

Gluten-Free Decision Factors:
- Ensure stocks and broths are not made from bouillon which may contain gluten

- Ensure clean water is used to cook rice

Arroz (Rice)

Food Allergen Preparation Considerations:
- May contain corn from bouillon and vegetable oil

- May contain peanuts from vegetable oil

- May contain soy from bouillon and vegetable oil

Frijoles (Beans)
Pinto beans are the most popular variety in Northern Mexico, while black beans are mostly enjoyed in southern Mexico. Dried beans are boiled until soft, then mashed and fried with lard or oil to make *Frijoles*. This preparation style is called *Frijoles Refritos* or "refried beans" and is typically topped with cheese. Beans can also be served whole in their own broth and may be flavored with salted pork.

Gluten-Free Decision Factors:
- Ensure no wheat flour in beans

Food Allergen Preparation Considerations:
- May contain corn from cheese and vegetable oil
- May contain dairy from cheese
- May contain peanuts from vegetable oil
- May contain soy from cheese and vegetable oil

Desserts
Arroz con Leche (Rice Pudding)

Mexican rice pudding is a great dessert choice. Rice is boiled with cinnamon until soft. Milk or cream, raisins, sugar and vanilla beans or extract are then added. This is heated for a few minutes, then eggs and more cinnamon are added. This dessert can be served chilled or warm.

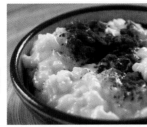
Arroz con Leche (Rice Pudding)

Gluten-Free Decision Factors:
- Ensure clean water is used to cook rice

Food Allergen Preparation Considerations:
- Contains dairy from cream and milk
- Contains eggs as an ingredient
- May contain corn from vanilla extract

Flan (Custard)

Flan is the national dessert of Spain and it is a common dessert in most Latin cuisines. Its ingredients are simple: cream, eggs, sugar and vanilla beans or extract. You may see it on the menu as *"Flan con Dulce de Leche,"* which means it is topped with caramel sauce.

9

Gluten-Free Decision Factors:
- Ensure no wheat flour as an ingredient

Food Allergen Preparation Considerations:
- Contains dairy from cream

- Contains eggs as an ingredient

- May contain corn from caramel sauce and vanilla extract

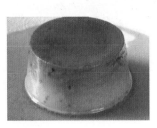
Flan

Helados (Ice Cream, Sherbet or Sorbet)
Helados are usually available in Mexican restaurants. Many establishments make these items in-house, yet others prefer to offer pre-fabricated *Helados*. It is generally best to keep your flavor choices simple. In either case, inquire about the ingredients.

Gluten-Free Decision Factors:
- Ensure no malt or wheat as ingredients

- Ensure no stabilizers which may contain gluten

- Ensure no cookie/biscuit

Food Allergen Preparation Considerations:
- May contain corn from caramel sauce and colors or flavors

- May contain dairy as an ingredient and from chocolate and cookie/biscuit

- May contain eggs from cookie/biscuit

- May contain peanuts from colors or flavors and cookie/biscuit

- May contain soy from chocolate, colors or flavors and cookie/biscuit

- May contain tree nuts from colors or flavors and cookie/biscuit

9

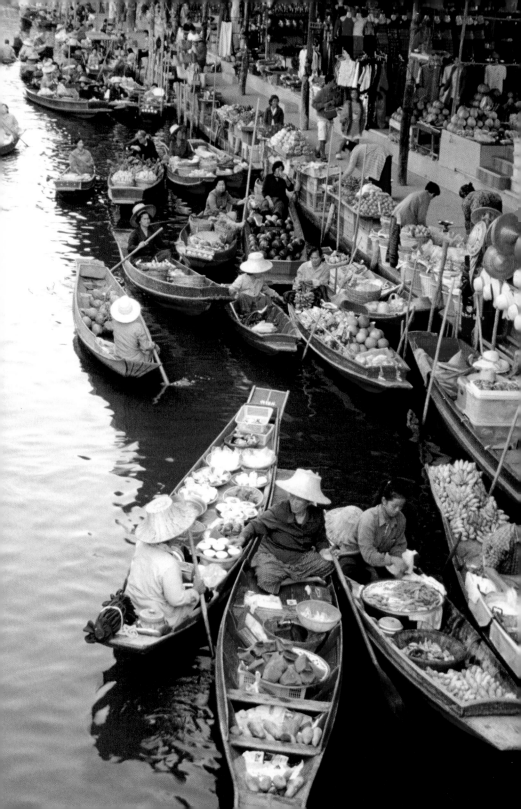

*If you knew what I know about the power of giving,
you would not let a single meal pass without
sharing it in some way.*
—Buddha

Chapter 10
Let's Eat Thai Cuisine

Cuisine Overview

Thailand lies in the heart of Southeast Asia and encompasses a land mass slightly larger than Spain or Italy and two times the size of Wyoming. The country has 76 provinces and almost 65 million inhabitants, 95% of which are Buddhist.

A unified Thai kingdom was established in the mid-14th century and was known as Siam until 1939 when a bloodless coup instituted a constitutional monarchy and the name The Kingdom of Thailand. Thailand is the only Southeast Asian country never to have been conquered by a European power.

Thai food is unique among the cuisines of Southeast Asia. Its colorful and aromatic nature is uncommon in both appearance and flavor. It is a distinct cuisine in its own right; largely due to the ability of the Thai people to absorb outside influences or culinary practices and develop them into something uniquely their own.

The skill of blending the five flavors—sweet, sour, salty, bitter and hot—is the hallmark of this cuisine. Thai food has the texture of Chinese food, minus the complicated sauces, and the spiciness of Indian food without the use of dairy products.

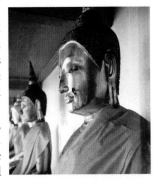
Line of Golden Buddhas

Although gluten is often found in other Asian noodle dishes and hidden in soy sauce, Thai food differs in this respect. Most noodle dishes have rice flour-based noodles and soy sauce is rarely used. Regardless of the dish, the influence of Buddhism on Thai cuisine requires a harmony of tastes and textures, both within a dish and throughout the meal.

Like most Asian cuisines, chefs in Thai restaurants use Chinese cooking techniques. These techniques of preparing food grew out of an economic need rather than an aesthetic aspiration, as there were periods in history of famine and fuel shortage.

Stir frying eliminated food waste and reduced the amount of fuel necessary to prepare a meal, which ultimately solved two problems at the same time. Cooking foods for a short time at a high temperature also allows vegetables to remain crisp, thereby retaining a greater amount of their raw nutritional value.

10

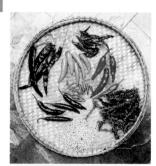

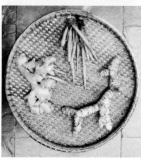

Chili Peppers (top); Galangal, Ginger and Lemongrass (bottom)

Traditional Ingredients

Thailand's culinary palate is similar to other Asian cuisines in its use of vegetables, proteins and starch. Protein and vegetable dishes are balanced with noodle and rice dishes at every meal. Soups are also an important source of daily nutrition.

Vegetables used in Thai cooking are similar to those used in most cuisines in Southeast Asia. Bamboo shoots, bean sprouts, broccoli, celery, eggplant, mushrooms, onions and shallots are common, along with fruits such as coconut, lime and pineapple. Thai cooking's use of fresh aromatic herbs and spices is unique and includes basil, chili pepper, coriander, cumin, garlic, galangal, ginger, lemongrass and turmeric.

There are many different types of protein featured in Thai cuisine. Meats such as beef, chicken, duck and pork are commonly used. Other sources of protein include bean curd, eggs, fish, nuts and shellfish.

Rice is the main form of starch. In addition to eating the whole grain, rice is also converted into flour used to make noodles, rice paper and dumpling skins. The influence of China has also brought wheat flour-based noodles into many Thai kitchens; however, most still prefer to use traditional rice noodles.

Beverages in Thailand are quite interesting. In addition to tropical fruit juices, thick Thai style iced coffee and tea are very popular. Both are prepared in a similar fashion with lots of sugar and topped with sweet condensed milk. Beers such as Singha malt beverage are very common and are not gluten-free.

Gluten Awareness

Since gluten can be found in some areas of Thai cuisine, we have outlined 20 items in our sample menu. There are eight primary points that you need to consider when dining at a Thai restaurant. To ensure a gluten-free experience, the areas of food preparation that you need to inquire about with your server or chef are listed below.

Fish Sauce	Ensure no wheat as ingredient
Soy Sauce	Although an unusual additive in Thai food, ensure no soy sauce
Flour Dusting	Tapioca, potato or corn starch is typically used—ensure no wheat flour
Stocks and Broths	Ensure all are made fresh or from allergen-free mixes and not from bouillon, which may contain gluten
Cooking Oil	Ensure frying oil has not been used to fry battered foods that may contain gluten
Noodles and Dumplings	Rice flour is typically used—ensure no wheat flour
Battering	Request plain-cooked food—ensure no batter
Cross-Contamination	Ensure all utensils and cooking surfaces have been cleaned prior to the preparation of your meal

Fish Sauce

Fish sauce, rather than soy sauce, is used in Thai cuisine to add the flavor of salt to a dish. Called *"nam pla"* in Thai, or literally, "fish water," genuine fish sauce is the juice in the flesh of fish and is extracted via prolonged salting and fermentation. It is made from small

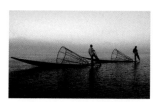
Thai Fishermen

saltwater or freshwater fish that would otherwise have little value for consumption. Today, most fish sauce is made from saltwater fish, as pollution and dams have drastically reduced the once plentiful supply of freshwater fish in the heartlands of Southeast Asia. Top quality fish sauce is naturally gluten-free.

When you are planning to go to a Thai restaurant, you may want to call in advance to inquire about the fish sauce. If you are at a restaurant and have not called in advance, ask your waiter what brand they use and request to see the bottle.

To help you to discern whether the fish sauce is gluten/wheat-free, safe to eat and a good quality brand, you need to:

1. Review the product label

2. Assess specific characteristics

If the restaurant presents you with a bottle of fish sauce, read the label for each of the ingredients which should include fish, salt, sugar and water. Due to country-specific labeling regulations, the ingredients may or may not be listed on the product.

If the ingredients are not listed or if they are written in a foreign language, look for the following characteristics:

- Color - Clear, reddish brown (similar to a good whiskey or sherry) without any sediment

- Smell - Pleasant aroma without an intense fish smell

- Source - Product of Thailand

- Processing - Processed in Thailand

Note: If the product is processed outside of Thailand, it may indicate a lower quality sauce due to higher manufacturing processing and may or may not be gluten/wheat-free.

Soy Sauce
Although it is uncommon, soy sauce may be used in some Thai restaurants. Soy sauce has a stronger flavor than fish sauce, so some chefs incorporate it into vegetarian dishes. Occasionally, it may also be used in a marinade for *Gai Yang* (roasted chicken). Black sauce *(siew dam)* is a thick sweet sauce made by fermenting soy beans with molasses. It may be present in noodle dishes; however, most brands produced in Thailand do not contain wheat. If used, request to see the bottle to verify the ingredients. Since most establishments prepare dishes made to order, soy sauce can easily be omitted from the few dishes where it is possibly present.

Flour Dusting
Flour dusting is common in Thai cuisine. Most restaurants prefer to dust meat or fish with tapioca, potato or corn starch—rather than wheat flour—for texture prior to pan-frying, allowing a sauce to be evenly distributed. Ensure that wheat flour is not used to dust meat or fish in the preparation of your meal.

10

Stocks and Broths
Stocks and broths are used frequently in Thai cuisines and are present in sauces and soups. Ensure all are made fresh or from allergen-free mixes and not from bouillon, which may contain gluten.

Cooking Oil
Canola oil is typically used in Thai restaurants; however, peanut oil and other vegetable oils may be used from time to time. Oil is used to fry or sauté foods. When ordering food that is prepared by frying, ensure that there is a dedicated fryer in the kitchen for non-battered menu items. Since battered foods may contain wheat flour, this practice minimizes the potential of gluten cross-contamination from frying.

Noodles and Dumplings

Rice flour is used for most dumpling skins and noodles. Although it is uncommon for Thai restaurants to serve wheat flour-based noodles and dumpling skins, lack of availability or non-traditional culinary practices may cause these ingredients to be present in some establishments. It is important to ensure with your server or chef that only rice flour is used.

Battering

Battering of meats is uncommon in Thai cuisine. Some restaurants use tempura battering for a few dishes, so it important to ensure that the oil used for frying is fresh and has not been used to fry other foods whose batter may contain gluten.

Cross-Contamination

Cross-contamination occurs in two primary instances and should be considered at any restaurant you choose to dine in. One may occur when your meal is prepared in the same frying oil as foods containing other possible allergens. The second may occur when food particles are transferred from one food to another by using the same knife, cutting board, pots, pans or other utensils without washing the surfaces or tools in between uses. In the case of open flamed grills, the extreme temperature turns most food particles into carbon. Use of a wire brush designed for grill racks typically removes residual contaminants.

To avoid cross-contamination, restaurants need to dedicate fryers for specific foods and wash all materials that may come in contact with food in hot, soapy water prior to preparing items for those with special dietary requirements. It is important to ensure that the restaurant follows these procedures for an allergen-free dining experience.

Other Allergy Considerations

If you have other food allergies or sensitivities, it is important to remain diligent in your approach to dining out. Because Thai cuisine is complex, there are many common food allergens used on a regular basis. As previously noted, canola oil is typically used in Thai restaurants; however, corn, peanut and vegetable oil (which may contain corn, peanuts or soy) can also be used. If used, bouillon may contain Hydrolyzed Vegetable Protein (HVP) that can be derived from corn, soy or wheat. We have indicated the potential presence of bouillon and oils.

From the 20 items we have listed in our sample menu, we have identified each common allergen typically included in the dish as an ingredient. We have also indicated other potential allergens that may be present based upon varied culinary practices. The chances of encountering common food allergens in items specific to our sample menu are outlined below.

High Likelihood   Fish, peanuts, shellfish and tree nuts

Moderate Likelihood Corn, eggs and soy

Low Likelihood   Dairy, gluten and wheat

10

In addition, your sensitivity to spice levels can be an important concern. If you see the words *"prik"* or *"kra prow,"* you can be sure that the dish is going to be spiced with chili peppers or curry powder. The term *"pet mak"* indicates that a dish is made especially spicy. You can have almost any Thai dish made spicier by requesting that it be prepared in one of these styles. If you are especially sensitive, it is important to discuss these concerns with your server or chef.

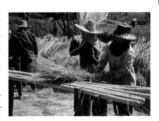
Rice Harvest in Thailand

Dining Considerations

Menus in Thai restaurants tend to be presented in the language that you're dining in. Since the Thai language has a different alphabet than the English language, menus may have the name of a dish spelled phonetically in English. With this in mind, you will soon realize that there are many different ways to phonetically spell a Thai dish. *Pad Thai*, whether it is spelled *Phad Thai, Phat Thai* or *Pat Thai,* are all the same delicious rice noodle dish.

As is the case with most Asian cuisines, Thai food is designed to be enjoyed family style. Most food is brought to the table at one time in Thailand and they do not follow a course structure. Restaurants outside of Thailand allow you to eat your meal in a Western fashion. Finding a balance between dishes and sharing them with your table is a very important part of the Thai gastronomic experience. Due to the influences of Buddhism, Hinduism and Taoism on Thai culture, it is customary to order a combination of dishes that compliment each other, balancing noodle and rice dishes with meat and vegetable dishes.

Gkin Kao!
(Bon Appetit in Thai, literally means "Eat Rice!")

10

Sample Thai Menu

Starters
Kanom Jeeb (Shrimp Dumplings)
Satay (Skewered Beef, Chicken or Shrimp)
Som Tam (Papaya Salad)
Summer Rolls

Soups
Tom Kha Gai (Chicken and Coconut Soup)
Tom Yum Groong (Spicy Shrimp Soup)

Noodle and Rice Dishes
Kaw Pad (Thai Fried Rice)
Pad See Yu
Pad Thai
Sticky Rice

Curries (Kang)
Kang Dang or Malay (Red Curry)
Kang Khiao Wan (Green Curry)
Kang Massaman (Tamarind Curry)
Kang Panang (Peanut Curry)

Beef Dishes
Braised Beef Short Ribs

Chicken Dishes
Gai Yang (Thai Barbeque Chicken)

Seafood Dishes
Pla Rad Prik (Crispy Whole Fish)

Desserts
Fresh Tropical Fruits
Sweet Sticky Rice
Tropical Fruit Sorbets

10

We would like to thank Chef Pam Panyasiri of Pam Real Thai in New York, New York for her valuable contribution in reviewing the following menu items.

Thai Menu Item Descriptions

Starters
Kanom Jeeb (Shrimp Dumplings)

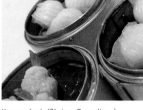

Kanom Jeeb (Shrimp Dumplings)

Dumplings are a regular starter at Asian restaurants. *Kanom Jeeb* differ from other Southeast Asian dumplings in that rice flour skins made of rice flour and eggs are almost always used. The dumplings are usually steamed; however, you can get them pan fried in oil if you prefer the texture and flavor. Inside the dumpling skin is a combination of ground shrimp, garlic, ginger and chives, with a little fish sauce for seasoning. A touch of egg is usually used to seal the dumpling. The accompanying dipping sauce, *nam pla prik*, is made from fish sauce, garlic and chili peppers.

Gluten-Free Decision Factors:
- Ensure no wheat in fish sauce
- Ensure no soy sauce in dumplings
- Ensure no soy sauce in dipping sauce
- Ensure no wheat flour—rice flour is typically used

Food Allergen Preparation Considerations:
- Contains fish from fish sauce
- Contains shellfish from shrimp
- May contain corn from vegetable oil
- May contain eggs from dumpling skin and egg seal
- May contain peanuts from vegetable oil
- May contain soy from soy sauce and vegetable oil

10

Satay (Skewered Beef, Chicken or Shrimp)

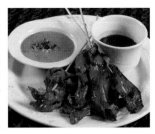
Beef Satay

Satay is a starter that you will find in virtually every Thai restaurant. There are three basic types of *satay*: beef, chicken and shrimp. *Chicken Satay* is prepared by marinating slices of chicken breast in coconut milk, yellow curry, coriander, cumin, turmeric and possibly fish sauce for seasoning. The marinade for *Beef* and *Shrimp Satay* is fish sauce, rice vinegar, garlic and onions. The beef, chicken or shrimp is then skewered and grilled. *Satays* are served with a peanut dipping sauce that is made from puréed peanuts and tamarind juice. Sometimes chili is added to give the sauce a little kick. *Satays* are usually garnished with a side of cucumber and onion salad with rice wine vinegar.

Gluten-Free Decision Factors:

- Ensure no wheat in fish sauce

- Ensure no soy sauce or wheat flour in marinade

- Ensure no soy sauce in dipping sauce

Food Allergen Preparation Considerations:

- Contains fish from fish sauce

- Contains peanuts from dipping sauce

- May contain shellfish from shrimp if ordered

- May contain soy from soy sauce in dipping sauce and marinade

Som Tam (Papaya Salad)

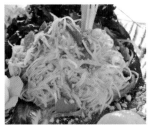
Som Tam (Papaya Salad)

This salad is made from either unripened green papaya or ripe papaya. It contains chili, green beans, tomatoes, garlic, onions and peanuts. It is then tossed in fish sauce, tamarind juice and lime. Some restaurants may include dried shrimp to add a saltier flavor and crunchy texture. Sometimes there is a garnish of ground nuts that may contain tree nuts in addition to peanuts. The flavor profile of *som tam* is sweet, tangy and spicy.

Gluten-Free Decision Factors:
- Ensure no wheat in fish sauce
- Ensure no soy sauce as an ingredient

Food Allergen Preparation Considerations:
- Contains fish from fish sauce
- Contains peanuts as an ingredient
- May contain shellfish from shrimp
- May contain soy from soy sauce
- May contain tree nuts from garnish

Summer Rolls

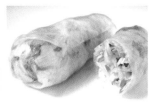

Summer Rolls

A cold starter, summer rolls are a light choice to begin your Thai meal. Julienned carrots, cucumber, onions, scallions and ginger are wrapped in a thin layer of rice paper. Fish sauce may be used for seasoning. The vegetables can either be steamed or boiled in fresh chicken stock prior to wrapping. Sometimes the vegetables are left raw, giving a nice, crunchy texture. The dipping sauce is usually a plum sauce and may be mild or spicy. Its ingredients are puréed plums, ginger and sometimes chili pepper. Although most restaurants will make fresh plum sauce, some may opt for the prefabricated variety. If the restaurant cannot verify the nature of the plum sauce, *nam pla prik* or peanut sauce may be substituted.

Gluten-Free Decision Factors:
- Ensure no wheat in fish sauce
- Ensure no soy sauce as seasoning
- Ensure no soy sauce in dipping sauce
- Ensure no wheat flour—rice flour paper is typically used
- Ensure stocks and broths are not made from bouillon which may contain gluten

10

Food Allergen Preparation Considerations:
- May contain corn from bouillon

- May contain fish from fish sauce

- May contain peanuts from peanut sauce

- May contain soy from bouillon, soy sauce as seasoning and in dipping sauce

Soups
Tom Kha Gai (Chicken and Coconut Soup)

Tom Kha Gai is a very popular Thai soup. At first glance, it appears to be a dairy-based soup but in reality, coconut milk gives *Tom Kha Gai* its look and texture. The broth is made with fresh chicken stock, coconut milk, lime juice and possibly fish sauce. Slices of chicken breast, fresh mushrooms, bamboo shoots, lemon grass and galangal root provide the bulk of the soup. *Tom Kha Gai* is usually garnished with a kaffir lime leaf or coriander leaf (cilantro) and sliced Thai chili peppers. It may also be garnished with crushed peanuts or tree nuts. This soup is moderately spicy, but you can most likely have it made mild because Thai soups are almost always made to order.

Gluten-Free Decision Factors:
- Ensure no wheat in fish sauce

- Ensure no soy sauce as an ingredient

- Ensure stocks and broths are not made from bouillon which may contain gluten

Food Allergen Preparation Considerations:
- May contain corn from bouillon

- May contain fish from fish sauce

- May contain peanuts from garnish

- May contain soy from bouillon and soy sauce

- May contain tree nuts from garnish

10

Tom Yum Groong (Spicy Shrimp Soup)

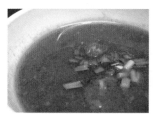
Tom Yum Groong (Spicy Shrimp Soup)

Tom Yum Groong is another common soup found on most Thai menus. It is similar to hot and sour soup found in Chinese restaurants. Shrimp, straw mushrooms, lemon grass, galangal root, Thai chili peppers, coriander and garlic are simmered in fresh chicken broth with lime juice and a touch of fish sauce. *Tom Yum Groong* is usually garnished with a kaffir lime leaf or coriander leaf and sliced Thai chili peppers. It may also be garnished with crushed peanuts or tree nuts. This soup can be very spicy, but since Thai soups are usually made to order, you will likely have the opportunity to request it mild, if you prefer.

Gluten-Free Decision Factors:
- Ensure no wheat in fish sauce
- Ensure no soy sauce as an ingredient
- Ensure stocks and broths are not made from bouillon which may contain gluten

Food Allergen Preparation Considerations:
- Contains fish from fish sauce
- Contains shellfish from shrimp
- May contain corn from bouillon
- May contain peanuts from garnish
- May contain soy from bouillon and soy sauce
- May contain tree nuts from garnish

Noodle and Rice Dishes
Kaw Pad (Thai Fried Rice)

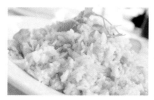
Kaw Pad (Thai Fried Rice)

There are literally hundreds of recipes for *Kaw Pad*. Luckily, they are all variations on one theme so you may be fairly certain of the ingredients. Whether you want chicken, beef, pork, shrimp, vegetarian or even pineapple *Kaw Pad,* the base of all of these dishes is the same. Steamed jasmine, white or brown rice—preferably a day old—is tossed in a wok with fish sauce,

10

garlic, scallions, eggs and tomatoes. Bean curd is also typically included in this dish. Fresh basil is added to give it that authentic Southeast Asian flavor and the dish is garnished with kaffir lime wedges and bean sprouts. Occasionally, ground peanuts or tree nuts are also used as a garnish. If you see the words *"prik"* or *"kra prow"* after *Kaw Pad,* you can be sure that the rice is going to be spiced with chili pepper or red curry powder.

Gluten-Free Decision Factors:
- Ensure no wheat in fish sauce

- Ensure no soy sauce as an ingredient

Food Allergen Preparation Considerations:
- Contains eggs as an ingredient

- Contains fish from fish sauce

- Contains soy from bean curd and possibly from soy sauce and vegetable oil

- May contain corn from vegetable oil

- May contain peanuts from garnish, peanut oil and vegetable oil

- May contain shellfish from shrimp

- May contain tree nuts from garnish

10

Pad See Yu
Pad See Yu is very prevalent in Thai restaurants. At the center of this simple stir-fried dish are broad rice noodles, similar to *chow fun* noodles found in Chinese restaurants. *Pad See Yu* comes with sliced chicken or beef and contains Chinese broccoli, onions and egg. The sauce is made from canola oil, fish sauce, garlic and palm sugar. Black sauce *(siew dam)* may also be used as a substitution for fish sauce and palm sugar. It is usually garnished with kaffir lime wedges and basil, and may additionally be garnished with chopped peanuts or tree nuts. Though Thai noodle dishes are generally lighter than most Asian noodle dishes, *Pad*

See Yu is definitely a hearty meal. It is easily shared as an accompaniment to other menu items when eating family style.

Gluten-Free Decision Factors:
- Ensure no wheat in fish sauce

- Ensure no soy sauce as an ingredient

- Ensure black sauce *(siew dam)* does not list wheat as an ingredient

- Ensure no wheat flour—rice flour noodles are typically used

Food Allergen Preparation Considerations:
- Contains eggs as an ingredient and possibly from noodles

- Contains fish from fish sauce

- May contain corn from vegetable oil

- May contain peanuts from garnish, peanut oil and vegetable oil

- May contain soy from black sauce *(siew dam),* soy sauce and vegetable oil

- May contain tree nuts from garnish

Pad Thai

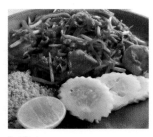
Pad Thai

Pad Thai is by far the most popular Thai noodle dish worldwide. It is difficult to find a Thai menu that does not include this classic. *Pad Thai* is typically made of bean curd, bean sprouts, cabbage, carrots, chicken, chili powder, fish sauce, garlic, ground peanuts, lime, onions, palm sugar, pickled radish, rice vinegar, canola oil and narrow rice noodles. Black sauce *(siew dam)* may also be used as a substitution for fish sauce and palm sugar. Depending on the restaurant, shrimp may also be included. The chef sautés garlic and onions with oil, adds eggs, then the other ingredients. The contents of the dish are then tossed in the wok and plated. *Pad Thai* is garnished with chopped peanuts or tree nuts, bean sprouts, cabbage, carrots and sliced lime. Due to the nature of its preparation, *Pad Thai* is always made to order. With this in mind, it is easy to omit any ingredients.

Gluten-Free Decision Factors:
- Ensure no wheat in fish sauce

- Ensure no soy sauce as an ingredient

- Ensure black sauce *(siew dam)* does not list wheat as an ingredient

- Ensure no wheat flour—rice flour noodles are typically used

Food Allergen Preparation Considerations:
- Contains eggs as an ingredient and possibly from noodles

- Contains fish from fish sauce

- Contains peanuts from garnish and possibly from peanut oil and vegetable oil

- Contains soy from bean curd and possibly from black sauce *(siew dam)*, soy sauce and vegetable oil

- May contain corn from vegetable oil

- May contain shellfish from shrimp

- May contain tree nuts from garnish

10

Sticky Rice

Sticky rice is a fun, hands-on experience. It is prepared by first letting the rice sit in water for a day or so. This process allows the starch of the rice to expand through the shell of the grain. As a result, the rice sticks together when steamed and can be formed into any shape desired. The Thai use sticky rice to soak up the sauces or curries in their meals. This custom is sure to lighten the atmosphere of any Thai dining experience, especially when eating family style.

Gluten-Free Decision Factors:
- Ensure clean water is used to cook rice

Food Allergen Preparation Considerations:
- None

Curries (Kang)
Kang Dang or Malay (Red Curry)

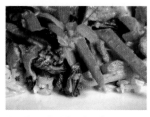

Kang Dang (Thai Red Curry)

Shrimp is the most common protein item in *Kang Dang*, but you can also have sliced chicken, pork or beef. The sauce is made of red curry paste and coconut milk. Thai long beans, bamboo shoots and fresh basil are usually present, as are onions, pineapple, tomato, sliced chili peppers and possibly fish sauce for seasoning. Because coconut milk is at the base of this curry, it will look like a bowl of soup. It is meant to be spooned over steamed rice, but diners often dip chunks of sticky rice straight into the bowl. The garnish is usually basil and sliced chili peppers, but crushed peanuts and tree nuts may also be used.

Gluten-Free Decision Factors:
- Ensure no wheat in fish sauce
- Ensure no soy sauce as an ingredient
- Ensure chicken is not battered or dusted with wheat flour

Food Allergen Preparation Considerations:
- May contain corn from vegetable oil
- May contain eggs from batter
- May contain fish from fish sauce
- May contain peanuts from garnish, peanut oil and vegetable oil
- May contain shellfish from shrimp if ordered
- May contain soy from soy sauce and vegetable oil
- May contain tree nuts from garnish

10

Kang Khiao Wan (Green Curry)

Like all Thai curries, *Kang Khiao Wan* can be made with your choice of chicken, pork, beef or shrimp; however, chicken is usually the meat of choice. Be sure to request plain, sliced chicken because of the tendency to tempura-fry chicken in curry dishes. The sauce for this dish is made up of green curry paste, coconut milk and possibly fish sauce for seasoning. Bamboo shoots and fresh basil are staple ingredients, and sometimes Japanese eggplant and sliced chili peppers are included. *Kang Khiao Wan* is a little milder than kang dang, but it is still spicy. It is difficult to adjust the level of spiciness in curry dishes, but some chefs suggest adding pineapple to even out the flavor profile. The garnish is usually Thai basil and sliced chili peppers, but crushed peanuts and tree nuts may also be used.

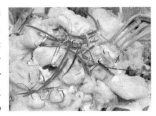

Kang Khiao Wan Gai (Thai Green Curry with Chicken)

Gluten-Free Decision Factors:

- Ensure no wheat in fish sauce

- Ensure no soy sauce as an ingredient

- Ensure chicken is not battered or dusted with wheat flour

Food Allergen Preparation Considerations:

- May contain corn from vegetable oil

- May contain eggs from batter

- May contain fish from fish sauce

- May contain peanuts from garnish, peanut oil and vegetable oil

- May contain shellfish from shrimp if ordered

- May contain soy from soy sauce and vegetable oil

- May contain tree nuts from garnish

Kang Massaman (Tamarind Curry)

Kang Massaman is a delicacy, combining almost all the spices featured in Thai cuisine. This complex, brown curry is moderately spicy to very spicy, depending on the restaurant, and resembles a stew. The usual ingre-

10

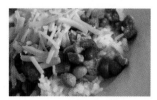

Kang Massaman (Tamarind Curry)

dients are cardamom, coconut milk, coriander, cumin, curry powder, galangal root, garlic, lemon grass, lime zest, palm sugar, peanuts and tamarind juice. Fish sauce may be added for seasoning. Whole shallots, potatoes and cherry tomatoes round out the bulk of the dish. Although chicken or beef is commonly ordered, duck is preferred by some since the richness of the sauce is considered the perfect complement to its bold flavor. Shrimp may also be ordered if available. The garnish is usually basil, though crushed peanuts and tree nuts may also be used.

Gluten-Free Decision Factors:
- Ensure no wheat in fish sauce
- Ensure no soy sauce as an ingredient
- Ensure chicken is not battered or dusted with wheat flour

Food Allergen Preparation Considerations:
- Contains peanuts as an ingredient and possibly from peanut oil and vegetable oil
- May contain corn from vegetable oil
- May contain eggs from batter
- May contain fish from fish sauce
- May contain shellfish from shrimp if ordered
- May contain soy from soy sauce and vegetable oil
- May contain tree nuts from garnish

Kang Panang (Peanut Curry)
This mild curry contains chopped peanuts, so it is often referred to as peanut curry. It is brownish green in color and more like a thick sauce, as opposed to a soupy curry. Beef is the meat of choice for this dish; however, chicken, duck, pork or shrimp can also be ordered. Thin slices of beef are tossed in the peanut curry with one or two vegetables, usually Chinese broccoli and onions. Sometimes pineapple is added to balance out the flavor and fish sauce may be added

for seasoning. The garnish is usually basil, though crushed peanuts and tree nuts may also be used. If your stomach is sensitive to spicy foods, the relatively mild *Kang Panang* curry is your best bet.

Gluten-Free Decision Factors:
- Ensure no wheat in fish sauce
- Ensure no soy sauce as an ingredient
- Ensure chicken is not battered or dusted with wheat flour

Food Allergen Preparation Considerations:
- Contains peanuts as an ingredient and possibly from peanut oil and vegetable oil
- May contain corn from vegetable oil
- May contain eggs from batter
- May contain fish from fish sauce
- May contain shellfish from shrimp if ordered
- May contain soy from soy sauce and vegetable oil
- May contain tree nuts from garnish

10

Beef Dishes
Braised Beef Short Ribs
Braised beef short ribs are a delicacy served at many upscale Thai restaurants and can be prepared a number of different ways. The most common is with traditional green curry. First, the short ribs are removed from the bone and pan seared. They are then marinated in green curry and coconut milk for six to 24 hours. After this, the ribs are braised in a wok with green curry and served with vegetables, usually Thai eggplant (which resembles a green tomato), onions and tomatoes. The dish is usually garnished with a large sprig of basil and sometimes crushed peanuts or tree nuts. Additional ingredients may include cardamom, coriander, cumin, fish sauce, galangal root, garlic, lemon grass and sliced Thai chili pepper. The result of this process is beef so tender and savory, a fork slices through it with ease.

Gluten-Free Decision Factors:
- Ensure no wheat in fish sauce
- Ensure no soy sauce as an ingredient
- Ensure no soy sauce or wheat flour in marinade

Food Allergen Preparation Considerations:
- May contain fish from fish sauce
- May contain peanuts from garnish
- May contain soy from soy sauce
- May contain tree nuts from garnish

Chicken Dishes
Gai Yang (Thai Barbeque Chicken)
Gai Yang can be prepared in many different ways, due to the fact that there are hundreds of recipes for the marinade. The most common style is usually some variation of the following recipe. Half a chicken is marinated in a combination of coconut milk, rice vinegar and fish sauce for two to twenty-four hours. It is seasoned with cilantro, curry powder, garlic, palm sugar, chili pepper and turmeric. The chicken is then removed from the marinade and cooked on the grill. The garnish for this dish is usually basil or coriander leaf. The most common dipping sauces provided are a sweet chili dipping sauce made with fish sauce, vinegar, palm sugar, garlic and chili pepper; or a garlic and rice vinegar sauce with sliced chili peppers and shallots.

Gluten-Free Decision Factors:
- Ensure no wheat in fish sauce
- Ensure no soy sauce in dipping sauce
- Ensure no soy sauce or wheat flour in marinade

Food Allergen Preparation Considerations:
- Contains fish from fish sauce
- May contain soy from soy sauce in dipping sauce and marinade

Seafood Dishes
Pla Rad Prik (Crispy Whole Fish)

Having a cooked whole fish staring at you during your dinner may be a bit hard for some to handle. Even though this type of presentation is, at the very least, "foreign" to many in the Western world, *Pla Rad Prik* is an amazing treat. Although a two to three pound red snapper is usually the fish of choice, any fish of similar size can be used. The fish is deeply scored at an angle on both sides and then dredged in corn, potato or tapioca starch with salt and pepper. The fish is then, typically, pan fried in canola oil until golden brown. An accompanying spicy, tangy tamarind sauce combines chopped garlic, shallots and chili peppers with tamarind juice, fish sauce and palm sugar. It is reduced in a hot wok to the consistency of maple syrup. The sauce is then poured over the whole fried fish and garnished with basil or coriander leaves. The texture and flavor of the fish combined with the sweet, sour and spicy flavor of the sauce is heaven to Thai food aficionados.

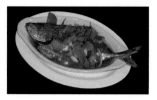
Pla Rad Prik (Crispy Whole Fish)

10

Gluten-Free Decision Factors:
- Ensure no wheat in fish sauce

- Ensure no soy sauce as an ingredient

- Ensure fish is not dusted with wheat flour

Food Allergen Preparation Considerations:
- Contains fish as an ingredient

- May contain corn from corn starch and vegetable oil

- May contain peanuts from peanut oil and vegetable oil

- May contain soy from soy sauce and vegetable oil

Desserts

Fresh Tropical Fruits

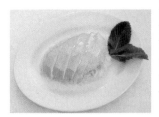

Sweet Sticky Rice served with a mango

Fresh tropical fruit makes a light choice for dessert. Bite-sized chunks of pineapple, guava, papaya and banana are the most common fruits served. Some restaurants serve "fruit sushi," which is sweet sticky rice topped with slices of tropical fruit and drizzled with liquid palm sugar.

Gluten-Free Decision Factors:
- Ensure no cookie/biscuit

Food Allergen Preparation Considerations:
- May contain dairy from cookie/biscuit

- May contain eggs from cookie/biscuit

- May contain peanuts from cookie/biscuit

- May contain soy from cookie/biscuit

- May contain tree nuts from cookie/biscuit

Sweet Sticky Rice

Sweet sticky rice is prepared like regular sticky rice except that palm sugar is added to the rice during the soaking process. It can be served plain or rolled into balls and served with coconut milk.

Gluten-Free Decision Factors:
- Ensure clean water is used to cook rice

Food Allergen Preparation Considerations:
- None

10

Tropical Fruit Sorbets

Sorbet is great for cleansing the palate after a Thai dining experience. If the restaurant offers sorbets, tropical flavors such as mango, guava and banana will usually be available. Raspberry, lemon and lime sorbets are also common.

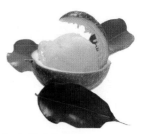

Tropical Fruit Sorbets

Gluten-Free Decision Factors:
- Ensure no colors or flavors containing gluten
- Ensure no stabilizers which may contain gluten
- Ensure no cookie/biscuit

Food Allergen Preparation Considerations:
- May contain corn from colors or flavors
- May contain dairy from colors or flavors and cookie/biscuit
- May contain eggs from colors or flavors and cookie/biscuit
- May contain peanuts from cookie/biscuit
- May contain soy from colors or flavors and cookie/biscuit
- May contain tree nuts from cookie/biscuit

10

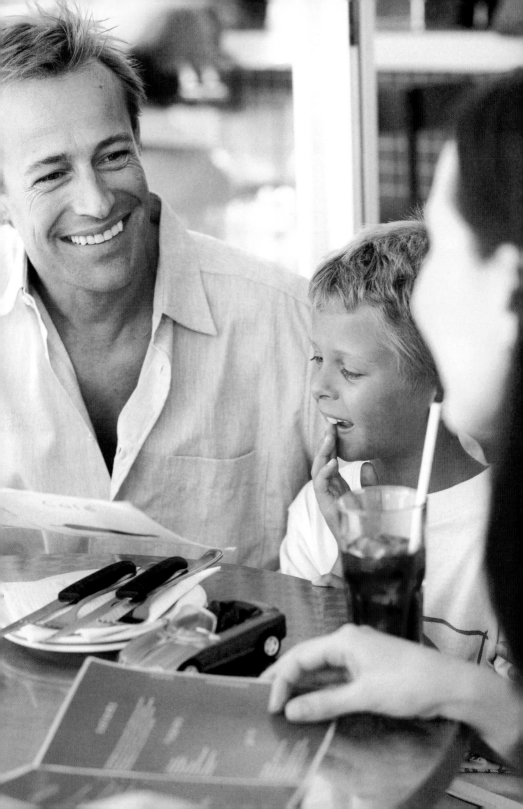

He who would learn to fly,
one day must learn to stand and walk
and run and climb and dance;
one cannot fly into flying.
—Friedrich Nietzsche

Chapter 11
Allergen-Free Preparation Checklists

Chapter Overview

The allergen-free preparation checklists represent each of the seven international cuisines detailed in this book including:

11

- American Steak and Seafood

- Chinese

- French

- Indian

- Italian

- Mexican

- Thai

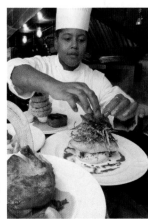

The checklists have been designed to assist in simplifying the ordering process between guests and restaurants by quickly identifying the questions to ask to ensure that meals are allergen-free. They allow guests to walk into any restaurant that serves these cuisines, scan the menu and quickly spot the safest allergen-free choices. Restaurants can use the checklists to identify potential ingredients and hidden food allergens in various menu items.

These are intended to refresh your memory, providing you with quick and easy access to the detailed information outlined in each of the cuisine chapters.

Color Key for the Preparation Checklists

Corn–dark brown
Soy–light brown
Gluten/Wheat–dark yellow
Dairy–light yellow
Fish–dark blue
Shellfish–light blue
Peanuts–dark green
Tree Nuts–light green
Eggs–pink

Allergen-Free Preparation Checklist Descriptions

The checklists are organized by the seven international cuisines and associated sample menu items detailed in Chapters 4–10. Each dish for the specific cuisine identifies ingredients and food preparation techniques to be aware of based upon common food allergens. These ten allergens are color-coded and highlighted in the chart to the left.

The *Allergen-Free Preparation Checklists* indicate where each allergen may be found by menu item. The items reflect if the dish "typically contains the allergen – ●" or if the dish "may contain the allergen – ○". Additionally, up to 25 codes by allergen are further detailed in this easy-to-follow format as outlined below and on the next page.

At first, the level of detail may seem overwhelming and complex. Keep in mind that every effort has been made to incorporate both traditional and non-traditional culinary practices which may vary by country and/or geographic region. The preparation checklists are designed to be as thorough as possible while taking into consideration cultural variations to ensure safe eating anywhere.

11

Corn
- (Al) Almonds or Almond Extract
- (Am) Artificial Mashed Potato Mix
- (Ba) Batter
- (Bb) Artificial Bacon Bits
- (Bd) Breading
- (Bo) Bouillon
- (Br) Bread or Bread Crumbs
- (C) Corn
- (Cf) Colors or Flavors
- (Ch) Cheese
- (Cr) Croutons
- (Cs) Corn Flour, Meal, Starch or Syrup
- (Dr) Salad Dressing

Corn, continued
- (Ic) Imitation Crabmeat or Seafood
- (Ms) Masa
- (Mv) Malt / Malt Vinegar
- (Sa) Sauce
- (Se) Seasonings
- (Tc) Tortillas or Tortilla Chips
- (Ve) Vanilla Extract
- (Vo) Vegetable Oil

Dairy
- (Am) Artificial Mashed Potato Mix
- (Bd) Breading
- (Br) Bread or Bread Crumbs
- (Bu) Butter

Dairy, continued
- (Cc) Chocolate
- (Cf) Colors or Flavors
- (Ch) Cheese
- (Ck) Cake, Cookie or Biscuit
- (Cm) Cream, Sour Cream or Whipped Cream
- (Cr) Croutons
- (D) Dairy
- (Dr) Salad Dressing
- (Mk) Milk or Buttermilk
- (Pr) Prosciutto
- (Sa) Sauce
- (Se) Seasonings
- (Yo) Yogurt, Curd or Sauce

Eggs

- (Ba) Batter
- (Bd) Breading
- (Br) Bread or Bread Crumbs
- (Cf) Colors or Flavors
- (Ck) Cake, Cookie or Biscuit
- (Cr) Croutons
- (Dr) Salad Dressing
- (Ds) Dumpling Skin
- (E) Eggs
- (Es) Egg Sealer
- (Ey) Egg Yolk
- (Ic) Imitation Crabmeat or Seafood
- (Mo) Mayonnaise
- (No) Noodles or Pasta
- (Sa) Sauce

Fish

- (An) Anchovies
- (Dr) Salad Dressing
- (F) Fish
- (Fs) Fish Sauce
- (Ic) Imitation Crabmeat or Seafood
- (Sl) Salmon
- (St) Stock or Broth
- (Tu) Tuna

Gluten / Wheat

- (Am) Artificial Mashed Potato Mix
- (Ba) Batter
- (Bb) Artificial Bacon Bits
- (Bd) Breading
- (Be) Beans
- (Bo) Bouillon
- (Br) Bread or Bread Crumbs
- (Cf) Colors or Flavors
- (Ck) Cake, Cookie or Biscuit
- (Cl) Clean Water
- (Cr) Croutons

Gluten / Wheat, continued

- (Df) Dedicated Fryer and/or Fresh Cooking Oil
- (Dr) Salad Dressing
- (Fd) Wheat Flour Dusting
- (Fs) Fish Sauce
- (Ga) Garnish
- (Ic) Imitation Crabmeat or Seafood
- (Mv) Malt / Malt Vinegar
- (No) Noodles or Pasta
- (Sa) Sauce
- (Sb) Stabilizers
- (Se) Seasonings
- (Ss) Soy Sauce
- (Tc) Tortillas or Tortilla Chips
- (Wf) Wheat Flour

Peanuts

- (Am) Artificial Mashed Potato Mix
- (Br) Bread or Bread Crumb
- (Cf) Colors or Flavors
- (Ck) Cake, Cookie or Biscuit
- (Cr) Croutons
- (Ga) Garnish
- (P) Peanuts
- (Po) Peanut Oil
- (Sa) Sauce
- (Vo) Vegetable Oil

Shellfish

- (Ca) Calamari
- (Cb) Crab
- (Es) Escargot (Snails)
- (Lo) Lobster
- (Mu) Mussels
- (Oy) Oysters
- (Sf) Shellfish
- (Sh) Shrimp
- (St) Stock or Broth

Soy

- (Am) Artificial Mashed Potato Mix
- (Bb) Artificial Bacon Bits
- (Bc) Bean Curd
- (Bd) Breading
- (Bo) Bouillon
- (Br) Bread or Bread Crumbs
- (Cc) Chocolate
- (Cf) Colors or Flavors
- (Ch) Cheese
- (Ck) Cake, Cookie or Biscuit
- (Cr) Croutons
- (Cs) Corn Flour, Meal, Starch or Syrup
- (Dr) Salad Dressing
- (Ic) Imitation Crabmeat or Seafood
- (Kt) Ketchup
- (Mo) Mayonnaise
- (Ms) Masa
- (Sa) Sauce
- (Se) Seasonings
- (Ss) Soy Sauce
- (To) Tofu
- (Tc) Tortillas or Tortilla Chips
- (Vo) Vegetable Oil

Tree Nuts

- (Al) Almonds or Almond Extract
- (Br) Bread or Bread Crumbs
- (Cf) Colors or Flavors
- (Ck) Cake, Cookie or Biscuit
- (Cr) Croutons
- (Cw) Cashews or Cashew Powder
- (Ga) Garnish
- (Pi) Pistachios
- (Sa) Sauce
- (T) Tree Nuts
- (Wn) Walnuts

11

These checklists are intended to provide a level of comfort while eating outside the home. With key information at your finger tips, guests and restaurants can effectively understand the presence of hidden allergens, communicate special needs, ensure concerns are addressed and concentrate on safe allergen-free experiences.

American Steak & Seafood: Starters, Soups and Salads

	Corn	Dairy	Eggs	Fish
Starters				
Oysters on the Half Shell	(Bo)(Cs)	(Sa)	(Sa)	(St)
Shrimp Cocktail	(Bo)(Cs)		(Sa)	(St)
Soups				
Bisque (Cream Soup)	(Bo)(Cr)(Ic)	**(Bu)(Cm)**(Cr)	(Cr)(Ic)	(F)(Ic)(St)
Salads				
Buffalo Mozzarella and Tomato Salad	(Vo)	**(Ch)**		
Chopped Salad	(Bb)(Ch)(Cr) (Dr)(Vo)	(Ch)(Cr)(Dr)	(Cr)(Dr)	(Dr)
Cobb Salad	(Bb)(Ch)(Cr) (Dr)(Vo)	**(Ch)**(Cr)(Dr)	(Cr)(Dr)**(E)**	(Dr)
Hearts of Palm Salad	(Vo)		(E)	
Mixed Green Salad	(Bb)(Ch)(Cr) (Dr)(Vo)	(Ch)(Cr)(Dr)	(Cr)(Dr)	(Dr)

Ensure no cross-contaminaton in food preparation. Food allergens vary depending upon type of accompaniment, garnish or side.

● Typically contains allergen   ○ May contain allergen

Corn	**Dairy**	**Eggs**	**Fish**
(Bb) Artificial Bacon Bits	(Bu) Butter	(Cr) Croutons	(Dr) Salad Dressing
(Bo) Bouillon	(Ch) Cheese	(Dr) Salad Dressing	(F) Fish
(Ch) Cheese	(Cm) Cream, Sour Cream or	(E) Eggs	(Ic) Imitation Crabmeat or
(Cr) Croutons	Whipped Cream	(Ic) Imitation Crabmeat or	Seafood
(Cs) Corn Flour, Meal, Starch	(Cr) Croutons	Seafood	(St) Stock or Broth
or Syrup	(Dr) Salad Dressing	(Sa) Sauce	
(Dr) Salad Dressing	(Sa) Sauce		
(Ic) Imitation Crabmeat or			
Seafood			
(Vo) Vegetable Oil			

11

	Gluten/Wheat	Peanuts	Shellfish	Soy	Tree Nuts
Starters					
Oysters on the Half Shell	(Bo)(Sa)		(Oy)	(Bo)	
Shrimp Cocktail	(Bo)		(Sh)	(Bo)(Sa)	
Soups					
Bisque (Cream Soup)	(Bo)(Cr)(Ga)(Ic)(Wf)	(Cr)(P)	(Sf)(St)	(Bo)(Cr)(Ic)	(Cr)(T)
Salads					
Buffalo Mozzarella and Tomato Salad		(Vo)		(Vo)	
Chopped Salad	(Bb)(Cr)(Dr)(Ga)	(Cr)(Vo)		(Bb)(Ch)(Cr)(Dr)(Vo)	(Cr)
Cobb Salad	(Bb)(Cr)(Dr)(Ga)	(Cr)(Vo)		(Bb)(Ch)(Cr)(Dr)(Vo)	(Cr)
Hearts of Palm Salad		(Vo)		(Vo)	
Mixed Green Salad	(Bb)(Cr)(Dr)(Ga)	(Cr)(Vo)		(Bb)(Ch)(Cr)(Dr)(Vo)	(Cr)

11

Ensure no cross-contaminaton in food preparation. Food allergens vary depending upon type of accompaniment, garnish or side.

● Typically contains allergen   ○ May contain allergen

Gluten / Wheat
(Bb) Artificial Bacon Bits
(Bo) Bouillon
(Cr) Croutons
(Dr) Salad Dressing
(Ga) Garnish
(Ic) Imitation Crabmeat or Seafood
(Sa) Sauce
(Wf) Wheat Flour

Peanuts
(Cr) Croutons
(P) Peanuts
(Vo) Vegetable Oil

Shellfish
(Oy) Oysters
(Sf) Shellfish
(Sh) Shrimp
(St) Stock or Broth

Soy
(Bb) Artificial Bacon Bits
(Bo) Bouillon
(Ch) Cheese
(Cr) Croutons
(Dr) Salad Dressing
(Ic) Imitation Crabmeat or Seafood
(Sa) Sauce
(Vo) Vegetable Oil

Tree Nuts
(Cr) Croutons
(T) Tree Nuts

American Steak & Seafood: Meat, Chicken and Seafood Dishes

	Corn	Dairy	Eggs	Fish
Meat Dishes				
Hamburgers	(Br)(Cs)(Se)(Vo)	(Br)(Se)	(Br)(Mo)	
Pork Chops	(Vo)	(Bu)		
Lamb Chops	(Br)(Vo)	(Br)(Bu)	(Br)	
Steaks	(Vo)	(Bu)(Sa)	(Sa)	
Chicken Dishes				
Grilled Chicken Breast	(Vo)	(Bu)(Mk)		
Roasted Chicken	(Vo)	(Bu)		
Seafood Dishes				
Crab	(Bo)(Br)(Vo)	(Br)(Bu)	(Br)	(St)
Fish Filet	(Bo)(Vo)	(Ba)(Bu)(Fd)	(Ba)	●
Lobster	(Bo)(Br)(Vo)	(Br)(Bu)	(Br)	(St)

Ensure no cross-contaminaton in food preparation. Food allergens vary depending upon type of accompaniment, garnish or side.

● Typically contains allergen   ○ May contain allergen

Corn	**Dairy**	**Eggs**	**Fish**
(Bo) Bouillon	(Br) Bread or Bread Crumbs	(Ba) Batter	(F) Fish
(Br) Bread or Bread Crumbs	(Bu) Butter	(Br) Bread or Bread Crumbs	(St) Stock or Broth
(Cs) Corn Flour, Meal, Starch or Syrup	(Mk) Milk or Buttermilk	(Mo) Mayonnaise	
(Se) Seasonings	(Sa) Sauce	(Sa) Sauce	
(Vo) Vegetable Oil	(Se) Seasonings		

	Gluten/ Wheat	Peanuts	Shellfish	Soy	Tree Nuts
Meat Dishes					
Hamburgers	(Br)(Df)(Fd)(Se)	(Br)(Po)(Vo)		(Br)(Kt)(Mo)(Se)(Vo)	(Br)
Pork Chops	(Fd)(Sa)(Ss)(Wf)	(Vo)		(Ss)(Vo)	
Lamb Chops	(Br)(Fd)(Sa)(Ss)(Wf)	(Br)(Vo)		(Br)(Ss)(Vo)	(Br)
Steaks	(Fd)(Sa)(Ss)(Wf)	(Vo)		(Ss)(Vo)	
Chicken Dishes					
Grilled Chicken Breast	(Fd)(Sa)(Ss)(Wf)	(Vo)		(Ss)(Vo)	
Roasted Chicken	(Fd)(Sa)(Ss)(Wf)	(Vo)		(Ss)(Vo)	
Seafood Dishes					
Crab	(Bo)(Br)	(Br)(Vo)	(Cb)	(Bo)(Br)(Vo)	(Br)
Fish Filet	(Ba)(Bo)(Fd)(Sa)	(Vo)		(Bo)(Vo)	
Lobster	(Bo)(Br)	(Br)(Vo)	(Lo)	(Bo)(Br)(Vo)	(Br)

Ensure no cross-contaminaton in food preparation. Food allergens vary depending upon type of accompaniment, garnish or side.

● Typically contains allergen   ◯ May contain allergen

Gluten / Wheat
(Ba) Batter
(Bo) Bouillon
(Br) Bread or Bread Crumbs
(Df) Dedicated Fryer and/or Fresh Cooking Oil
(Fd) Wheat Flour Dusting
(Sa) Sauce
(Se) Seasonings
(Ss) Soy Sauce
(Wf) Wheat Flour

Peanuts
(Br) Bread or Bread Crumbs
(Po) Peanut Oil
(Vo) Vegetable Oil

Shellfish
(Cb) Crab
(Lo) Lobster

Soy
(Bo) Bouillon
(Br) Bread or Bread Crumbs
(Kt) Ketchup
(Mo) Mayonnaise
(Se) Seasonings
(Ss) Soy Sauce
(Vo) Vegetable Oil

Tree Nuts
(Br) Bread or Bread Crumbs

11

American Steak & Seafood: Sides

Sides	Corn	Dairy	Eggs	Fish
Asparagus	(Vo)	(Bu)(Sa)	(Sa)	
Baked Potato	(Bb)(Sa)	(Bu)(Ch)(Cm)		
Broccoli	(Sa)(Vo)	(Bu)(Sa)		
French Fried Potatoes	(Cs)(Se)(Vo)	(Se)		
Green Beans	(Vo)	(Bu)(Sa)	(Sa)	
Hash Browns	(Se)(Vo)	(Bu)(Se)		
Mashed Potatoes	(Am)	(Am)(Bu)(Ch)(Mk)		
Potatoes Lyonnaise	(Vo)	(Bu)		
Spinach	(Vo)	(Bu)(Cm)		

Ensure no cross-contaminaton in food preparation. Food allergens vary depending upon type of accompaniment, garnish or side.

● Typically contains allergen   ○ May contain allergen

Corn
- (Am) Artificial Mashed Potato Mix
- (Bb) Artificial Bacon Bits
- (Cs) Corn Flour, Meal, Starch or Syrup
- (Sa) Sauce
- (Se) Seasonings
- (Vo) Vegetable Oil

Dairy
- (Am) Artificial Mashed Potato Mix
- (Bu) Butter
- (Ch) Cheese
- (Cm) Cream, Sour Cream or Whipped Cream
- (Mk) Milk or Buttermilk
- (Sa) Sauce
- (Se) Seasonings

Eggs
- (Sa) Sauce

11

Sides

	Gluten/Wheat	Peanuts	Shellfish	Soy	Tree Nuts
Asparagus	(Sa)	(Vo)		(Vo)	
Baked Potato	(Bb)(Sa)			(Bb)(Sa)	
Broccoli	(Sa)	(Vo)		(Sa)(Vo)	
French Fried Potatoes	(Df)(Fd)(Se)	(Po)(Vo)		(Kt)(Se)(Vo)	
Green Beans	(Sa)	(Vo)		(Vo)	(Al)
Hash Browns	(Se)(Wf)	(Vo)		(Se)(Vo)	
Mashed Potatoes	(Am)(Wf)	(Am)		(Am)	
Potatoes Lyonnaise	(Wf)	(Vo)		(Vo)	
Spinach	(Wf)	(Vo)		(Vo)	

11

Ensure no cross-contaminaton in food preparation. Food allergens vary depending upon type of accompaniment, garnish or side.

● Typically contains allergen   ○ May contain allergen

Gluten / Wheat
(Am) Artificial Mashed Potato Mix
(Bb) Artificial Bacon Bits
(Df) Dedicated Fryer and/or Fresh Cooking Oil
(Fd) Wheat Flour Dusting
(Sa) Sauce
(Se) Seasonings
(Wf) Wheat Flour

Peanuts
(Am) Artificial Mashed Potato Mix
(Po) Peanut Oil
(Vo) Vegetable Oil

Soy
(Am) Artificial Mashed Potato Mix
(Bb) Artificial Bacon Bits
(Kt) Ketchup
(Sa) Sauce
(Se) Seasonings
(Vo) Vegetable Oil

Tree Nuts
(Al) Almonds or Almond Extract

American Steak & Seafood: Desserts

Desserts	Corn	Dairy	Eggs	Fish
Chocolate Mousse	(Cf)	(Cc)(Ck)(Cm)(Mk)	(Ck) ●	
Crème Brulée (Baked Custard)	(Al)(Ve)	(Ck)(Cm)	(Ck) ●	
Flourless Chocolate Torte	(Br)	(Br)(Bu)(Cc)	(Br) ●	
Fresh Berries with Whipped Cream		(Ck)(Cm)	(Ck)	
Ice Cream	(Cf)(Mv)	(Cc)(Cf)(Ck) ●	(Ck)	
Sorbet	(Cf)	(Cc)(Cf)(Ck)	(Ck)	

Ensure no cross-contaminaton in food preparation. Food allergens vary depending upon type of accompaniment, garnish or side.

● Typically contains allergen   ◯ May contain allergen

11

Corn
(Al) Almonds or Almond Extract
(Br) Bread or Bread Crumbs
(Cf) Colors or Flavors
(Mv) Malt / Malt Vinegar
(Ve) Vanilla Extract

Dairy
(Br) Bread or Bread Crumbs
(Bu) Butter
(Cc) Chocolate
(Cf) Colors or Flavors
(Ck) Cake, Cookie or Biscuit
(Cm) Cream, Sour Cream or Whipped Cream
(D) Dairy
(Mk) Milk or Buttermilk

Eggs
(Br) Bread or Bread Crumbs
(Ck) Cake, Cookie or Biscuit
(E) Eggs
(Ey) Egg Yolk

Desserts	Gluten/Wheat	Peanuts	Shellfish	Soy	Tree Nuts
Chocolate Mousse	(Cf)(Ck)(Wf)	(Cf)(Ck)		(Cc)(Cf)(Ck)	(Cf)(Ck)
Crème Brulée (Baked Custard)	(Ck)(Wf)	(Ck)		(Cc)(Ck)	(Al)(Ck)
Flourless Chocolate Torte	(Br)(Fd)(Wf)	(Br)		(Br)(Cc)	(Br)
Fresh Berries with Whipped Cream	(Ck)	(Ck)		(Ck)	(Ck)
Ice Cream	(Cf)(Ck)(Mv)(Sb)(Wf)	(Cf)(Ck)		(Cc)(Cf)(Ck)	(Cf)(Ck)
Sorbet	(Ck)(Sb)(Wf)	(Cf)(Ck)		(Cc)(Cf)(Ck)	(Cf)(Ck)

Ensure no cross-contaminaton in food preparation. Food allergens vary depending upon type of accompaniment, garnish or side.

● Typically contains allergen   ○ May contain allergen

Gluten / Wheat
(Br) Bread or Bread Crumbs
(Cf) Colors or Flavors
(Ck) Cake, Cookie or Biscuit
(Fd) Wheat Flour Dusting
(Mv) Malt / Malt Vinegar
(Sb) Stabilizers
(Wf) Wheat Flour

Peanuts
(Br) Bread or Bread Crumb
(Cf) Colors or Flavors
(Ck) Cake, Cookie or Biscuit

Soy
(Br) Bread or Bread Crumbs
(Cc) Chocolate
(Cf) Colors or Flavors
(Ck) Cake, Cookie or Biscuit

Tree Nuts
(Al) Almonds or Almond Extract
(Br) Bread or Bread Crumbs
(Cf) Colors or Flavors
(Ck) Cake, Cookie or Biscuit

11

Chinese Cuisine: Soups, Dishes (Chicken, Seafood, Vegetarian, Rice) and Desserts

	Corn	Dairy	Eggs	Fish
Soups				
Egg Drop Soup	(Bo) (Cs) (Vo)		● E	
Sizzling Rice Soup	(Bo) (Cs) (Vo)		(E)	
Chicken Dishes				
Lemon Chicken	(Bo) (Cs) (Vo)		(Ba)	
Steamed Chicken and Broccoli				
Seafood Dishes				
Steamed Fish				● F
Vegetarian Dishes				
Buddha's Feast	(Bo) (C) (Vo)			
Rice Dishes				
Steamed Rice				
Desserts				
Fresh Tropical Fruits		(Ck)	(Ck)	

Ensure no cross-contaminaton in food preparation. Food allergens vary depending upon type of accompaniment, garnish or side.

● Typically contains allergen   ○ May contain allergen

Corn
(Bo) Bouillon
(C) Corn
(Cs) Corn Flour, Meal, Starch or Syrup
(Vo) Vegetable Oil

Dairy
(Ck) Cake, Cookie or Biscuit

Eggs
(Ba) Batter
(Ck) Cake, Cookie or Biscuit
(E) Eggs

Fish
(F) Fish

	Gluten/Wheat	Peanuts	Shellfish	Soy	Tree Nuts
Soups					
Egg Drop Soup	(Bo)(No)(Ss)(Wf)	(Po)(Vo)		(Bo)(Ss)(To)(Vo)	
Sizzling Rice Soup	(Bo)(Cl)(No)(Ss)(Wf)	(Po)(Vo)	(Sh)	(Bo)(Ss)(To)(Vo)	
Chicken Dishes					
Lemon Chicken	(Ba)(Bo)(Df)(Fd)(Ss)	(Po)(Vo)		(Bo)(Ss)(Vo)	
Steamed Chicken and Broccoli	(Ss)			(Ss)	
Seafood Dishes					
Steamed Fish	(Ss)			(Ss)	
Vegetarian Dishes					
Buddha's Feast	(Bo)(Ss)	(Po)(Vo)		(Bc)(Bo)(Ss)(To)(Vo)	
Rice Dishes					
Steamed Rice	(Cl)				
Desserts					
Fresh Tropical Fruits	(Ck)	(Ck)		(Ck)	(Ck)

Ensure no cross-contaminaton in food preparation. Food allergens vary depending upon type of accompaniment, garnish or side.

● Typically contains allergen ○ May contain allergen

Gluten / Wheat
(Ba) Batter
(Bo) Bouillon
(Ck) Cake, Cookie or Biscuit
(Cl) Clean Water
(Df) Dedicated Fryer and/or Fresh Cooking Oil
(Fd) Wheat Flour Dusting
(No) Noodles or Pasta

Gluten / Wheat, cont.
(Ss) Soy Sauce
(Wf) Wheat Flour

Peanuts
(Ck) Cake, Cookie or Biscuit
(Po) Peanut Oil
(Vo) Vegetable Oil

Shellfish
(Sh) Shrimp

Soy
(Bc) Bean Curd
(Bo) Bouillon
(Ck) Cake, Cookie or Biscuit
(Ss) Soy Sauce

Soy, cont.
(To) Tofu
(Vo) Vegetable Oil

Tree Nuts
(Ck) Cake, Cookie or Biscuit

11

French Cuisine: Starters and Soups

	Corn	Dairy	Eggs	Fish
Starters				
Crevette Cocktail (Shrimp Cocktail)	(Bo)(Cs)		(Sa)	(St)
Escargot (Snails)	(Br)	(Br)(Bu)	(Br)	
Foies Gras (Fat Liver)	(Br)	(Br)(Mk)	(Br)(E)	
Les Huîtres (Oysters on the Half Shell)	(Bo)(Cs)	(Sa)	(Sa)	(St)
Steak Tartare (Beef Tartar)	(Br)(Cs)(Vo)	(Br)	(Br)(E)(Mo)	(An)
Tartare de Saumon (Salmon Tartar)	(Vo)		(Mo)	●(Sl)
Soups				
Bisque (Cream Soup)	(Bo)(Cr)(Ic)	●(Bu)●(Cm)(Cr)	(Cr)(Ic)	(F)(Ic)(St)
Vichyssoise (Potato Leek Soup)	(Bo)	●(Bu)●(Cm)		

11

Ensure no cross-contaminaton in food preparation. Food allergens vary depending upon type of accompaniment, garnish or side.

● Typically contains allergen   ○ May contain allergen

Corn	**Dairy**	**Eggs**	**Fish**
(Bo) Bouillon	(Br) Bread or Bread Crumbs	(Br) Bread or Bread Crumbs	(An) Anchovies
(Br) Bread or Bread Crumbs	(Bu) Butter	(Cr) Croutons	(F) Fish
(Cr) Croutons	(Cm) Cream, Sour Cream or Whipped Cream	(E) Eggs	(Ic) Imitation Crabmeat or Seafood
(Cs) Corn Flour, Meal, Starch or Syrup	(Cr) Croutons	(Ic) Imitation Crabmeat or Seafood	(Sl) Salmon
(Ic) Imitation Crabmeat or Seafood	(Mk) Milk or Buttermilk	(Mo) Mayonnaise	(St) Stock or Broth
(Vo) Vegetable Oil	(Sa) Sauce	(Sa) Sauce	

	Gluten/Wheat	Peanuts	Shellfish	Soy	Tree Nuts
Starters					
Crevette Cocktail (Shrimp Cocktail)	(Bo)(Sa)		(Sh)	(Bo)(Sa)	
Escargot (Snails)	(Br)	(Br)	(Es)	(Br)	(Br)
Foies Gras (Fat Liver)	(Br)	(Br)		(Br)	(Br)
Les Huîtres (Oysters on the Half Shell)	(Bo)(Sa)		(Oy)	(Bo)	
Steak Tartare (Beef Tartar)	(Br)	(Br)(Vo)		(Mo)(Vo)	(Br)
Tartare de Saumon (Salmon Tartar)		(Vo)		(Mo)(Vo)	
Soups					
Bisque (Cream Soup)	(Bo)(Cr)(Ga)(Ic)(Wf)	(Cr)(P)	(Sf)(St)	(Bo)(Cr)(Ic)	(Cr)(T)
Vichyssoise (Potato Leek Soup)	(Bo)(Wf)			(Bo)	

11

Ensure no cross-contaminaton in food preparation. Food allergens vary depending upon type of accompaniment, garnish or side.

● Typically contains allergen   ○ May contain allergen

Gluten / Wheat
(Bo) Bouillon
(Br) Bread or Bread Crumbs
(Cr) Croutons
(Ga) Garnish
(Ic) Imitation Crabmeat or Seafood
(Sa) Sauce
(Wf) Wheat Flour

Peanuts
(Br) Bread or Bread Crumbs
(Cr) Croutons
(P) Peanuts
(Vo) Vegetable Oil

Shellfish
(Es) Escargot (Snails)
(Oy) Oysters
(Sf) Shellfish
(Sh) Shrimp
(St) Stock or Broth

Soy
(Bo) Bouillon
(Br) Bread or Bread Crumbs
(Cr) Croutons
(Ic) Imitation Crabmeat or Seafood
(Mo) Mayonnaise
(Sa) Sauce
(Vo) Vegetable Oil

Tree Nuts
(Br) Bread or Bread Crumbs
(Cr) Croutons
(T) Tree Nuts

French Cuisine: Salads, Egg and Beef Dishes

	Corn	Dairy	Eggs	Fish
Salads				
Artichauts à la Vinaigrette (Artichoke Salad)	(Vo)			
Asperge à la Vinaigrette (Asparagus Salad)	(Vo)		(E)	
Mesclun de Salade (Mixed Green Salad)	(Cr)(Vo)	(Cr)	(Cr)	
Salade Niçoise (Nice Style Salad)	(Cr)(Vo)	(Cr)	(Cr)●	●●●
Egg Dishes				
Les Oeufs (Fried Eggs)	(Vo)	(Bu)	●	
Les Omelettes (Omelets)	(Vo)	(Bu)(Ch)	●	
Beef Dishes				
Filet de Boeuf (Beef Filet)	(Bd)(Vo)	(Bd)(Bu)(Sa)	(Bd)(Sa)	
Fondue Bourguignon (Beef Fondue)	(Cs)(Vo)	(Bu)(Sa)	(Mo)(Sa)	
Steak au Poivre (Peppered Steak)	(Vo)	●		
Steak Frites (Steak and French Fried Potatoes)	(Cs)(Vo)	(Bu)(Sa)	(Mo)(Sa)	

Ensure no cross-contaminaton in food preparation. Food allergens vary depending upon type of accompaniment, garnish or side.

● Typically contains allergen   ◯ May contain allergen

Corn	**Dairy**	**Eggs**	**Fish**
(Bd) Breading	(Bd) Breading	(Bd) Breading	(An) Anchovies
(Cr) Croutons	(Bu) Butter	(Cr) Croutons	(Sl) Salmon
(Cs) Corn Flour, Meal, Starch or Syrup	(Ch) Cheese	(E) Eggs	(Tu) Tuna
(Vo) Vegetable Oil	(Cr) Croutons	(Mo) Mayonnaise	
	(Sa) Sauce	(Sa) Sauce	

11

	Gluten/ Wheat	Peanuts	Shellfish	Soy	Tree Nuts
Salads					
Artichauts à la Vinaigrette (Artichoke Salad)		(Vo)		(Vo)	
Asperge à la Vinaigrette (Asparagus Salad)		(Vo)		(Vo)	
Mesclun de Salade (Mixed Green Salad)	(Cr)(Ga)	(Cr)(Vo)		(Cr)(Vo)	(Cr)(Wn)
Salade Niçoise (Nice Style Salad)	(Cr)(Ga)	(Cr)(Vo)		(Cr)(Vo)	(Cr)
Egg Dishes					
Les Oeufs (Fried Eggs)	(Df)	(Po)(Vo)		(Vo)	
Les Omelettes (Omelets)	(Df)(Wf)	(Po)(Vo)		(Vo)	
Beef Dishes					
Filet de Boeuf (Beef Filet)	(Bd)(Fd)(Sa)	(Vo)		(Bd)(Vo)	
Fondue Bourguignon (Beef Fondue)	(Fd)(Sa)	(Po)(Vo)		(Mo)(Vo)	
Steak au Poivre (Peppered Steak)	(Fd)(Sa)	(Vo)		(Vo)	
Steak Frites (Steak and French Fried Potatoes)	(Df)(Fd)(Mv)(Sa)	(Po)(Vo)		(Mo)(Vo)	

11

Ensure no cross-contaminaton in food preparation. Food allergens vary depending upon type of accompaniment, garnish or side.

● Typically contains allergen   ◯ May contain allergen

Gluten / Wheat	Peanuts	Soy	Tree Nuts
(Bd) Breading	(Cr) Croutons	(Bd) Breading	(Cr) Croutons
(Cr) Croutons	(Po) Peanut Oil	(Cr) Croutons	(Wn) Walnuts
(Df) Dedicated Fryer and/or Fresh Cooking Oil	(Vo) Vegetable Oil	(Mo) Mayonnaise	
(Fd) Wheat Flour Dusting		(Vo) Vegetable Oil	
(Ga) Garnish			
(Mv) Malt / Malt Vinegar			
(Sa) Sauce			
(Wf) Wheat Flour			

French Cuisine: Chicken & Seafood Dishes and Sides

	Corn	Dairy	Eggs	Fish
Chicken Dishes				
Poulet Provençal (Roasted Chicken with Herbs)				
Seafood Dishes				
Bouillabaisse (Seafood Stew)	(Bo)(Br)(Cr)	(Br)(Cr)	(Br)(Cr)	● (F)
Moules Frites (Mussels and French Fried Potatoes)	(Bo)(Br)(Cs)(Vo)	(Br)(Bu)(Sa)	(Br)(Mo)(Sa)	
Saumon en Papillote (Baked Salmon)	(Vo)	(Bu)	(Eg)	● (Sl)
Sides				
Gratin Dauphinois (Creamed Potatoes)	(Br)	(Br)(Bu)(Ch)(Cm)(Mk)	(Br)	
Haricots Verts (French Green Beans)	(Vo)	(Bu)(Sa)	(Sa)	
Pommes Frites (French Fried Potatoes)	(Cs)(Vo)	(Bu)(Sa)	(Mo)(Sa)	
Ratatouille (Vegetable Stew)	(Bo)(Vo)	(Ch)		

Ensure no cross-contaminaton in food preparation. Food allergens vary depending upon type of accompaniment, garnish or side.

● Typically contains allergen   ○ May contain allergen

Corn	**Dairy**	**Eggs**	**Fish**
(Bo) Bouillon	(Br) Bread or Bread Crumbs	(Br) Bread or Bread Crumbs	(F) Fish
(Br) Bread or Bread Crumbs	(Bu) Butter	(Cr) Croutons	(Sl) Salmon
(Cr) Croutons	(Ch) Cheese	(Eg) Egg Sealer	
(Cs) Corn Flour, Meal, Starch or Syrup	(Cm) Cream, Sour Cream or Whipped Cream	(Mo) Mayonnaise	
(Vo) Vegetable Oil	(Cr) Croutons	(Sa) Sauce	
	(Mk) Milk or Buttermilk		
	(Sa) Sauce		

11

	Gluten/Wheat	Peanuts	Shellfish	Soy	Tree Nuts
Chicken Dishes					
Poulet Provençal (Roasted Chicken with Herbs)	(Ss)(Wf)			(Ss)	
Seafood Dishes					
Bouillabaisse (Seafood Stew)	(Bo)(Br)(Cr)(Wf)	(Br)(Cr)	● (Sf)	(Bo)(Br)(Cr)	(Br)(Cr)
Moules Frites (Mussels and French Fried Potatoes)	(Bo)(Br)(Df)(Fd)(Mv)(Sa)	(Br)(Po)(Vo)	● (Mu)	(Bo)(Br)(Vo)	(Br)
Saumon en Papillote (Baked Salmon)	(Fd)	(Po)(Vo)		(Vo)	
Sides					
Gratin Dauphinois (Creamed Potatoes)	(Br)(Wf)	(Br)		(Br)	(Br)
Haricots Verts (French Green Beans)	(Sa)	(Po)(Vo)		(Vo)	(Al)
Pommes Frites (French Fried Potatoes)	(Df)(Fd)(Mv)	(Po)(Vo)		(Mo)(Vo)	
Ratatouille (Vegetable Stew)	(Bo)(Wf)	(Vo)		(Bo)(Vo)	

11

Ensure no cross-contaminaton in food preparation. Food allergens vary depending upon type of accompaniment, garnish or side.

● Typically contains allergen   ○ May contain allergen

Gluten / Wheat
(Bo) Bouillon
(Br) Bread or Bread Crumbs
(Cr) Croutons
(Df) Dedicated Fryer and/or Fresh Cooking Oil
(Fd) Wheat Flour Dusting
(Mv) Malt / Malt Vinegar
(Sa) Sauce
(Ss) Soy Sauce
(Wf) Wheat Flour

Peanuts
(Br) Bread or Bread Crumbs
(Cr) Croutons
(Po) Peanut Oil
(Vo) Vegetable Oil

Shellfish
(Mu) Mussels
(Sf) Shellfish

Soy
(Bo) Bouillon
(Br) Bread or Bread Crumbs
(Cr) Croutons
(Mo) Mayonnaise
(Ss) Soy Sauce
(Vo) Vegetable Oil

Tree Nuts
(Al) Almonds or Almond Extract
(Br) Bread or Bread Crumbs
(Cr) Croutons

French Cuisine: Desserts

Desserts	Corn	Dairy	Eggs	Fish
Assiette de Fromage (Cheese Plate)	(Br)	(Br)(Ch)	(Br)(E)	
Crème Brulée (Baked Custard)	(Al)(Ve)	(Ck)(Cm)	(Ck)(Ey)	
Fruits à la Crème (Fresh Fruit with Cream)		(Ck)(Cm)	(Ck)	
Mousse au Chocolat (Chocolate Mousse)		(Cc)(Ck)(Cm)(Mk)	(Ck)(E)	
Les Sorbets (Sorbet)	(Cf)	(Ck)	(Ck)	

Ensure no cross-contaminaton in food preparation. Food allergens vary depending upon type of accompaniment, garnish or side.

● Typically contains allergen   ○ May contain allergen

Corn
(Al) Almonds or Almond Extract
(Br) Bread or Bread Crumbs
(Cf) Colors or Flavors
(Ve) Vanilla Extract

Dairy
(Br) Bread or Bread Crumbs
(Cc) Chocolate
(Ch) Cheese
(Ck) Cake, Cookie or Biscuit
(Cm) Cream, Sour Cream or Whipped Cream
(Mk) Milk or Buttermilk

Eggs
(Br) Bread or Bread Crumbs
(Ck) Cake, Cookie or Biscuit
(E) Eggs
(Ey) Egg Yolk

11

Desserts	Gluten/Wheat	Peanuts	Shellfish	Soy	Tree Nuts
Assiette de Fromage (Cheese Plate)	(Br)	(Br)		(Br)	(Br)
Crème Brulée (Baked Custard)	(Ck)(Wf)	(Ck)		(Cc)(Ck)	(Al)(Ck)
Fruits à la Crème (Fresh Fruit with Cream)	(Ck)	(Ck)		(Ck)	(Ck)
Mousse au Chocolat (Chocolate Mousse)	(Ck)(Wf)	(Cf)(Ck)		(Ck)	(Cf)(Ck)
Les Sorbets (Sorbet)	(Ck)(Sb)(Wf)	(Cf)(Ck)		(Cc)(Cf)(Ck)	(Cf)(Ck)

Ensure no cross-contaminaton in food preparation. Food allergens vary depending upon type of accompaniment, garnish or side.

● Typically contains allergen   ○ May contain allergen

Gluten / Wheat
(Br) Bread or Bread Crumbs
(Ck) Cake, Cookie or Biscuit
(Sb) Stabilizers
(Wf) Wheat Flour

Peanuts
(Br) Bread or Bread Crumbs
(Cf) Colors or Flavors
(Ck) Cake, Cookie or Biscuit

Soy
(Br) Bread or Bread Crumbs
(Cc) Chocolate
(Cf) Colors or Flavors
(Ck) Cake, Cookie or Biscuit

Tree Nuts
(Al) Almonds or Almond Extract
(Br) Bread or Bread Crumbs
(Cf) Colors or Flavors
(Ck) Cake, Cookie or Biscuit

11

Indian Cuisine: Starters, Soups and Salads

	Corn	Dairy	Eggs	Fish
Starters				
Aloo Tikki (Potato Patty)	(Cs)(Vo)	(Bu)(Yo)		
Kabobs (Skewered Meat)	(Vo)	**(Yo)**		(F)
Pakoras (Vegetable Fritters)	(Cs)(Vo)	(Bu)		
Papadam (Spicy Crackers)	(Cs)(Vo)	(Bu)(Yo)		
Soups				
Curried Coconut Soup		(Bu)**(Mk)**	(Ey)	
Mulligatawny (Chicken and Vegetable Soup)	(Bo)(Vo)	(Bu)(Cm)(Mk)		
Sambar (Lentil and Vegetable Stew)	(Bo)(Cs)(Vo)	(Bu)		
Salads				
Kachumber (Chopped Salad)	(Vo)			

Ensure no cross-contaminaton in food preparation. Food allergens vary depending upon type of accompaniment, garnish or side.

● Typically contains allergen   ○ May contain allergen

Corn	**Dairy**	**Eggs**	**Fish**
(Bo) Bouillon	(Bu) Butter	(Ey) Egg Yolk	(F) Fish
(Cs) Corn Flour, Meal, Starch or Syrup	(Cm) Cream, Sour Cream or Whipped Cream		
(Vo) Vegetable Oil	(Mk) Milk or Buttermilk		
	(Yo) Yogurt, Curd or Sauce		

11

	Gluten/Wheat	Peanuts	Shellfish	Soy	Tree Nuts
Starters					
Aloo Tikki (Potato Patty)	(Sa)(Wf)	(Po)(Vo)		(Vo)	
Kabobs (Skewered Meat)	(Sa)(Ss)(Wf)	(Po)(Vo)	(Sf)	(Ss)(Vo)	
Pakoras (Vegetable Fritters)	(Sa)(Wf)	(Po)(Vo)		(Vo)	
Papadam (Spicy Crackers)	(Sa)(Wf)	(Po)(Vo)		(Vo)	
Soups					
Curried Coconut Soup	(Wf)				(Al)(Pi)
Mulligatawny (Chicken and Vegetable Soup)	(Bo)(Wf)	(Po)(Vo)		(Bo)(Vo)	(Al)(Pi)
Sambar (Lentil and Vegetable Stew)	(Bo)(Wf)	(Po)(Vo)		(Bo)(Vo)	
Salads					
Kachumber (Chopped Salad)		(Po)(Vo)		(Vo)	

Ensure no cross-contaminaton in food preparation. Food allergens vary depending upon type of accompaniment, garnish or side.

● Typically contains allergen ○ May contain allergen

Gluten / Wheat
(Bo) Bouillon
(Sa) Sauce
(Ss) Soy Sauce
(Wf) Wheat Flour

Peanuts
(Po) Peanut Oil
(Vo) Vegetable Oil

Shellfish
(Sf) Shellfish

Soy
(Bo) Bouillon
(Ss) Soy Sauce
(Vo) Vegetable Oil

Tree Nuts
(Al) Almonds or Almond Extract
(Pi) Pistachios

11

Indian Cuisine: Curry Dishes

Curry Dishes	Corn	Dairy	Eggs	Fish
Channa Masala (Chickpeas in Tomato Curry)	(Bo)(Vo)	(Bu)		
Gosht Vindaloo (Spicy Lamb Curry)	(Vo)	(Bu)		
Jhinga Masala (Shrimp in Coconut Curry)	(Vo)	(Bu)		
Malai Kofta (Vegetarian Croquettes in Mild Curry)	(Vo)	(Bu)(Ch)(Cm)(Yo)		
Murg Korma (Chicken in Cream Curry)	(Vo)	(Bu)(Cm)(Yo)		
Murg Tikki Masala (Chicken in Tomato Curry)	(Cf)(Vo)	(Bu)(Cm)(Yo)		
Rogan Josh (Mild Lamb Curry)	(Vo)	(Bu)(Yo)		
Saag Paneer (Indian Cheese and Spinach Curry)	(Vo)	(Bu)(Ch)(Cm)(Mk)(Yo)		

11

Ensure no cross-contaminaton in food preparation. Food allergens vary depending upon type of accompaniment, garnish or side.

● Typically contains allergen   ○ May contain allergen

Corn
(Bo) Bouillon
(Cf) Colors or Flavors
(Vo) Vegetable Oil

Dairy
(Bu) Butter
(Ch) Cheese
(Cm) Cream, Sour Cream or Whipped Cream
(Mk) Milk or Buttermilk
(Yo) Yogurt, Curd or Sauce

Curry Dishes	Gluten/Wheat	Peanuts	Shellfish	Soy	Tree Nuts
Channa Masala (Chickpeas in Tomato Curry)	(Bo) (Sa)	(Po) (Vo)		(Bo) (Vo)	
Gosht Vindaloo (Spicy Lamb Curry)	(Sa) (Ss) (Wf)	(Po) (Vo)		(Ss) (Vo)	
Jhinga Masala (Shrimp in Coconut Curry)	(Sa)	(Po) (Vo)	**(Sh)**	(Vo)	
Malai Kofta (Vegetarian Croquettes in Mild Curry)	(Fd) (Sa) (Wf)	(Po) (Vo)		(Vo)	**(Cw)**
Murg Korma (Chicken in Cream Curry)	(Sa)	(Po) (Vo)		(Vo)	(Al)
Murg Tikki Masala (Chicken in Tomato Curry)	(Sa) (Ss) (Wf)	(Po) (Vo)		(Cf) (Ss) (Vo)	(Al) (Cw)
Rogan Josh (Mild Lamb Curry)	(Sa) (Ss) (Wf)	(Po) (Vo)		(Ss) (Vo)	
Saag Paneer (Indian Cheese and Spinach Curry)	(Sa)	(Po) (Vo)		(Vo)	

Ensure no cross-contaminaton in food preparation. Food allergens vary depending upon type of accompaniment, garnish or side.

● Typically contains allergen   ◯ May contain allergen

11

Gluten / Wheat
(Bo) Bouillon
(Fd) Wheat Flour Dusting
(Sa) Sauce
(Ss) Soy Sauce
(Wf) Wheat Flour

Peanuts
(Po) Peanut Oil
(Vo) Vegetable Oil

Shellfish
(Sh) Shrimp

Soy
(Bo) Bouillon
(Cf) Colors or Flavors
(Ss) Soy Sauce
(Vo) Vegetable Oil

Tree Nuts
(Al) Almonds or Almond Extract
(Cw) Cashews or Cashew Powder

Indian Cuisine: Tandoor Specialties, Dosas and Desserts

	Corn	Dairy	Eggs	Fish
Tandoor Specialties				
Boti Kabob (Skewered Lamb)	(Vo)	(Yo)		
Murg Tandoori (Tandoori Barbeque Chicken)	(Vo)	(Bu)(Yo)		
Murg Tikka (Yogurt Marinated Chicken)	(Cf)(Vo)	(Bu)(Yo)		
Seekh Kabob (Skewered Minced Lamb)	(Cf)	(Yo)	(E)	
Dosas (South Indian Specialties)				
Masala Dosa (Spicy Vegetable Filled Crepe)	(Bo)(Vo)	(Bu)(Yo)		
Sada Dosa (Lentil and Rice Crepe)	(Bo)(Vo)	(Bu)(Yo)		
Uthappam (Lentil and Rice Pancake)	(Bo)(Vo)	(Bu)(Yo)		
Desserts				
Kheer (Rice Pudding)		(Mk)		
Kulfi (Indian Ice Cream)		(Cm)(Mk)		
Rasmalai (Cheese Balls in Sweet Cream)	(Ve)	(Ch)(Cm)		

Ensure no cross-contaminaton in food preparation. Food allergens vary depending upon type of accompaniment, garnish or side.

● Typically contains allergen   ○ May contain allergen

Corn
(Bo) Bouillon
(Cf) Colors or Flavors
(Ve) Vanilla Extract
(Vo) Vegetable Oil

Dairy
(Bu) Butter
(Ch) Cheese
(Cm) Cream, Sour Cream or Whipped Cream
(Mk) Milk or Buttermilk
(Yo) Yogurt, Curd or Sauce

Eggs
(E) Eggs

	Gluten/Wheat	Peanuts	Shellfish	Soy	Tree Nuts
Tandoor Specialties					
Boti Kabob (Skewered Lamb)	(Ss)(Wf)	(Po)(Vo)		(Ss)(Vo)	
Murg Tandoori (Tandoori Barbeque Chicken)	(Ss)(Wf)	(Po)(Vo)		(Ss)(Vo)	
Murg Tikka (Yogurt Marinated Chicken)	(Ss)(Wf)	(Po)(Vo)		(Cf)(Ss)(Vo)	
Seekh Kabob (Skewered Minced Lamb)	(Sa)			(Cf)	●Cw
Dosas (South Indian Specialties)					
Masala Dosa (Spicy Vegetable Filled Crepe)	(Bo)(Sa)(Wf)	(Po)(Vo)		(Bo)(Vo)	
Sada Dosa (Lentil and Rice Crepe)	(Bo)(Sa)(Wf)	(Po)(Vo)		(Bo)(Vo)	
Uthappam (Lentil and Rice Pancake)	(Bo)(Sa)(Wf)	(Po)(Vo)		(Bo)(Vo)	●Cw
Desserts					
Kheer (Rice Pudding)	(Wf)				●Al ●Cw ●Pi
Kulfi (Indian Ice Cream)	(Wf)				●T
Rasmalai (Cheese Balls in Sweet Cream)					●Al ●Cw ●Pi

11

Ensure no cross-contaminaton in food preparation. Food allergens vary depending upon type of accompaniment, garnish or side.

● Typically contains allergen   ○ May contain allergen

Gluten / Wheat
(Bo) Bouillon
(Sa) Sauce
(Ss) Soy Sauce
(Wf) Wheat Flour

Peanuts
(Po) Peanut Oil
(Vo) Vegetable Oil

Soy
(Bo) Bouillon
(Cf) Colors or Flavors
(Ss) Soy Sauce
(Vo) Vegetable Oil

Tree Nuts
(Al) Almonds or Almond Extract
(Cw) Cashews or Cashew Powder
(Pi) Pistachios
(T) Tree Nuts

Italian Cuisine: Starters, Soups and Salads

	Corn	Dairy	Eggs	Fish
Starters				
Calamari alla Griglia (Grilled Calamari)	(Ba)(Br)(Sa)(Vo)	(Br)(Sa)	(Ba)(Br)(Sa)	
Carpaccio di Manzo (Beef Carpaccio)	(Vo)	**(Ch)**		
Carpaccio di Salmone (Salmon Carpaccio)	(Vo)			**(Sl)**
Cocktail di Gamberi (Shrimp Cocktail)	(Bo)(Cs)		(Sa)	(St)
Cozze al Vapore (Steamed Mussels)	(Bo)(Br)	(Br)**(Bu)**	(Br)(No)	
Prosciutto e Melone (Cured Ham and Melon)		(Ch)(Pr)		
Soups				
Gazpaccio	(C)(Cr)	(Cr)	(Cr)	
Salads				
Insalata Caprese (Mozzarella Tomato Salad)	(Vo)	**(Ch)**		
Insalata Mista (Mixed Green Salad)	(Vo)		(Cr)	(An)

Ensure no cross-contaminaton in food preparation. Food allergens vary depending upon type of accompaniment, garnish or side.

● Typically contains allergen ○ May contain allergen

Corn	Dairy	Eggs	Fish
(Ba) Batter	(Br) Bread or Bread Crumbs	(Ba) Batter	(An) Anchovies
(Bo) Bouillon	(Bu) Butter	(Br) Bread or Bread Crumbs	(Sl) Salmon
(Br) Bread or Bread Crumbs	(Ch) Cheese	(Cr) Croutons	(St) Stock or Broth
(C) Corn	(Cr) Croutons	(No) Noodles or Pasta	
(Cr) Croutons	(Pr) Prosciutto	(Sa) Sauce	
(Cs) Corn Flour, Meal, Starch or Syrup	(Sa) Sauce		
(Sa) Sauce			
(Vo) Vegetable Oil			

	Gluten/Wheat	Peanuts	Shellfish	Soy	Tree Nuts
Starters					
Calamari alla Griglia (Grilled Calamari)	(Ba)(Br)(Fd)(Sa)	(Br)(Sa)(Vo)	● (Ca)	(Br)(Vo)	(Br)(Sa)
Carpaccio di Manzo (Beef Carpaccio)	(Ga)	(Vo)		(Vo)	
Carpaccio di Salmone (Salmon Carpaccio)	(Be)	(Vo)		(Vo)	
Cocktail di Gamberi (Shrimp Cocktail)	(Bo)		● (Sh)	(Bo)(Sa)	
Cozze al Vapore (Steamed Mussels)	(Bo)(Br)(No)	(Br)	● (Mu)	(Bo)(Br)	(Br)
Prosciutto e Melone (Cured Ham and Melon)					
Soups					
Gazpaccio	(Cr)(Wf)	(Cr)		(Cr)	(Cr)
Salads					
Insalata Caprese (Mozzarella Tomato Salad)		(Vo)		(Vo)	
Insalata Mista (Mixed Green Salad)	(Cr)(Ga)	(Vo)		(Vo)	

11

Ensure no cross-contaminaton in food preparation. Food allergens vary depending upon type of accompaniment, garnish or side.

● Typically contains allergen   ○ May contain allergen

Gluten / Wheat
(Ba) Batter
(Be) Beans
(Bo) Bouillon
(Br) Bread or Bread Crumbs
(Cr) Croutons
(Fd) Wheat Flour Dusting
(Ga) Garnish
(No) Noodles or Pasta
(Sa) Sauce
(Wf) Wheat Flour

Peanuts
(Br) Bread or Bread Crumbs
(Cr) Croutons
(Sa) Sauce
(Vo) Vegetable Oil

Shellfish
(Ca) Calamari
(Mu) Mussels
(Sh) Shrimp

Soy
(Bo) Bouillon
(Br) Bread or Bread Crumbs
(Cr) Croutons
(Sa) Sauce
(Vo) Vegetable Oil

Tree Nuts
(Br) Bread or Bread Crumbs
(Cr) Croutons
(Sa) Sauce

Italian Cuisine: Italian Specialities, Meat and Chicken Dishes

	Corn	Dairy	Eggs	Fish
Italian Specialties				
Risotto ai Frutti di Mare (Arborio Rice and Seafood Dish)	(Bo)(Vo)	(Bu)(Ch)		● F
Risotto ai Funghi (Arborio Rice and Mushroom Dish)	(Bo)(Vo)	(Bu)(Ch)		
Risotto ai Quattro Formaggi (Arborio Rice and Cheese Dish)	(Bo)(Vo)	(Bu)(Ch)		
Risotto al Pollo (Arborio Rice and Chicken Dish)	(Bo)(Vo)	(Bu)(Ch)		
Meat Dishes				
Costatella D'Agnello (Rack of Lamb)	(Br)(Vo)	(Br)	(Br)(No)	
Fileto di Manzo (Filet Mignon)	(Vo)	(Bu)	(No)	
Medalione di Manzo (Beef Tenderloin Medallions)	(Vo)	(Bu)(Sa)	(No)	
Vitello (Veal)	(Bd)(Br)(Vo)	(Bd)(Br)(Bu)(Ch)(Sa)	(Bd)(Br)(No)	
Chicken Dishes				
Petti di Pollo (Chicken Breast)	(Bd)(Br)(Vo)	(Bd)(Br)(Bu)(Ch)(Cm)(Sa)	(Bd)(Br)(No)	
Pollo Arrosto Rosmarino (Rosemary Roasted Chicken)	(Br)(Vo)	(Br)	(Br)(No)	

Ensure no cross-contaminaton in food preparation. Food allergens vary depending upon type of accompaniment, garnish or side.

● Typically contains allergen   ○ May contain allergen

Corn	**Dairy**	**Eggs**	**Fish**
(Bd) Breading	(Bd) Breading	(Bd) Breading	(F) Fish
(Bo) Bouillon	(Br) Bread or Bread Crumbs	(Br) Bread or Bread Crumbs	
(Br) Bread or Bread Crumbs	(Bu) Butter	(No) Noodles or Pasta	
(Vo) Vegetable Oil	(Ch) Cheese		
	(Cm) Cream, Sour Cream or Whipped Cream		
	(Sa) Sauce		

11

	Gluten/Wheat	Peanuts	Shellfish	Soy	Tree Nuts
Italian Specialties					
Risotto ai Frutti di Mare (Arborio Rice and Seafood Dish)	(Bo)(Cl)	(Vo)	● (Sf)	(Bo)(Vo)	
Risotto ai Funghi (Arborio Rice and Mushroom Dish)	(Bo)(Cl)	(Vo)		(Bo)(Vo)	
Risotto ai Quattro Formaggi (Arborio Rice and Cheese Dish)	(Bo)(Cl)	(Vo)		(Bo)(Vo)	
Risotto al Pollo (Arborio Rice and Chicken Dish)	(Bo)(Cl)	(Vo)		(Bo)(Vo)	
Meat Dishes					
Costatella D'Agnello (Rack of Lamb)	(Br)(Fd)(No)	(Br)(Vo)		(Br)(Vo)	(Br)
Fileto di Manzo (Filet Mignon)	(Fd)(No)	(Vo)		(Vo)	
Medalione di Manzo (Beef Tenderloin Medallions)	(Fd)(No)(Sa)	(Vo)		(Vo)	(Sa)
Vitello (Veal)	(Bd)(Br)(Fd)(No)(Sa)	(Br)(Vo)		(Bd)(Br)(Vo)	(Br)(Sa)
Chicken Dishes					
Petti di Pollo (Chicken Breast)	(Bd)(Br)(Fd)(No)(Sa)	(Br)(Vo)		(Bd)(Br)(Vo)	(Br)(Sa)
Pollo Arrosto Rosmarino (Rosemary Roasted Chicken)	(Br)(No)	(Br)(Vo)		(Br)(Vo)	(Br)

11

Ensure no cross-contaminaton in food preparation. Food allergens vary depending upon type of accompaniment, garnish or side.

● Typically contains allergen ◯ May contain allergen

Gluten / Wheat
(Bd) Breading
(Bo) Bouillon
(Br) Bread or Bread Crumbs
(Cl) Clean Water
(Fd) Wheat Flour Dusting
(No) Noodles or Pasta
(Sa) Sauce

Peanuts
(Br) Bread or Bread Crumbs
(Vo) Vegetable Oil

Shellfish
(Sf) Shellfish

Soy
(Bd) Breading
(Bo) Bouillon
(Br) Bread or Bread Crumbs
(Vo) Vegetable Oil

Tree Nuts
(Br) Bread or Bread Crumbs
(Sa) Sauce

Italian Cuisine: Seafood Dishes, Sides and Desserts

	Corn	Dairy	Eggs	Fish
Seafood Dishes				
Salmone alla Griglia (Grilled Salmon)	(Vo)	(Bu)(Sa)	(No)	**(Sl)**
Scampi (Prawns)	(Br)(Vo)	(Br)(Bu)(Ch)(Cm)(Sa)	(Br)(No)	
Sides				
Broccoli Rabe (Broccoli Florets)	(Vo)	(Bu)		
Funghi all' Aglio e Olio (Mushrooms in Garlic and Olive Oil)	(Br)(Vo)	(Br)(Bu)	(Br)	
Melanzane alla Griglia (Grilled Eggplant)	(Br)(Vo)	(Br)	(Br)	
Polenta (Boiled Corn Meal)	**(C)**(Vo)	(Bu)(Ch)(Sa)		
Desserts				
Gelato (Italian Ice Cream or Sherbet)	(Cf)	(Ck)**(D)**	(Cf)(Ck)	
Granita (Italian Ice)	(Cf)			
Zabaglione (Italian Custard)		(Ck)	(Ck)**(Ey)**	

Ensure no cross-contaminaton in food preparation. Food allergens vary depending upon type of accompaniment, garnish or side.

● Typically contains allergen   ○ May contain allergen

Corn	**Dairy**	**Eggs**	**Fish**
(Br) Bread or Bread Crumbs	(Br) Bread or Bread Crumbs	(Br) Bread or Bread Crumbs	(Sl) Salmon
(C) Corn	(Bu) Butter	(Cf) Colors or Flavors	
(Cf) Colors or Flavors	(Ch) Cheese	(Ck) Cake, Cookie or Biscuit	
(Vo) Vegetable Oil	(Ck) Cake, Cookie or Biscuit	(Ey) Egg Yolk	
	(Cm) Cream, Sour Cream or Whipped Cream	(No) Noodles or Pasta	
	(D) Dairy		
	(Sa) Sauce		

11

	Gluten/Wheat	Peanuts	Shellfish	Soy	Tree Nuts
Seafood Dishes					
Salmone alla Griglia (Grilled Salmon)	(No)(Sa)	(Vo)		(Vo)	(Sa)
Scampi (Prawns)	(Br)(No)(Sa)	(Br)(Vo)	● (Sh)	(Br)(Vo)	(Br)(Sa)
Sides					
Broccoli Rabe (Broccoli Florets)		(Vo)		(Vo)	
Funghi all' Aglio e Olio (Mushrooms in Garlic and Olive Oil)	(Br)(Wf)	(Br)(Vo)		(Br)(Vo)	(Br)
Melanzane alla Griglia (Grilled Eggplant)	(Br)(Fd)	(Br)(Vo)		(Br)(Vo)	(Br)
Polenta (Boiled Corn Meal)	(Df)(Sa)	(Vo)		(Vo)	(Sa)
Desserts					
Gelato (Italian Ice Cream or Sherbet)	(Ck)(Sb)	(Cf)(Ck)		(Cf)(Ck)	(Cf)(Ck)
Granita (Italian Ice)	(Mv)(Sb)			(Cf)	
Zabaglione (Italian Custard)	(Ck)	(Ck)		(Ck)	(Ck)

Ensure no cross-contaminaton in food preparation. Food allergens vary depending upon type of accompaniment, garnish or side.

● Typically contains allergen ○ May contain allergen

Gluten / Wheat
(Br) Bread or Bread Crumbs
(Ck) Cake, Cookie or Biscuit
(Df) Dedicated Fryer and/or Fresh Cooking Oil
(Fd) Wheat Flour Dusting
(Mv) Malt / Malt Vinegar
(No) Noodles or Pasta
(Sa) Sauce
(Sb) Stabilizers
(Wf) Wheat Flour

Peanuts
(Br) Bread or Bread Crumbs
(Cf) Colors or Flavors
(Ck) Cake, Cookie or Biscuit
(Vo) Vegetable Oil

Shellfish
(Sh) Shrimp

Soy
(Br) Bread or Bread Crumbs
(Cf) Colors or Flavors
(Ck) Cake, Cookie or Biscuit
(Vo) Vegetable Oil

Tree Nuts
(Br) Bread or Bread Crumbs
(Cf) Colors or Flavors
(Ck) Cake, Cookie or Biscuit
(Sa) Sauce

11

Mexican Cuisine: Starters, Soups and Salads

	Corn	Dairy	Eggs	Fish
Starters				
Ceviche (Raw Fish Salad)	(Tc)(Vo)			**(F)**
Chile con Queso (Chili Cheese Dip)	(Ch)(Tc)(Vo)	**(Bu)(Ch)**		
Guacamole (Avocado Dip)	(Tc)(Vo)			
Queso Fundido (Cheese Dip)	(Ch)(Tc)(Vo)	**(Bu)(Ch)**		
Tortillas y Salsa (Chips and Salsa)	(Sa)(Tc)(Vo)			
Soups				
Posole (Chili Corn Soup)	(Bo)**(C)**(Vo)			
Sopa Azteca (Lime Chicken Soup)	(Bo)(Ch)(Tc)(Vo)	**(Ch)(Cm)**		
Salads				
Ensalada (House Salad)	(Vo)			
Taco Salad	(Ch)(Sa)(Tc)(Vo)	**(Ch)(Cm)**		

Ensure no cross-contaminaton in food preparation. Food allergens vary depending upon type of accompaniment, garnish or side.

● Typically contains allergen   ○ May contain allergen

Corn	**Dairy**	**Fish**
(Bo) Bouillon	(Bu) Butter	(F) Fish
(C) Corn	(Ch) Cheese	
(Ch) Cheese	(Cm) Cream, Sour Cream or	
(Sa) Sauce	Whipped Cream	
(Tc) Tortillas or Tortilla Chips		
(Vo) Vegetable Oil		

11

	Gluten/Wheat	Peanuts	Shellfish	Soy	Tree Nuts
Starters					
Ceviche (Raw Fish Salad)	(Df)(Tc)	(Vo)	(Sf)	(Tc)(Vo)	
Chile con Queso (Chili Cheese Dip)	(Df)(Sa)(Tc)	(Vo)		(Ch)(Tc)(Vo)	
Guacamole (Avocado Dip)	(Df)(Tc)	(Vo)		(Tc)(Vo)	
Queso Fundido (Cheese Dip)	(Df)(Sa)(Tc)	(Vo)		(Ch)(Tc)(Vo)	
Tortillas y Salsa (Chips and Salsa)	(Df)(Sa)(Tc)	(Vo)		(Tc)(Vo)	
Soups					
Posole (Chili Corn Soup)	(Bo)(Wf)	(Vo)		(Bo)(Vo)	
Sopa Azteca (Lime Chicken Soup)	(Bo)(Df)(Tc)(Wf)	(Vo)		(Bo)(Ch)(Tc)(Vo)	
Salads					
Ensalada (House Salad)	(Ga)	(Vo)		(Vo)	
Taco Salad	(Be)(Df)(Sa)(Ss)(Tc)(Wf)	(Vo)		(Ch)(Ss)(Tc)(Vo)	

11

Ensure no cross-contaminaton in food preparation. Food allergens vary depending upon type of accompaniment, garnish or side.

● Typically contains allergen   ○ May contain allergen

Gluten / Wheat
- (Be) Beans
- (Bo) Bouillon
- (Df) Dedicated Fryer and/or Fresh Cooking Oil
- (Ga) Garnish
- (Sa) Sauce
- (Ss) Soy Sauce
- (Tc) Tortillas or Tortilla Chips
- (Wf) Wheat Flour

Peanuts
- (Vo) Vegetable Oil

Shellfish
- (Sf) Shellfish

Soy
- (Bo) Bouillon
- (Ch) Cheese
- (Ss) Soy Sauce
- (Tc) Tortillas or Tortilla Chips
- (Vo) Vegetable Oil

Mexican Cuisine: Egg Dishes and Antojos

	Corn	Dairy	Eggs	Fish
Egg Dishes				
Huevos Mexicanos (Mexican Eggs)	(Ch)(Sa)(Tc)(Vo)	(Bu)(Ch)	● E	
Huevos Rancheros (Ranch Style Eggs)	(Ch)(Sa)(Tc)(Vo)	(Bu)●Ch	● E	
Antojos (Mexican Specialties)				
Enchiladas	(Ch)(Tc)(Vo)	●Ch(Cm)	○ E	
Enfrijoladas	(Ch)(Sa)(Tc)(Vo)	●Ch●Cm	○ E	
Tacos	(Ch)(Sa)(Tc)(Vo)	●Ch●Cm		○ F
Tamales (Stuffed Corn Meal)	●Ms(Vo)			
Tostadas Compuestas (Filled Corn Tortillas)	(Ch)(Sa)(Tc)(Vo)	●Ch(Cm)		

11

Ensure no cross-contaminaton in food preparation. Food allergens vary depending upon type of accompaniment, garnish or side.

● Typically contains allergen ○ May contain allergen

Corn
(Ch) Cheese
(Ms) Masa
(Sa) Sauce
(Tc) Tortillas or Tortilla Chips
(Vo) Vegetable Oil

Dairy
(Bu) Butter
(Ch) Cheese
(Cm) Cream, Sour Cream or Whipped Cream

Eggs
(E) Eggs

Fish
(F) Fish

	Gluten/Wheat	Peanuts	Shellfish	Soy	Tree Nuts
Egg Dishes					
Huevos Mexicanos (Mexican Eggs)	(Be)(Df)(Sa)(Tc)	(Vo)		(Ch)(Tc)(Vo)	
Huevos Rancheros (Ranch Style Eggs)	(Be)(Df)(Sa)(Tc)	(Vo)		(Ch)(Tc)(Vo)	
Antojos (Mexican Specialties)					
Enchiladas	(Df)(Sa)(Tc)	(Sa)(Vo)		(Ch)(Sa)(Tc)(Vo)	(Sa)
Enfrijoladas	(Df)(Sa)(Tc)	(Vo)		(Ch)(Tc)(Vo)	
Tacos	(Df)(Sa)(Tc)	(Vo)	(Sf)	(Ch)(Tc)(Vo)	
Tamales (Stuffed Corn Meal)	(Sa)	(Vo)		(Ms)(Vo)	
Tostadas Compuestas (Filled Corn Tortillas)	(Be)(Df)(Sa)(Ss)(Tc)(Wf)	(Vo)		(Ch)(Ss)(Tc)(Vo)	

Ensure no cross-contaminaton in food preparation. Food allergens vary depending upon type of accompaniment, garnish or side.

● Typically contains allergen ◯ May contain allergen

11

Gluten / Wheat
(Be) Beans
(Df) Dedicated Fryer and/or Fresh Cooking Oil
(Sa) Sauce
(Ss) Soy Sauce
(Tc) Tortillas or Tortilla Chips
(Wf) Wheat Flour

Peanuts
(Sa) Sauce
(Vo) Vegetable Oil

Shellfish
(Sf) Shellfish

Soy
(Ch) Cheese
(Ms) Masa
(Ss) Soy Sauce
(Sa) Sauce
(Tc) Tortillas or Tortilla Chips
(Vo) Vegetable Oil

Tree Nuts
(Sa) Sauce

Mexican Cuisine: Meat, Chicken and Turkey Dishes

	Corn	Dairy	Eggs	Fish
Meat Dishes				
Arracheras (Flank or Skirt Steak)	(Ch)(Sa)(Tc)(Vo)	(Ch)		
Bistek (Steak)	(Ch)(Sa)(Vo)	(Ch)		
Carne Asada (Broiled Beef)	(Ch)(Sa)(Tc)(Vo)	(Ch)		
Carnitas (Simmered Pork)	(Ch)(Sa)(Tc)(Vo)	(Ch)		
Machaca (Shredded Beef)	(Ch)(Sa)(Tc)(Vo)	(Ch)		
Chicken and Turkey Dishes				
Mole	(Ch)(Tc)(Vo)	(Ch)		
Pechuga de Pollo (Chicken Breast)	(Ch)(Sa)(Tc)(Vo)	(Ch)		
Pollo Asado (Broiled Chicken)	(Ch)(Sa)(Tc)(Vo)	(Ch)		

Ensure no cross-contaminaton in food preparation. Food allergens vary depending upon type of accompaniment, garnish or side.

● Typically contains allergen   ○ May contain allergen

Corn
(Ch) Cheese
(Sa) Sauce
(Tc) Tortillas or Tortilla Chips
(Vo) Vegetable Oil

Dairy
(Ch) Cheese

11

	Gluten/Wheat	Peanuts	Shellfish	Soy	Tree Nuts
Meat Dishes					
Arracheras (Flank or Skirt Steak)	(Be)(Sa)(Ss)(Tc)(Wf)	(Vo)		(Ch)(Ss)(Tc)(Vo)	
Bistek (Steak)	(Be)(Df)(Sa)(Ss)(Wf)	(Vo)		(Ch)(Ss)(Vo)	
Carne Asada (Broiled Beef)	(Be)(Sa)(Ss)(Tc)(Wf)	(Vo)		(Ch)(Ss)(Tc)(Vo)	
Carnitas (Simmered Pork)	(Be)(Sa)(Tc)	(Vo)		(Ch)(Tc)(Vo)	
Machaca (Shredded Beef)	(Be)(Sa)(Tc)	(Vo)		(Ch)(Tc)(Vo)	
Chicken and Turkey Dishes					
Mole	(Be)(Sa)(Tc)	(Sa)(Vo)		(Ch)(Sa)(Tc)(Vo)	(Sa)
Pechuga de Pollo (Chicken Breast)	(Be)(Sa)(Ss)(Tc)(Wf)	(Vo)		(Ch)(Ss)(Tc)(Vo)	
Pollo Asado (Broiled Chicken)	(Be)(Sa)(Ss)(Tc)(Wf)	(Vo)		(Ch)(Ss)(Tc)(Vo)	

11

Ensure no cross-contaminaton in food preparation. Food allergens vary depending upon type of accompaniment, garnish or side.

● Typically contains allergen   ○ May contain allergen

Gluten / Wheat
(Be) Beans
(Df) Dedicated Fryer and/or Fresh Cooking Oil
(Sa) Sauce
(Ss) Soy Sauce
(Tc) Tortillas or Tortilla Chips
(Wf) Wheat Flour

Peanuts
(Sa) Sauce
(Vo) Vegetable Oil

Soy
(Ch) Cheese
(Sa) Sauce
(Ss) Soy Sauce
(Tc) Tortillas or Tortilla Chips
(Vo) Vegetable Oil

Tree Nuts
(Sa) Sauce

Mexican Cuisine: Seafood Dishes, Sides and Desserts

	Corn	Dairy	Eggs	Fish
Seafood Dishes				
Langosta (Lobster)	(Bo)(Sa)(Tc)(Vo)	(Bu)		(St)
Paella Mariscos (Seafood and Rice)	(Bo)(Vo)			●F
Sides				
Arroz (Rice)	(Bo)(Vo)			
Frijoles (Beans)	(Ch)(Vo)	(Ch)		
Desserts				
Arroz con Leche (Rice Pudding)	(Ve)	●Cm ●Mk	●E	
Flan (Custard)	(Sa)(Ve)	●Cm	●E	
Helados (Ice Cream, Sherbet or Sorbet)	(Cf)(Sa)	(Cc)(Ck)(D)	(Ck)	

11

Ensure no cross-contaminaton in food preparation. Food allergens vary depending upon type of accompaniment, garnish or side.

● Typically contains allergen   ○ May contain allergen

Corn	**Dairy**	**Eggs**	**Fish**
(Bo) Bouillon	(Bu) Butter	(Ck) Cake, Cookie or Biscuit	(F) Fish
(Cf) Colors or Flavors	(Cc) Chocolate	(E) Eggs	(St) Stock or Broth
(Ch) Cheese	(Ch) Cheese		
(Sa) Sauce	(Ck) Cake, Cookie or Biscuit		
(Tc) Tortillas or Tortilla Chips	(Cm) Cream, Sour Cream or Whipped Cream		
(Ve) Vanilla Extract	(D) Dairy		
(Vo) Vegetable Oil	(Mk) Milk or Buttermilk		

	Gluten/ Wheat	Peanuts	Shellfish	Soy	Tree Nuts
Seafood Dishes					
Langosta (Lobster)	(Bo)(Sa)(Tc)	(Vo)	●(St)	(Bo)(Tc)(Vo)	
Paella Mariscos (Seafood and Rice)	(Bo)	(Vo)	●	(Bo)(Vo)	
Sides					
Arroz (Rice)	(Bo)(Cl)	(Vo)		(Bo)(Vo)	
Frijoles (Beans)	(Be)	(Vo)		(Ch)(Vo)	
Desserts					
Arroz con Leche (Rice Pudding)	(Cl)				
Flan (Custard)	(Wf)				
Helados (Ice Cream, Sherbet or Sorbet)	(Ck)(Mv)(Sb)(Wf)	(Cf)(Ck)		(Cc)(Cf)(Ck)	(Cf)(Ck)

Ensure no cross-contaminaton in food preparation. Food allergens vary depending upon type of accompaniment, garnish or side.

● Typically contains allergen ○ May contain allergen

Gluten / Wheat
(Be) Beans
(Bo) Bouillon
(Ck) Cake, Cookie or Biscuit
(Cl) Clean Water
(Mv) Malt / Malt Vinegar
(Sa) Sauce
(Sb) Stabilizers
(Tc) Tortillas or Tortilla Chips
(Wf) Wheat Flour

Peanuts
(Cf) Colors or Flavors
(Ck) Cake, Cookie or Biscuit
(Vo) Vegetable Oil

Shellfish
(Lo) Lobster
(Sf) Shellfish
(St) Stock or Broth

Soy
(Bo) Bouillon
(Cc) Chocolate
(Cf) Colors or Flavors
(Ch) Cheese
(Ck) Cake, Cookie or Biscuit
(Tc) Tortillas or Tortilla Chip
(Vo) Vegetable Oil

Tree Nuts
(Cf) Colors or Flavors
(Ck) Cake, Cookie or Biscuit

11

Thai Cuisine: Starters and Soups

	Corn	Dairy	Eggs	Fish
Starters				
Kanom Jeeb (Shrimp Dumplings)	(Vo)		(Ds)(Eg)	● Fs
Satay (Skewered Beef, Chicken or Shrimp)				● Fs
Som Tam (Papaya Salad)				● Fs
Summer Rolls	(Bo)			(Fs)
Soups				
Tom Kha Gai (Chicken and Coconut Soup)	(Bo)			(Fs)
Tom Yum Groong (Spicy Shrimp Soup)	(Bo)			● Fs

Ensure no cross-contaminaton in food preparation. Food allergens vary depending upon type of accompaniment, garnish or side.

● Typically contains allergen   ○ May contain allergen

11

Corn	**Eggs**	**Fish**
(Bo) Bouillon	(Ds) Dumpling Skin	(Fs) Fish Sauce
(Vo) Vegetable Oil	(Eg) Egg Sealer	

	Gluten/ Wheat	Peanuts	Shellfish	Soy	Tree Nuts
Starters					
Kanom Jeeb (Shrimp Dumplings)	(Fs)(Sa)(Ss)(Wf)	(Vo)	(Sh)	(Ss)(Vo)	
Satay (Skewered Beef, Chicken or Shrimp)	(Fs)(Sa)(Ss)(Wf)	(Sa)	(Sh)	(Ss)	
Som Tam (Papaya Salad)	(Fs)(Ss)	(P)	(Sh)	(Ss)	(Ga)
Summer Rolls	(Bo)(Fs)(Sa)(Se)(Wf)	(Sa)		(Bo)(Ss)	
Soups					
Tom Kha Gai (Chicken and Coconut Soup)	(Bo)(Fs)(Ss)	(Ga)		(Bo)(Ss)	(Ga)
Tom Yum Groong (Spicy Shrimp Soup)	(Bo)(Fs)(Ss)	(Ga)	(Sh)	(Bo)(Ss)	(Ga)

Ensure no cross-contaminaton in food preparation. Food allergens vary depending upon type of accompaniment, garnish or side.

● Typically contains allergen   ○ May contain allergen

Gluten / Wheat
(Bo) Bouillon
(Fs) Fish Sauce
(Sa) Sauce
(Se) Seasonings
(Ss) Soy Sauce
(Wf) Wheat Flour

Peanuts
(Ga) Garnish
(P) Peanuts
(Sa) Sauce
(Vo) Vegetable Oil

Shellfish
(Sh) Shrimp

Soy
(Bo) Bouillon
(Ss) Soy Sauce
(Vo) Vegetable Oil

Tree Nuts
(Ga) Garnish

11

Thai Cuisine: Noodle & Rice Dishes and Curries

	Corn	Dairy	Eggs	Fish
Noodle and Rice Dishes				
Kaw Pad (Thai Fried Rice)	(Vo)		● E	(Fs)
Pad See Yu	(Vo)		● E (No)	(Fs)
Pad Thai	(Vo)		● E (No)	(Fs)
Sticky Rice				
Curries (Kang)				
Kang Dang or Malay (Red Curry)	(Vo)		(Ba)	(Fs)
Kang Khiao Wan (Green Curry)	(Vo)		(Ba)	(Fs)
Kang Massaman (Tamarind Curry)	(Vo)		(Ba)	(Fs)
Kang Panang (Peanut Curry)	(Vo)		(Ba)	(Fs)

Ensure no cross-contaminaton in food preparation. Food allergens vary depending upon type of accompaniment, garnish or side.

● Typically contains allergen ○ May contain allergen

Corn
(Vo) Vegetable Oil

Eggs
(Ba) Batter
(E) Eggs
(No) Noodles or Pasta

Fish
(Fs) Fish Sauce

11

	Gluten/Wheat	Peanuts	Shellfish	Soy	Tree Nuts
Noodle and Rice Dishes					
Kaw Pad (Thai Fried Rice)	(Fs)(Ss)	(Ga)(Po)(Vo)	(Sh)	(Bc)(Ss)(Vo)	(Ga)
Pad See Yu	(Fs)(Sa)(Ss)(Wf)	(Ga)(Po)(Vo)		(Sa)(Ss)(Vo)	(Ga)
Pad Thai	(Fs)(Sa)(Ss)(Wf)	(Ga)(Po)(Vo)	(Sh)	(Bc)(Sa)(Ss)(Vo)	(Ga)
Sticky Rice	(Cl)				
Curries (Kang)					
Kang Dang or Malay (Red Curry)	(Ba)(Fd)(Fs)(Ss)	(Ga)(Po)(Vo)	(Sh)	(Ss)(Vo)	(Ga)
Kang Khiao Wan (Green Curry)	(Ba)(Fd)(Fs)(Ss)	(Ga)(Po)(Vo)	(Sh)	(Ss)(Vo)	(Ga)
Kang Massaman (Tamarind Curry)	(Ba)(Fd)(Fs)(Ss)	(P)(Po)(Vo)	(Sh)	(Ss)(Vo)	(Ga)
Kang Panang (Peanut Curry)	(Ba)(Fd)(Fs)(Ss)	(P)(Po)(Vo)	(Sh)	(Ss)(Vo)	(Ga)

Ensure no cross-contaminaton in food preparation. Food allergens vary depending upon type of accompaniment, garnish or side.

● Typically contains allergen   ○ May contain allergen

Gluten / Wheat
(Ba) Batter
(Cl) Clean Water
(Fd) Wheat Flour Dusting
(Fs) Fish Sauce
(Sa) Sauce
(Ss) Soy Sauce
(Wf) Wheat Flour

Peanuts
(Ga) Garnish
(P) Peanuts
(Po) Peanut Oil
(Vo) Vegetable Oil

Shellfish
(Sh) Shrimp

Soy
(Bc) Bean Curd
(Sa) Sauce
(Ss) Soy Sauce
(Vo) Vegetable Oil

Tree Nuts
(Ga) Garnish

11

Thai Cuisine: Dishes (Beef, Chicken, Seafood) and Desserts

	Corn	Dairy	Eggs	Fish
Beef Dishes				
Braised Beef Short Ribs				(Fs)
Chicken Dishes				
Gai Yang (Thai Barbeque Chicken)				● Fs
Seafood Dishes				
Pla Rad Prik (Crispy Whole Fish)	(Cs)(Vo)			● F
Desserts				
Fresh Tropical Fruits		(Ck)	(Ck)	
Sweet Sticky Rice				
Tropical Fruit Sorbets	(Cf)	(Cf)(Ck)	(Cf)(Ck)	

Ensure no cross-contaminaton in food preparation. Food allergens vary depending upon type of accompaniment, garnish or side.

● Typically contains allergen ◯ May contain allergen

Corn	**Dairy**	**Eggs**	**Fish**
(Cf) Colors or Flavors	(Cf) Colors or Flavors	(Cf) Colors or Flavors	(F) Fish
(Cs) Corn Flour, Meal, Starch or Syrup	(Ck) Cake, Cookie or Biscuit	(Ck) Cake, Cookie or Biscuit	(Fs) Fish Sauce
(Vo) Vegetable Oil			

11

	Gluten/Wheat	Peanuts	Shellfish	Soy	Tree Nuts
Beef Dishes					
Braised Beef Short Ribs	(Fs)(Ss)(Wf)	(Ga)		(Ss)	(Ga)
Chicken Dishes					
Gai Yang (Thai Barbeque Chicken)	(Fs)(Sa)(Ss)(Wf)			(Ss)	
Seafood Dishes					
Pla Rad Prik (Crispy Whole Fish)	(Fd)(Fs)(Ss)	(Po)(Vo)		(Ss)(Vo)	
Desserts					
Fresh Tropical Fruits	(Ck)	(Ck)		(Ck)	(Ck)
Sweet Sticky Rice	(Cl)				
Tropical Fruit Sorbets	(Cf)(Ck)(Sb)	(Ck)		(Cf)(Ck)	(Ck)

11

Ensure no cross-contaminaton in food preparation. Food allergens vary depending upon type of accompaniment, garnish or side.

● Typically contains allergen   ○ May contain allergen

Gluten / Wheat	**Peanuts**	**Soy**	**Tree Nuts**
(Cf) Colors or Flavors	(Ck) Cake, Cookie or Biscuit	(Cf) Colors or Flavors	(Ck) Cake, Cookie or Biscuit
(Ck) Cake, Cookie or Biscuit	(Ga) Garnish	(Ck) Cake, Cookie or Biscuit	(Ga) Garnish
(Cl) Clean Water	(Po) Peanut Oil	(Ss) Soy Sauce	
(Fd) Wheat Flour Dusting	(Vo) Vegetable Oil	(Vo) Vegetable Oil	
(Fs) Fish Sauce			
(Sa) Sauce			
(Sb) Stabilizers			
(Ss) Soy Sauce			
(Wf) Wheat Flour			

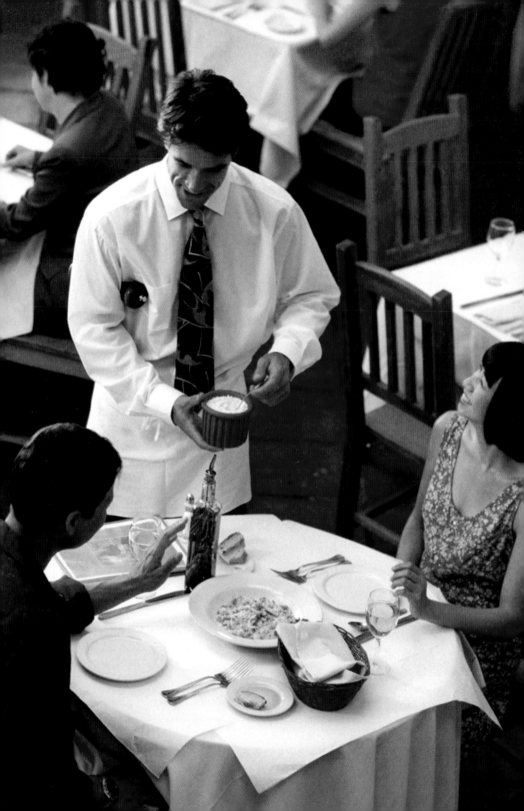

What the caterpillar calls the end of the world,
the master calls a butterfly.
—Richard Bach

Chapter 12

Gluten-Free Preparation Checklists

Chapter Overview

The gluten-free preparation checklists represent each of the seven international cuisines detailed in this book including:

12

- American Steak and Seafood

- Chinese

- French

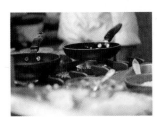

- Indian

- Italian

- Mexican

- Thai

The checklists have been designed to assist in simplifying the ordering process between guests and restaurants by quickly identifying the questions to ask to ensure that meals are gluten/wheat-free. They allow guests to walk into any restaurant that serves these cuisines, scan the menu and quickly spot the safest gluten/wheat-free choices. Restaurants can use the checklists to identify potential ingredients and hidden food allergens in various menu items.

These are intended to refresh your memory, providing you with quick and easy access to the detailed information outlined in each of the cuisine chapters for safe gluten/wheat-free eating anywhere.

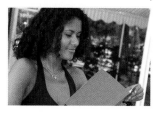

Gluten-Free Preparation Checklist Descriptions

The checklists are organized by sample menu items and highlight areas that you need to ensure are safe from gluten-containing ingredients and food preparation techniques that may affect your needs.

These ingredients and techniques are categorized into the following primary key concerns:

- Battering and Breading
- Bread, Bread Crumbs & Croutons
- Cooking Oil
- Dosas
- Flour Dusting
- Ingredients
- Malt Vinegar

- Marinades
- Noodles and Dumplings
- Pastas
- Sauces
- Stocks and Broths
- Tortillas
- Other

At first, the level of detail may seem overwhelming and complex. Keep in mind that every effort has been made to incorporate both traditional and non-traditional culinary practices which may vary by country and/or geographic region. The preparation checklists are designed to be as thorough as possible while taking into consideration cultural variations to ensure safe eating anywhere.

On the next page, key concerns associated with each of the 7 cuisines are further detailed in an easy-to-follow format. Guests and eating establishments need to ensure that each menu item is prepared gluten/wheat-free and safe to eat.

12

Gluten-Free Preparation Checklist Key

(Am) Ensure no artificial mashed potato mix

(Ba) Ensure no wheat flour in batter—request plain

(Bb) Ensure no artificial bacon bits

(Bd) Ensure no wheat flour in breading—request plain or gluten-free

(Bo) Ensure no packaged bouillon

(Br) Ensure no bun or bread crumbs

(Cf) Ensure no gluten in artificial colors or flavors

(Ck) Ensure no gluten in cake, cookie or biscuit

(Cl) Ensure clean water is used to cook rice

(Cr) Ensure no croutons

(Df) Ensure dedicated fryer

(Dr) Ensure no gluten in salad dressing

(Fd) Ensure no dusting with wheat flour

(Fo) Ensure fresh cooking oil

(Fs) Ensure no wheat in fish sauce

(Ga) Ensure no gluten-containing garnish

(Ic) Ensure no imitation crabmeat or seafood

(Ma) Ensure no wheat flour in marinade

(Mv) Ensure no malt or malt vinegar

(No) Ensure no wheat flour in noodles or pasta—request gluten-free

(Sa) Ensure no wheat flour in sauce

(Sb) Ensure no gluten in stabilizers

(Se) Ensure no gluten in packaged seasonings

(Ss) Ensure no soy sauce

(Tc) Ensure no wheat flour tortillas or tortilla chips

(Th) Ensure no wheat flour as thickening agent

(Wf) Ensure no wheat flour as ingredient

12

American Steak & Seafood: Starters, Soups, Salads and Meat Dishes

	Sauces	Flour Dusting	Stocks & Broths	Cooking Oil	Bread, Bread Crumbs & Croutons	Marinades	Ingredients	Other
Starters								
Oysters on the Half Shell	(Sa)		(Bo)					
Shrimp Cocktail			(Bo)					
Soups								
Bisque (Cream Soup)			(Bo)(Th)		(Cr)(Ga)			(Ic)
Salads								
Buffalo Mozzarella and Tomato Salad								
Chopped Salad	(Dr)				(Cr)(Ga)			(Bb)
Cobb Salad	(Dr)				(Cr)(Ga)			(Bb)
Hearts of Palm Salad								
Mixed Green Salad	(Dr)				(Cr)(Ga)			(Bb)
Meat Dishes								
Hamburgers		(Fd)		(Df)	(Br)			(Se)
Pork Chops	(Sa)	(Fd)				(Ss)(Wf)		
Lamb Chops	(Sa)	(Fd)			(Br)	(Ss)(Wf)		
Steaks	(Sa)	(Fd)				(Ss)(Wf)		

(Bb) Ensure no artificial bacon bits
(Bo) Ensure no packaged bouillon
(Br) Ensure no bun or bread crumbs
(Cr) Ensure no croutons
(Dr) Ensure no gluten in salad dressing

(Fd) Ensure no dusting with wheat flour
(Ga) Ensure no gluten-containing garnish
(Ic) Ensure no imitation crabmeat or seafood
(Sa) Ensure no wheat flour in sauce

(Se) Ensure no gluten in packaged seasonings
(Ss) Ensure no soy sauce
(Th) Ensure no wheat flour as thickening agent
(Wf) Ensure no wheat flour as ingredient

12

American Steak & Seafood: Chicken & Seafood Dishes and Sides

	Sauces	Flour Dusting	Stocks & Broths	Cooking Oil	Bread, Bread Crumbs & Croutons	Marinades	Ingredients	Other
Chicken Dishes								
Grilled Chicken Breast	(Sa)	(Fd)				(Ss)(Wf)		
Roasted Chicken	(Sa)	(Fd)				(Ss)(Wf)		
Seafood Dishes								
Crab			(Bo)		(Br)			
Fish Filet	(Sa)	(Fd)	(Bo)					(Ba)
Lobster			(Bo)		(Br)			
Sides								
Asparagus	(Sa)							
Baked Potato	(Sa)							(Bb)
Broccoli	(Sa)							
French Fried Potatoes		(Fd)		(Df)				(Se)
Green Beans	(Sa)							
Hash Browns								(Se)(Wf)
Mashed Potatoes							(Wf)	(Am)
Potatoes Lyonnaise							(Wf)	
Spinach							(Wf)	

12

(Am) Ensure no artificial mashed potato mix

(Ba) Ensure no wheat flour in batter—request plain

(Bb) Ensure no artificial bacon bits

(Bo) Ensure no packaged bouillon

(Br) Ensure no bun or bread crumbs

(Df) Ensure dedicated fryer

(Fd) Ensure no dusting with wheat flour

(Sa) Ensure no wheat flour in sauce

(Se) Ensure no gluten in packaged seasonings

(Ss) Ensure no soy sauce

(Wf) Ensure no wheat flour as ingredient

American Steak & Seafood: Desserts

Desserts	Sauces	Flour Dusting	Stocks & Broths	Cooking Oil	Bread, Bread Crumbs & Croutons	Marinades	Ingredients	Other
Chocolate Mousse							(Wf)	(Cf) (Ck)
Crème Brulée (Baked Custard)							(Wf)	(Ck)
Flourless Chocolate Torte		(Fd)			(Br)		(Wf)	
Fresh Berries with Whipped Cream								(Ck)
Ice Cream							(Mv) (Wf)	(Cf) (Ck) (Sb)
Sorbet							(Wf)	(Ck) (Sb)

(Br) Ensure no bun or bread crumbs
(Cf) Ensure no gluten in artificial colors or flavors

(Ck) Ensure no gluten in cake, cookie or biscuit
(Fd) Ensure no dusting with wheat flour
(Mv) Ensure no malt or malt vinegar

(Sb) Ensure no gluten in stabilizers
(Wf) Ensure no wheat flour as ingredient

12

Chinese Cuisine: Soups, Dishes (Chicken, Seafood, Vegetarian, Rice) and Desserts

	Sauces	Flour Dusting	Stocks & Broths	Cooking Oil	Noodles & Dumplings	Battering	Other
Soups							
Egg Drop Soup	(Ss)		(Bo)(Th)		(No)		
Sizzling Rice Soup	(Ss)		(Bo)(Th)		(No)		(Cl)
Chicken Dishes							
Lemon Chicken	(Ss)	(Fd)	(Bo)	(Fo)		(Ba)	
Steamed Chicken and Broccoli	(Ss)						
Seafood Dishes							
Steamed Fish	(Ss)						
Vegetarian Dishes							
Buddha's Feast	(Ss)		(Bo)				
Rice Dishes							
Steamed Rice							(Cl)
Desserts							
Fresh Tropical Fruits							(Ck)

(Ba) Ensure no wheat flour in batter—request plain

(Bo) Ensure no packaged bouillon

(Ck) Ensure no gluten in cake, cookie or biscuit

(Cl) Ensure clean water is used to cook rice

(Fd) Ensure no dusting with wheat flour

(Fo) Ensure fresh cooking oil

(No) Ensure no wheat flour in noodles or pasta—request gluten-free

(Ss) Ensure no soy sauce

(Th) Ensure no wheat flour as thickening agent

12

French Cuisine: Starters, Soups and Salads

	Sauces	Flour Dusting	Stocks & Broths	Cooking Oil	Bread, Bread Crumbs & Croutons	Malt Vinegar	Other
Starters							
Crevette Cocktail (Shrimp Cocktail)	(Sa)		(Bo)				
Escargot (Snails)					(Br)		
Foies Gras (Fat Liver)					(Br)		
Les Huîtres (Oysters on the Half Shell)	(Sa)		(Bo)				
Steak Tartare (Beef Tartar)					(Br)		
Tartare de Saumon (Salmon Tartar)							
Soups							
Bisque (Cream Soup)			(Bo)(Th)		(Cr)(Ga)		(Ic)
Vichyssoise (Potato Leek Soup)			(Bo)(Th)				
Salads							
Artichauts à la Vinaigrette (Artichoke Salad)							
Asperge à la Vinaigrette (Asparagus Salad)							
Mesclun de Salade (Mixed Green Salad)					(Cr)(Ga)		
Salade Niçoise (Nice Style Salad)					(Cr)(Ga)		

(Bo) Ensure no packaged bouillon

(Br) Ensure no bun or bread crumbs

(Cr) Ensure no croutons

(Ga) Ensure no gluten-containing garnish

(Ic) Ensure no imitation crabmeat or seafood

(Sa) Ensure no wheat flour in sauce

(Th) Ensure no wheat flour as thickening agent

12

French Cuisine: Dishes (Egg, Beef, Chicken, Seafood)

	Sauces	Flour Dusting	Stocks & Broths	Cooking Oil	Bread, Bread Crumbs & Croutons	Malt Vinegar	Other
Egg Dishes							
Les Oeufs (Fried Eggs)				(Fo)			
Les Omelettes (Omelets)				(Fo)			(Wf)
Beef Dishes							
Filet de Boeuf (Beef Filet)	(Sa)	(Fd)			(Bd)		
Fondue Bourguignon (Beef Fondue)	(Sa)	(Fd)					
Steak au Poivre (Peppered Steak)	(Sa)	(Fd)					
Steak Frites (Steak and French Fried Potatoes)	(Sa)	(Fd)		(Df)		(Mv)	
Chicken Dishes							
Poulet Provençal (Roasted Chicken with Herbs)							(Ma)(Ss)
Seafood Dishes							
Bouillabaisse (Seafood Stew)			(Bo)(Th)		(Br)(Cr)		
Moules Frites (Mussels and French Fried Potatoes)	(Sa)	(Fd)	(Bo)	(Df)	(Br)	(Mv)	
Saumon en Papillote (Baked Salmon)		(Fd)					

(Bd) Ensure no wheat flour in breading—request plain or gluten-free

(Bo) Ensure no packaged bouillon

(Br) Ensure no bun or bread crumbs

(Cr) Ensure no croutons

(Df) Ensure dedicated fryer

(Fd) Ensure no dusting with wheat flour

(Fo) Ensure fresh cooking oil

(Ma) Ensure no wheat flour in marinade

(Mv) Ensure no malt or malt vinegar

(Sa) Ensure no wheat flour in sauce

(Ss) Ensure no soy sauce

(Th) Ensure no wheat flour as thickening agent

(Wf) Ensure no wheat flour as ingredient

12

French Cuisine: Sides and Desserts

	Sauces	Flour Dusting	Stocks & Broths	Cooking Oil	Bread, Bread Crumbs & Croutons	Malt Vinegar	Other
Sides							
Gratin Dauphinois (Creamed Potatoes)					(Br)		(Wf)
Haricots Verts (French Green Beans)	(Sa)						
Pommes Frites (French Fried Potatoes)		(Fd)		(Df)		(Mv)	
Ratatouille (Vegetable Stew)			(Bo)				(Wf)
Desserts							
Assiette de Fromage (Cheese Plate)					(Br)		
Crème Brulée (Baked Custard)							(Ck)(Wf)
Fruits à la Crème (Fresh Fruit with Cream)							(Ck)
Mousse au Chocolat (Chocolate Mousse)							(Ck)(Wf)
Les Sorbets (Sorbet)							(Ck)(Sb)(Wf)

(Bo) Ensure no packaged bouillon
(Br) Ensure no bun or bread crumbs
(Ck) Ensure no gluten in cake, cookie or biscuit
(Df) Ensure dedicated fryer
(Fd) Ensure no dusting with wheat flour
(Mv) Ensure no malt or malt vinegar
(Sa) Ensure no wheat flour in sauce
(Sb) Ensure no gluten in stabilizers
(Wf) Ensure no wheat flour as ingredient

12

Indian Cuisine: Starters, Soups and Salads

	Sauces	Stocks & Broths	Cooking Oil	Bread & Dosas	Marinades	Other
Starters						
Aloo Tikki (Potato Patty)	(Sa)					(Wf)
Kabobs (Skewered Meat)	(Sa)					(Ss)(Wf)
Pakoras (Vegetable Fritters)	(Sa)					(Wf)
Papadam (Spicy Crackers)	(Sa)					(Wf)
Soups						
Curried Coconut Soup		(Th)				
Mulligatawny (Chicken and Vegetable Soup)		(Bo)(Th)				
Sambar (Lentil and Vegetable Stew)		(Bo)(Th)		(Wf)		
Salads						
Kachumber (Chopped Salad)						

(Bo) Ensure no packaged bouillon
(Sa) Ensure no wheat flour in sauce

(Ss) Ensure no soy sauce
(Th) Ensure no wheat flour as thickening agent

(Wf) Ensure no wheat flour as ingredient

12

Indian Cuisine: Curry Dishes and Tandoor Specialities

	Sauces	Stocks & Broths	Cooking Oil	Bread & Dosas	Marinades	Other
Curry Dishes						
Channa Masala (Chickpeas in Tomato Curry)	(Sa)	(Bo)				
Gosht Vindaloo (Spicy Lamb Curry)	(Sa)				(Ss)(Wf)	
Jhinga Masala (Shrimp in Coconut Curry)	(Sa)					
Malai Kofta (Vegetarian Croquettes in Mild Curry)	(Sa)					(Fd)(Wf)
Murg Korma (Chicken in Cream Curry)	(Sa)					
Murg Tikki Masala (Chicken in Tomato Curry)	(Sa)				(Ss)(Wf)	
Rogan Josh (Mild Lamb Curry)	(Sa)				(Ss)(Wf)	
Saag Paneer (Indian Cheese and Spinach Curry)	(Sa)					
Tandoor Specialties						
Boti Kabob (Skewered Lamb)					(Ss)(Wf)	
Murg Tandoori (Tandoori Barbeque Chicken)					(Ss)(Wf)	
Murg Tikka (Yogurt Marinated Chicken)					(Ss)(Wf)	
Seekh Kabob (Skewered Minced Lamb)	(Sa)					

(Bo) Ensure no packaged bouillon   (Sa) Ensure no wheat flour in sauce   (Wf) Ensure no wheat flour as ingredient
(Fd) Ensure no dusting with wheat flour   (Ss) Ensure no soy sauce

12

Indian Cuisine: Dosas and Desserts

	Sauces	Stocks & Broths	Cooking Oil	Bread & Dosas	Marinades	Other
Dosas (South Indian Specialties)						
Masala Dosa (Spicy Vegetable Filled Crepe)	(Sa)	(Bo)				(Wf)
Sada Dosa (Lentil and Rice Crepe)	(Sa)	(Bo)				(Wf)
Uthappam (Lentil and Rice Pancake)	(Sa)	(Bo)				(Wf)
Desserts						
Kheer (Rice Pudding)						(Wf)
Kulfi (Indian Ice Cream)						(Wf)
Rasmalai (Cheese Balls in Sweet Cream)						

(Bo) Ensure no packaged bouillon   (Sa) Ensure no wheat flour in sauce   (Wf) Ensure no wheat flour as ingredient

12

Italian Cuisine: Starters, Soups and Salads

	Sauces	Flour Dusting	Stocks & Broths	Cooking Oil	Pastas	Battering, Bread & Breading	Other
Starters							
Calamari alla Griglia (Grilled Calamari)	(Sa)	(Fd)				(Ba)(Br)	
Carpaccio di Manzo (Beef Carpaccio)							(Ga)
Carpaccio di Salmone (Salmon Carpaccio)							(Wf)
Cocktail di Gamberi (Shrimp Cocktail)			(Bo)				
Cozze al Vapore (Steamed Mussels)			(Bo)		(No)	(Br)	
Prosciutto e Melone (Cured Ham and Melon)							
Soups							
Gazpaccio			(Th)				(Cr)
Salads							
Insalata Caprese (Mozzarella Tomato Salad)							
Insalata Mista (Mixed Green Salad)							(Cr)(Ga)

(Ba) Ensure no wheat flour in batter—request plain

(Bo) Ensure no packaged bouillon

(Br) Ensure no bun or bread crumbs

(Cr) Ensure no croutons

(Fd) Ensure no dusting with wheat flour

(Ga) Ensure no gluten-containing garnish

(No) Ensure no wheat flour in noodles or pasta—request gluten-free

(Sa) Ensure no wheat flour in sauce

(Th) Ensure no wheat flour as thickening agent

(Wf) Ensure no wheat flour as ingredient

12

Italian Cuisine: Italian Specialities, Meat and Chicken Dishes

	Sauces	Flour Dusting	Stocks & Broths	Cooking Oil	Pastas	Battering, Bread & Breading	Other
Italian Specialties							
Risotto ai Frutti di Mare (Arborio Rice and Seafood Dish)			(Bo)				(Cl)
Risotto ai Funghi (Arborio Rice and Mushroom Dish)			(Bo)				(Cl)
Risotto ai Quattro Formaggi (Arborio Rice and Cheese Dish)			(Bo)				(Cl)
Risotto al Pollo (Arborio Rice and Chicken Dish)			(Bo)				(Cl)
Meat Dishes							
Costatella D'Agnello (Rack of Lamb)		(Fd)			(No)	(Br)	
Fileto di Manzo (Filet Mignon)		(Fd)			(No)		
Medalione di Manzo (Beef Tenderloin Medallions)	(Sa)	(Fd)			(No)		
Vitello (Veal)	(Sa)	(Fd)			(No)	(Bd)(Br)	
Chicken Dishes							
Petti di Pollo (Chicken Breast)	(Sa)	(Fd)			(No)	(Bd)(Br)	
Pollo Arrosto Rosmarino (Rosemary Roasted Chicken)					(No)	(Br)	

(Bd) Ensure no wheat flour in breading—request plain or gluten-free

(Bo) Ensure no packaged bouillon

(Br) Ensure no bun or bread crumbs

(Cl) Ensure clean water is used to cook rice

(Fd) Ensure no dusting with wheat flour

(No) Ensure no wheat flour in noodles or pasta—request gluten-free

(Sa) Ensure no wheat flour in sauce

12

Italian Cuisine: Seafood Dishes, Sides and Desserts

	Sauces	Flour Dusting	Stocks & Broths	Cooking Oil	Pastas	Battering, Bread & Breading	Other
Seafood Dishes							
Salmone alla Griglia (Grilled Salmon)	Sa				No		
Scampi (Prawns)	Sa				No	Br	
Sides							
Broccoli Rabe (Broccoli Florets)							
Funghi all' Aglio e Olio (Mushrooms in Garlic and Olive Oil)						Br	Wf
Melanzane alla Griglia (Grilled Eggplant)		Fd				Br	
Polenta (Boiled Corn Meal)	Sa			Df			
Desserts							
Gelato (Italian Ice Cream or Sherbet)							Ck Sb
Granita (Italian Ice)							Mv Sb
Zabaglione (Italian Custard)							Ck

Br Ensure no bun or bread crumbs

Ck Ensure no gluten in cake, cookie or biscuit

Df Ensure dedicated fryer

Fd Ensure no dusting with wheat flour

Mv Ensure no malt or malt vinegar

No Ensure no wheat flour in noodles or pasta—request gluten-free

Sa Ensure no wheat flour in sauce

Sb Ensure no gluten in stabilizers

Wf Ensure no wheat flour as ingredient

12

Mexican Cuisine: Starters, Soups and Salads

	Sauces	Stocks & Broths	Cooking Oil	Tortillas	Marinades	Other
Starters						
Ceviche (Raw Fish Salad)			(Df)(Fo)	(Tc)		
Chile con Queso (Chili Cheese Dip)	(Sa)		(Df)(Fo)	(Tc)		
Guacamole (Avocado Dip)			(Df)(Fo)	(Tc)		
Queso Fundido (Cheese Dip)	(Sa)		(Df)(Fo)	(Tc)		
Tortillas y Salsa (Chips and Salsa)	(Sa)		(Df)(Fo)	(Tc)		
Soups						
Posole (Chili Corn Soup)		(Bo)(Th)				
Sopa Azteca (Lime Chicken Soup)		(Bo)(Th)	(Df)(Fo)	(Tc)		
Salads						
Ensalada (House Salad)				(Ga)		
Taco Salad	(Sa)		(Df)(Fo)	(Tc)	(Ss)(Wf)	(Wf)

12

(Bo) Ensure no packaged bouillon

(Df) Ensure dedicated fryer

(Fo) Ensure fresh cooking oil

(Ga) Ensure no gluten-containing garnish

(Sa) Ensure no wheat flour in sauce

(Ss) Ensure no soy sauce

(Tc) Ensure no wheat flour tortillas or tortilla chips

(Th) Ensure no wheat flour as thickening agent

(Wf) Ensure no wheat flour as ingredient

Mexican Cuisine: Egg Dishes, Antojos and Meat Dishes

	Sauces	Stocks & Broths	Cooking Oil	Tortillas	Marinades	Other
Egg Dishes						
Huevos Mexicanos (Mexican Eggs)	(Sa)		(Df)(Fo)	(Tc)		(Wf)
Huevos Rancheros (Ranch Style Eggs)	(Sa)		(Df)(Fo)	(Tc)		(Wf)
Antojos (Mexican Specialties)						
Enchiladas	(Sa)		(Df)(Fo)	(Tc)		
Enfrijoladas	(Sa)		(Df)(Fo)	(Tc)		
Tacos	(Sa)		(Df)(Fo)	(Tc)		
Tamales (Stuffed Corn Meal)	(Sa)					
Tostadas Compuestas (Filled Corn Tortillas)	(Sa)		(Df)(Fo)	(Tc)	(Ss)(Wf)	(Wf)
Meat Dishes						
Arracheras (Flank or Skirt Steak)	(Sa)			(Tc)	(Ss)(Wf)	(Wf)
Bistek (Steak)	(Sa)		(Df)		(Ss)(Wf)	(Wf)
Carne Asada (Broiled Beef)	(Sa)			(Tc)	(Ss)(Wf)	(Wf)
Carnitas (Simmered Pork)	(Sa)			(Tc)		(Wf)
Machaca (Shredded Beef)	(Sa)			(Tc)		(Wf)

(Df) Ensure dedicated fryer
(Fo) Ensure fresh cooking oil

(Sa) Ensure no wheat flour in sauce
(Ss) Ensure no soy sauce

(Tc) Ensure no wheat flour tortillas or tortilla chips
(Wf) Ensure no wheat flour as ingredient

12

Mexican Cuisine: Dishes (Chicken, Turkey, Seafood) Sides and Desserts

	Sauces	Stocks & Broths	Cooking Oil	Tortillas	Marinades	Other
Chicken and Turkey Dishes						
Mole	(Sa)			(Tc)		(Wf)
Pechuga de Pollo (Chicken Breast)	(Sa)			(Tc)	(Ss)(Wf)	(Wf)
Pollo Asado (Broiled Chicken)	(Sa)			(Tc)	(Ss)(Wf)	(Wf)
Seafood Dishes						
Langosta (Lobster)	(Sa)	(Bo)		(Tc)		
Paella Mariscos (Seafood and Rice)		(Bo)				
Sides						
Arroz (Rice)		(Bo)				(Cl)
Frijoles (Beans)						(Wf)
Desserts						
Arroz con Leche (Rice Pudding)						(Cl)
Flan (Custard)						(Wf)
Helados (Ice Cream, Sherbet or Sorbet)						(Ck)(Mv)(Sb)(Wf)

(Bo) Ensure no packaged bouillon

(Ck) Ensure no gluten in cake, cookie or biscuit

(Cl) Ensure clean water is used to cook rice

(Mv) Ensure no malt or malt vinegar

(Sa) Ensure no wheat flour in sauce

(Sb) Ensure no gluten in stabilizers

(Ss) Ensure no soy sauce

(Tc) Ensure no wheat flour tortillas or tortilla chips

(Wf) Ensure no wheat flour as ingredient

12

Thai Cuisine: Starters, Soups and Noodle & Rice Dishes

	Sauces	Flour Dusting	Stocks & Broths	Cooking Oil	Noodles & Dumplings	Battering	Other
Starters							
Kanom Jeeb (Shrimp Dumplings)	(Fs)(Ss)				(Ss)		(Wf)
Satay (Skewered Beef, Chicken or Shrimp)	(Fs)(Ss)						(Ma)(Ss)
Som Tam (Papaya Salad)	(Fs)						(Ss)
Summer Rolls	(Fs)(Ss)		(Bo)				(Se)(Wf)
Soups							
Tom Kha Gai (Chicken and Coconut Soup)	(Fs)		(Bo)				(Ss)
Tom Yum Groong (Spicy Shrimp Soup)	(Fs)		(Bo)				(Ss)
Noodle and Rice Dishes							
Kaw Pad (Thai Fried Rice)	(Fs)						(Ss)
Pad See Yu	(Fs)(Sa)						(Ss)(Wf)
Pad Thai	(Fs)(Sa)						(Ss)(Wf)
Sticky Rice							(Cl)

(Bo) Ensure no packaged bouillon
(Cl) Ensure clean water is used to cook rice
(Fs) Ensure no wheat in fish sauce
(Ma) Ensure no wheat flour in marinade
(Sa) Ensure no wheat flour in sauce
(Se) Ensure no gluten in packaged seasonings
(Ss) Ensure no soy sauce
(Wf) Ensure no wheat flour as ingredient

12

Thai Cuisine: Curries, Dishes (Beef, Chicken, Seafood) and Desserts

	Sauces	Flour Dusting	Stocks & Broths	Cooking Oil	Noodles & Dumplings	Battering	Other
Curries (Kang)							
Kang Dang or Malay (Red Curry)	(Fs)	(Fd)				(Ba)	(Ss)
Kang Khiao Wan (Green Curry)	(Fs)	(Fd)				(Ba)	(Ss)
Kang Massaman (Tamarind Curry)	(Fs)	(Fd)				(Ba)	(Ss)
Kang Panang (Peanut Curry)	(Fs)	(Fd)				(Ba)	(Ss)
Beef Dishes							
Braised Beef Short Ribs	(Fs)						(Ma)(Ss)
Chicken Dishes							
Gai Yang (Thai Barbeque Chicken)	(Fs)(Ss)						(Ma)(Ss)
Seafood Dishes							
Pla Rad Prik (Crispy Whole Fish)	(Fs)	(Fd)					(Ss)
Desserts							
Fresh Tropical Fruits							(Ck)
Sweet Sticky Rice							(Cl)
Tropical Fruit Sorbets							(Cf)(Ck)(Sb)

(Ba) Ensure no wheat flour in batter—request plain

(Cf) Ensure no gluten in artificial colors or flavors

(Ck) Ensure no gluten in cake, cookie or biscuit

(Cl) Ensure clean water is used to cook rice

(Fd) Ensure no dusting with wheat flour

(Fs) Ensure no wheat in fish sauce

(Ma) Ensure no wheat flour in marinade

(Sb) Ensure no gluten in stabilizers

(Ss) Ensure no soy sauce

12

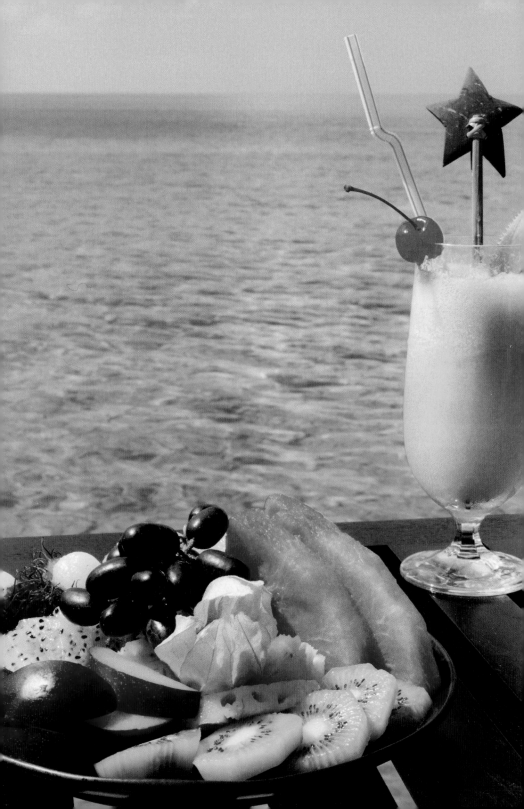

Friendships develop over food and wine.
—Prince Nicholas Romanoff

Chapter 13
Snacks, Breakfast and Beverage Suggestions

Chapter Overview

The suggestions for snacks, breakfast meals and beverages represent a variety of guidelines to help you both inside and outside your home. The snack ideas will satisfy your hunger while away from home for an extended period of time, whether at school, work, the airport, etc. The suggestions for breakfast meals provide you with the opportunity to enjoy breakfast in a restaurant, hotel room or even in your own home. The beverage guidelines will curb your thirst safely throughout the day anywhere you may be. The guidelines include:

13

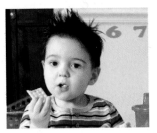

- On-the-road snack suggestions

- Breakfast meal overview

- Allergy awareness in beverages

- Non-alcoholic & alcoholic beverage ideas

On-The-Road Snack Suggestions

There are a wide variety of foods you can pack while traveling by car, train, boat or plane for an extended period of time. These snack ideas have been developed based upon years of personal global travel experiences, extensive research, focus group feedback and product ingredient analysis.

Remember to read each product label, review ingredients and use your best judgment to determine which snacks are safe for you.

Also, bring enough food to get you to your destination and for your excursions throughout your trip. For example, if you're flying eight hours to Hawaii, pack two to three meals worth of snacks in case of delays and/or mistakes.

The following snacks reflect products that can be readily eaten anywhere *without* a microwave, oven, stove, toaster or refrigerator. Some on-the-road snacks that you may want to consider are grouped into three basic categories:

- No preparation

- Hot water preparation

- Cooler required

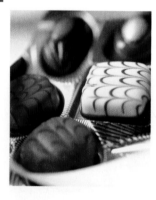

13

No Preparation Snack Tips

No preparation snacks can be easily carried in your backpack, school bag, purse and briefcase or stored in your school locker, office and car for extended periods of time. Depending upon your specific allergen concern(s), these suggestions may include the following:

- *Breads, Cereals, Cookies/Biscuits, Crackers and Rice Cakes*

- *Candy and Confectioneries*: bars, chocolates, gum, hard candies, lollipops, marshmallows

- *Canned/Packaged Fruits*: apple sauce, fruit cocktail, mandarin oranges, peaches, pears

- *Canned/Packaged Fish and Meats*: chicken, tuna

- *Chips and Crisps*: caramel corn, cheese snacks, chips (from corn, potato or rice), popcorn, pretzels

- *Dried Fruits*: apricots, dates, figs, fruit snacks, mango, pineapple, plantains, raisins

- *Fresh Fruits*: apples, bananas, cherries, grapes, oranges, peaches, pears, plums, strawberries

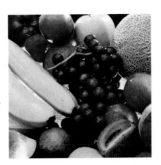

- *Fresh Vegetables*: broccoli, carrots, cauliflower, celery, cucumbers, edamame

- *Granola/Energy Bars*: fruit-filled bars, protein bars, vegan bars

- *Nuts*: almonds, cashews, peanuts, pecans, pistachios, walnuts

- *Prepared/Prepackaged Light Meals*: falafel, hard boiled eggs, sandwiches

- *Packaged Dressings/Sauces*: mayonnaise, olive oil, salad dressings, salsa, soy sauce

- *Seed Snacks*: pumpkin seeds, soy nuts, sunflower seeds

- *Trail Mixes*: combination of dried fruit, seeds and/ or nuts

Hot Water Preparation Tips

Hot water preparation snacks can also make tasty travel companions. Just ask for hot water in a cup or container, which can be found at convenience stores, restaurants, petrol stations, airports and on airplanes. Voilá! You can enjoy instant meals, such as:

- *Hot Cereals*: buckwheat, corn, oatmeal, quinoa, rice

- *Instant Soups/Meals*: beans, chicken, potato, rice, vegetable

- *Rice Noodle Dishes*: instant rice noodles

Cooler Required Snack Tips

Cooler required snacks can be transported and kept chilled in a small portable cooler, insulated lunch pack or insulated mug. These may include.

- *Dairy/Non-Dairy Alternatives*: cheese, cottage cheese, spreads, string cheese, yogurts

13

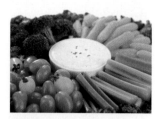

- *Deli/Packaged Meats*: chicken, corned beef, ham, pepperoni, prosciutto, roast beef, salami, sausage, turkey

- *Desserts*: flan, jello, mousse, pudding

- *Dips and Spreads*: bean dip, chutney, guacamole, hummus, jam, tapenade, pâtés, tzatziki

- *Fresh Fruits*: cantaloupe, honey dew, mango, melon, raspberries

- *Fresh Vegetables and Salads*

Additionally, some items can make eating snacks on-the-road a little easier. If there is room in your carry-on luggage or suitcase, consider packing the following as needed.

- Packets of dressings, condiments and/or sauces

- Re-sealable plastic baggies, toaster bags, oven sheets and/or aluminum foil

- Sterile wipes and/or napkins

- Disposable silverware, containers, cups and/or plates

Portable cold packs and a pocket knife can also come in handy. However, if you're traveling by air, they must be checked with baggage before entering security due to airport regulations.

Visit www.GlutenFreePassport.com or www.Allergy FreePassport.com for additional snack resources including:

- Downloadable shopping checklists by category with hundreds of snack ideas—Traveling section

- Store listings, by country, across the globe that carry gluten and allergen-free products— Reference Center

- Cookbooks around the world with recipes for preparing your own snacks—Book Corner

Breakfast Meal Overview

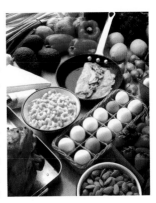

Over 125 breakfast meal suggestions have been outlined in a downloadable breakfast checklist to guide you in identifying meal options both inside and outside your home. You may use the checklist when shopping for groceries, dining at a restaurant or communicating your order to room service.

The checklist follows an easy-to-use format, allowing you to ask questions about ingredients and food preparation techniques. It encompasses categories such as breakfast specialties, egg dishes, omelets and bakery products. It also outlines yogurts, fruits, sides (meat, fish and potato) and spreads, jams and jellies that are safe for gluten and allergen-free breakfast meals.

Visit the Eating Out section at either www.Gluten FreePassport.com or www.AllergyFreePassport.com for a downloadable breakfast suggestions checklist. Visit www.GlutenFreeOnTheGo.com, the world's largest global on-line database of gluten-free eating establishments, to discover bakeries, cafés, coffee shops and restaurants catering to safe gluten-free meals.

Allergy Awareness in Beverages

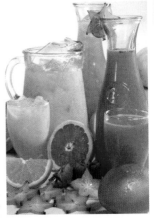

There are a variety of choices when it comes to gluten and allergen-free non-alcoholic and alcoholic beverages. At the same time, it is extremely important to ensure that there are no hidden allergens or ingredients used in the manufacturing process that you may have a reaction to. Non-alcoholic beverages label the specific ingredients found in their products, so it is necessary to read these labels carefully.

By contrast, alcohol manufacturers in some parts of the world are not required by law to list their ingredients. Some alcoholic products list what ingredients they are distilled from and some do not.

Actual contents of some ingredients may vary based upon your location and the geographic region of the manufacturer.

13

Below is a list of common ingredients that may contain hidden allergens in non-alcoholic and alcoholic beverages.

- Brown rice syrup (may contain barley/gluten)

- Caramel color (may contain corn, gluten/wheat or soy)

- Colors or flavors (may contain corn, gluten/wheat, soy, peanuts or tree nuts)

- Corn syrup (contains corn)

- Dextrin (made from corn or wheat)

- Hydrolyzed corn protein (contains corn)

- Hydrolyzed soy protein (contains soy)

- Hydrolyzed wheat protein (contains gluten/wheat)

- Malt or malt flavoring (made from barley/gluten or corn)

- Modified food starch (made from corn or gluten/wheat)

- Vegetable protein, hydrolyzed vegetable protein (HVP), hydrolyzed plant protein (HPP) or textured vegetable protein (TVP) (may contain corn, gluten/wheat or soy)

Non-Alcoholic Beverage Ideas

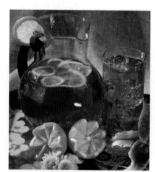

The following list reflects cold and hot non-alcoholic beverages to order around the corner or around the world.

Iced Coffee and Tea
Decaffeinated, flavored, herbal, iced cappuccino, iced coffee, iced tea, regular

Fruit Juice
Apple, banana, cherry, cranberry, grape, grapefruit, orange, peach, pear, pineapple, plum, prune

Vegetable Juice
Carrot, celery, aloe vera, tomato, vegetable

Mineral Water
Still and sparkling waters—some flavored waters may contain colors or flavors

13

Carbonated and Non-Carbonated Beverages
Cola, fruit punch, ginger ale, grape, lemonade, orange, root beer, soda water, sports drinks, tonic water

Dairy and Non-Dairy Beverages
Almond milk, cow's milk, hemp milk, protein drinks, rice milk, smoothie, soy drinks, soy milk, yogurt drinks

Hot Coffee
Café au lait, cappuccino, decaffeinated, espresso, flavored, instant, latte, regular

Hot Tea
Decaffeinated, flavored, herbal, regular

Hot Cider and Cocoa
Apple cider, hot chocolate

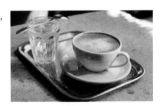

Alcoholic Beverage Ideas

In your gluten and allergen-free journeys, you may discover a broad spectrum of opinions on alcoholic beverages. Some sources advise you to stay away from alcohol, while others provide listings of products that may be gluten and allergen-free.

The distillation process removes all proteins from alcohol; thereby eliminating the substance in food that the body reacts to in an allergic response. The source of distilled alcohol in various types of beverages are noted for your reference in the following guide.

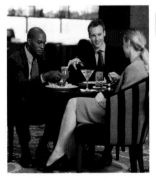

You need to consider whether colors or flavors are used in the production of the product. Colors and flavors may contain corn, dairy, eggs, gluten/wheat, peanuts, soy or tree nuts. In addition, some alcoholic beverages may be fortified with grain alcohol. Grain alcohol may be distilled from corn or wheat. Finally, some alcoholic beverages may contain malt which is derived from barley/gluten or corn.

The following charts reflect 10 categories of alcoholic beverages that you may consider ordering based upon the ingredients they are made from and their distillation process.

13

Quick Reference Guide: Vodka, Rum, Tequila, Mezcal, Gin, Jenever, Whiskey, Wine & Wine Beverages

Type of Beverage	Distilled / Made From

Vodka

Vodka, Flavored Vodka*	Corn, Grains, Grapes, Potato or Soy

May be mixed with artificial colors or flavors

Rum

Añejo Rum, Blanco (Clear) Rum, Dark Rum*, Flavored Rum*, Spiced Rum*	Sugar Cane

May be mixed with artificial colors or flavors

Tequila & Mezcal

Añejo Tequila - Aged at least one year* Blanco (Clear) or Gold Tequila - Aged no more than two months* Mezcal, Reposado - Aged at least six months*	Agave

Unless stated 100%, agave may be mixed with grain alcohol distilled from corn or sugar cane

Gin & Jenever

Gin (London Dry & Plymouth Styles), Flavored Gin*, Jenever (Dutch & European Styles), Flavored Jenever*	Grains

May be mixed with artificial colors or flavors

Whiskey

American (Bourbon, Sour Mash, Rye), Canadian (Rye), Irish, Scotch	Grains

Wine & Wine Beverages

Champagne and Sparkling Wine Red, White and Blush Wines Fortified Wine and Port (Madeira, Port, Sherry)* Vermouth (French Dry & Italian Sweet Styles)* Wine Coolers**	Grapes

May be fortified with grain alcohol or wine spirits
**May be mixed with artificial colors or flavors*

Quick Reference Guide: Beer, Cider, Sake, Brandy, Liqueur and Beverage Mixes

Type of Beverage	Distilled / Made From

Beer, Cider & Sake

Hard Cider	Apples and possibly Barley
Gluten-Free Beer	Gluten-Free Grains
Beer (Ale, Lager, Pilsner, Porter, Stout, Wheat-Beer), Non-Alcoholic Beer	Hops, Barley, Malt & Wheat
Sake (Known as rice wine, but fermented and brewed like beer)	Rice and Koji Enzymes grown on Miso (typically made from barley)

*For gluten-free beer manufacturers worldwide, visit the Eating Out section at **www.GlutenFreePassport.com***

Brandy

Calvados	Apples
Kirschwasser	Cherries
Eaux de Vie	Fruit
Brandy , Flavored Brandy*, Armagnac, Cognac, Flavored Cognac*	Grapes
Grappa	Grapes or Fruit

*May be mixed with artificial colors or flavors

Liqueur

Coffee Liqueur*	Coffee
Cream-Based Liqueur*	Cream
Fruit Flavored Liqueur*	Fruit
Schnapps*	Fruit and Herbs
Melon Liqueur*, Nut Flavored Liqueur*	Melon
Orange Flavored Liqueur*	Oranges

*May be mixed with alcohol distilled from corn or grain and/or artificial colors or flavors

Beverage Mixes

Colada Mixers*	Coconut-based mixture
Daiquiri Mixers*	Fruit-based mixture
Pre-Mixed Alcoholic Cocktails*	Ingredients vary
Margarita Mixers*	Lime-based mixture
Bloody Mary Mixers*	Tomato-based mixture

*Ingredients vary by manufacturer. Carefully review ingredients and labels.

13

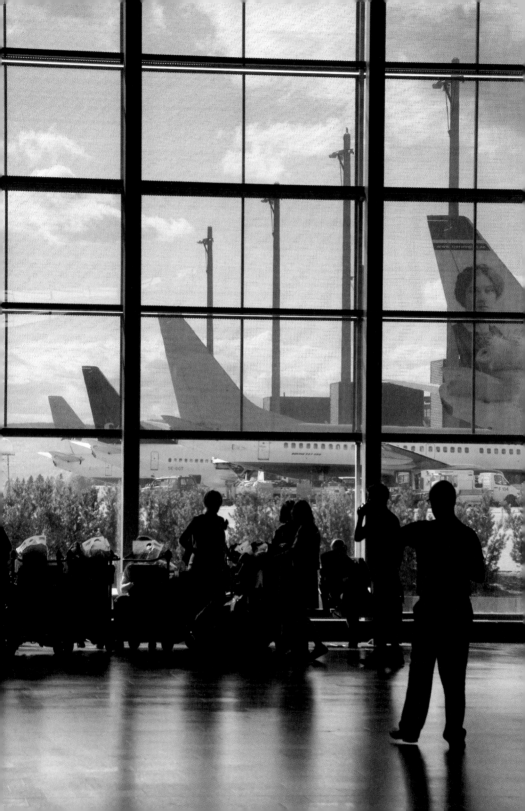

*The real voyage of discovery consists not in
seeking new landscapes, but in having new eyes.*
—Marcel Proust

Chapter 14

Airline, Hotel, Cruise and Travel Tips

Chapter Overview

The suggestions for airlines, accommodations and cruise ship travel represent a variety of guidelines to consider when planning a trip away from home. These travel tips may also assist you in choosing your preferred providers based upon your special dietary concerns and include:

14

- Overall travel considerations

- Airline guidelines and checklists

- Hotel and accommodations checklist

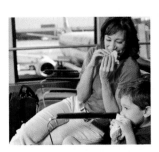

- Cruise line meals checklist

- International travel tips

- Foreign language translation cards

Overall Travel Considerations

Safely traveling while managing special diets is very doable and highly rewarding. You can discover new places and experience safe gluten and allergen-friendly journeys with careful planning and a little extra effort! The best way to expand your own personal comfort and reduce the stress associated with traveling is three-fold: education, preparation and communication.

Educate yourself on your travel and eating out options based upon what you can and cannot eat. Be prepared with snacks, medications and back-up plans in the event of a mistake, accident or emergency. Communicate your special dietary requirements effectively with airline, hotel, cruise line, restaurant and hospitality professionals as needed.

Achieving empowerment when eating out and traveling anywhere in the world requires due diligence, taking proper precautions and asking the right questions.

Airline Guidelines and Checklists

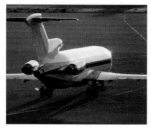

Eating gluten and allergen-free while traveling by air is possible. The best approach to gaining that often elusive comfort level when flying is a combination of at least three key areas of consideration, and possibly four if at risk to anaphylaxis.

These "how-to" guidelines and checklists are designed to assist you throughout your planning efforts, and while on board the airplane, to enjoy safe and comfortable flying experiences. The key four points, depending upon your concerns, include:

1. Bring your own carry-on snacks for your flight(s)

2. Understand standard airline meal codes

3. Order your special meal(s)

4. Communicate your life threatening condition, if applicable

Guidelines for Carry-On Snacks through Airport Security

Your first step, and your safest option, is to bring your own snacks to eat during your flight. You need to ensure that your snacks are portable and tasty as well as allowable based upon the respective airport security regulations for each departing and arriving country.

14

For example, when traveling within some countries, you may need to understand requirements such as:

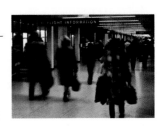

- If you are bringing packaged salad dressings or sauces, ensure that it falls within the liquid carry-on requirement.

- Remember to have liquid items available for inspection in an approved, re-sealable package.

- Products such as canned fruit may be considered liquid and may be confiscated at security.

- It is recommended that you do not bring cooling packs, as they are typically filled with chemical liquids or gels, and will likely be confiscated at security check points.

- Purchase your beverages for the flight after you have cleared security.

- Fill up your re-sealable baggy or travel-size cooler with ice, if needed, AFTER you go through security either at a food stand or on the airplane.

Standard Airline Meal Codes

Many airlines around the world are aware of and try to meet the needs of those who require special dietary meals when traveling by air. There are approximately 25 standard airline codes addressing various types of customer concerns. For your convenience, these codes are categorized as follows:

- Medically prescribed & recommended lifestyles

- Age considerations

- Religious considerations

- Health preferences

The special meal codes, their definitions and associated descriptions are defined on the following page. Many airline computer systems can only accept one standard airline code for special meal requests. For example, if you have multiple allergies and are allergic to both milk and gluten, you may have to choose one type of meal—either NLML or GFML.

Code	Definition	Description

Medically Prescribed & Recommended Lifestyles

Code	Definition	Description
GFML	Gluten-Free Meal	No wheat, rye, barley, oats or their derivatives
NLML	Non-Lactose Meal	No milk, cheese, dairy products or their derivatives
PFML	Peanut-Free Meal	No peanuts or its derivatives
DBML	Diabetic Meal	No refined sugars, syrups, jams, cakes, chocolates, etc.
LFML	Low-Fat/Cholesterol Meal	Limited amount of fat (particularly saturated fat)
PRML	Low-Purine Meal	No anchovies, crab, herring, liver, offal or shrimp
LPML	Low-Protein Meal	Limited amount of protein
LSML	Low-Sodium/Salt Meal	Little salt—Monosodium Glutamate (MSG) or baking soda/powder used

Age Considerations

Code	Definition	Description
BBML	Baby Meal	Soft and/or liquid foods—usually canned baby food or formula for infants under 2 years old
CHML	Child Meal	A combination of familiar foods for children 2–12 years old

Religious Considerations

Code	Definition	Description
HNML	Hindu Meal	No beef, veal, pork or their derivatives
JNML	Jain Meal	No root vegetables, onion or garlic
KSML	Kosher Meal	Prepared to comply with Jewish dietary laws
MOML	Muslim Meal	No pork, by-products of pork, shellfish or foodstuffs containing alcohol—all meat is Halal

Health Preferences

Code	Definition	Description
HFML	High-Fiber Meal	Unrefined flours are used over white flour products
LCML	Low-Calorie Meal	Limited amounts of fat, sugar and protein
AVML	Asian-Vegetarian Meal	No fish, shellfish, meat, poultry or eggs—typically spicy in content
VGML	Vegan Meal	No meat, fish, seafood, eggs, honey, dairy products or their derivatives
RVML	Raw-Vegetarian Meal	Combination of raw vegetables and fruit
VLML	Lacto-Ovo Vegetarian Meal	No meat, fish, or seafood—may contain dairy products such as milk, butter, cheese and eggs
ORML	Oriental Meal	Cooked in oriental or Chinese style—avoids meat, fish, milk, dairy products and root vegetables
FPML	Fruit Plate Meal	Contains a variety of fresh fruits and possibly a bakery item
SFML	Seafood Meal	Contains only seafood
BLML	Bland Meal	No spicy or acidic ingredients

14

For a list of 50-plus international airline carriers, visit the Traveling section at either www.GlutenFree Passport.com or www.AllergyFreePassport.com. Keep in mind that availability of airline meals and notification policies change frequently so contact your specific airline for the most up-to-date information.

Ordering Special Airline Meals Checklist

Different types of special meals are offered by specific airlines based on flight duration, destination and meal availability. Airlines typically require 24–96 hour advance notification to ensure that your designated meal is ready for the time of your departure. Meal selection and quality varies significantly from airline to airline. For those at risk to anaphylaxis, it is safest to bring your own meal—refer to the Anaphylaxis and Air Travel Checklist for more details.

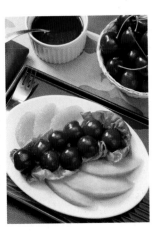

The following checklist is designed to guide you while ordering and eating special meals on board your flight.

1. Review the airline's website or call customer service before you book your flight to determine what foods are served and/or sold on board.

2. If you are booking directly through an airline carrier that offers special meals, request your special meal arrangements.

3. When booking your flight with a travel agent or through an on-line travel service, call the airline directly to request your special meal.

4. Provide the representative with one of the 25-plus standard codes used by the airline industry as previously outlined.

5. Re-confirm your meal request directly with the airline a minimum of 1 day prior to departure.

6. Remember that if you change flights, the special meal request does not necessarily remain in effect. In this case, you need to call the airline to request another special meal.

7. As a precautionary measure, pack snacks equivalent to at least one travel meal or enough food to

14

get you to your destination just in case your plane is delayed, plans change or a mistake happens.

8. If a special meal was ordered, notify the flight attendant of your request at the beginning of the meal service.

9. Once you receive your airline meal during your flight, review it to ensure that the food is safe to eat based upon your allergen concern.

10. Provide feedback to the flight attendant about your meal, as appropriate.

Anaphylaxis and Air Travel Checklist

Significant care and planning are critical to managing a potentially life threatening condition while away from home. To minimize the risks and expand your comfort zone, there are different considerations you need to think about when traveling by air with anaphylaxis.

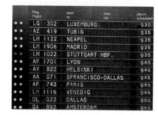

Some airlines and flight crews are more aware of food allergies and may accommodate your special requests while others may not. Keep in mind that airlines will not guarantee a "nut-free" flight and cannot prohibit other passengers from carrying peanuts or tree nuts onto your flight. However, some carriers and crews may refrain from serving the allergen on board your specific flight due to the severity of your condition.

Although the following checklist may seem a bit overwhelming with extensive precautions, thoroughness is a critical factor to ensuring safe travel journeys with severe food allergies.

1. Review the airlines in-flight food options, emergency protocol and allergy policy prior to booking your flight.

2. Call customer service and notify the representative and/or supervisor about the severity of your allergies.

3. Choose and book your airline based on your health and travel priorities.

4. Ideally, book the first non-stop flight of the day so that the plane has been cleaned from previous passengers.

14

5. Reserve your seating assignment with as few passengers in proximity to your seat as possible.

6. Re-confirm your allergen concerns directly with the airline a minimum of 1 day prior to departure.

7. Pack snacks equivalent to at least one travel meal or enough food to get you to your destination.

8. For security purposes, ensure all prescribed, non-expired medications that you are bringing on the plane include the respective passenger's name on the original labels.

9. Carry your medications, including several epinephrine auto-injectors, such as EpiPen® or TwinJect™, and any other related medicines.

10. Bring a doctor's note explaining the requirement to carry your medications on board.

11. Carry any other important medical records and wear a medical identification bracelet.

12. Notify airline staff at check-in and at the gate of the severity of your condition.

13. Request pre-boarding to wipe down and sterilize the seats, arm rests, tray tables, seat belt, windows, surfaces and surrounding areas.

14. Keep your medications and snacks with you at all times—do not store in the overhead bin.

15. Ask flight attendants to announce prior to take-off that there is a person on board with life threatening food allergies and to refrain from eating the allergen during the flight.

16. Carry extra snacks and offer them to other passengers in exchange for not consuming your allergen of concern or offer to buy them a different snack on board.

17. Bring your own pillow and blanket to avoid potential residual food particles from allergens.

18. Provide feedback to the flight crew about your experience as appropriate.

14

The bottom line is *always*:

- Be prepared with medication, documentation, snacks, plans and back-up plans.

- Communicate the severity of your anaphylaxis to each and every airline personnel.

Hotel and Accommodations Checklist

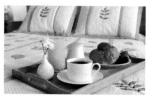

If you decide to stay on land, you need to ensure that you and your family are safe at your destination of choice. Your comfort level with managing your gluten and allergen-free lifestyle, the severity of your food allergies and your personal preferences are all key influencers in your choice of accommodations.

Various lodging alternatives may include hotels, resorts, bed & breakfasts, hostels, villas, apartments, cottages and even castles!

If you are looking to stay on land away from home, it is recommended that you:

1. Research your options to determine the best fit for your dietary needs and travel destinations.

2. Determine if you need a refrigerator and/or kitchen to prepare some of your meals. If desired, request a small refrigerator, which may result in an extra fee.

3. Contact the customer service department to address any unanswered questions prior to booking your reservation.

4. Inform the accommodation when making reservations of your allergen concerns.

5. Educate yourself on ingredients, food preparation techniques and hidden allergens to determine appropriate meals and restaurants, if applicable.

6. Discuss meal alternatives with the culinary specialists and order your allergen and gluten-free meals in advance, if appropriate.

14

7. Ideally, obtain in writing a mutually agreed upon meal plan and approach to ensure safe eating, especially if your accommodation is at an all-inclusive resort.

8. Determine what safe snacks you need to pack for excursions away from your accommodation.

9. Confirm your gluten and allergen-free meals with your accommodation 3- 5 days prior to your departure, if appropriate.

10. Prepare an emergency plan with medicine, location of closest medical facilities and instructions for others, if needed.

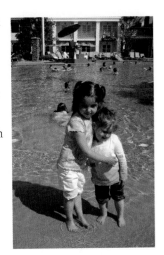

11. Research grocery stores and supermarkets close to your accommodation for some basic foods, if desired.

12. Check with your accommodation about restaurants nearby and contact them prior to your departure, if appropriate.

13. Stay within close proximity of the nearest hospital if at risk to anaphylaxis.

14. When you arrive, communicate your dietary concerns to the accommodation wait staff as required for safe eating.

Cruise Line Meals Checklist

Many cruise lines cater to guests with special dietary concerns, even identifying gluten and allergen-free meals as specific offerings in their promotional efforts.

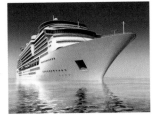

If you are looking to enjoy a cruise and explore various new destinations by sea, it is recommended that you:

1. Research cruise lines to determine the best fit for your dietary needs and desired travel plans.

2. Review the emergency medical facilities, medicines on board and procedures for life threatening reactions in the case of anaphylaxis.

3. Contact the customer service department of your preferred cruise line to address any unanswered questions prior to booking your reservation.

4. Inform the cruise line at the time of your reservation of your gluten and allergen concerns.

5. Educate yourself on ingredients, food preparation techniques and hidden allergens to determine appropriate meals and restaurants in your port cities, if desired.

6. Discuss meal alternatives with the culinary specialists from the cruise line and order your gluten and allergen-free meals in advance, if appropriate.

7. Ideally, obtain in writing a mutually agreed upon meal plan and approach to ensure safe eating on the cruise ship.

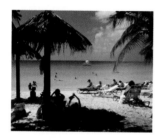

8. Determine if designated wait staff will serve each of your meals throughout the cruise.

9. Determine what safe snacks you need to pack for excursions away from the cruise ship.

10. Confirm your special meals with the cruise line 3- 5 days prior to your departure.

11. Meet with the Hotel Director (yes—on a cruise ship!), manager of the dining room, staff and/or chef once you have boarded the ship to reiterate your needs.

12. Communicate your dietary concerns to your designated wait staff and cabin crew, as required.

International Travel Tips

When venturing overseas, following these travel guidelines will help to make your journey more enjoyable and increase your comfort level while staying in both English and foreign-language speaking destinations.

1. Research on-line global databases and resources about eating out and traveling overseas.

2. Contact the local celiac / coeliac or food allergy associations for suggestions on eating gluten and allergen-free in that specific country.

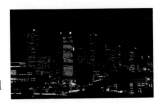

3. Understand country specific regulations regarding standards on allowable products packed in carry-on luggage.

4. Review food product labeling regulations for your destination, which may differ from your home country, to determine the availability of safe snacks for future purchase during your travels.

For those visiting foreign-speaking countries, it is also important to communicate your needs in the native language.

1. Ensure any medical documentation that may be needed has been translated into the language of each country included in your travels.

2. Carry pocket-size gluten and allergen-free translation cards which identify your special dietary requirements by allergen, key ingredients and critical food preparation techniques.

3. Pack a foreign language phrase guide such as the *Multi-Lingual Phrase Passport* for additional phrases such as common ingredients, dining requests, breakfast meals, health considerations and products.

14

Foreign Language Translation Cards

In order to navigate your way in foreign-speaking countries, it is important to effectively communicate your needs in the native language even if you can't pronounce the words or speak the language. Downloadable translation cards are available free of charge in various foreign languages ranging from Dutch, Portuguese and Spanish to Arabic, Greek and Russian.

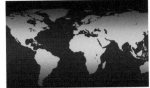

These cards are designed in an easy-to-use format so that you may refer to them when scanning a

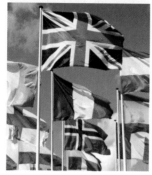

restaurant menu. You can also use them by pointing directly to the card to express your needs for safe gluten and allergen-free eating.

On the next page, sample gluten and allergen-free translation cards are included in the Italian and French languages. Electronic formats of these cards as well as many other languages are also provided in the Traveling section at either www.GlutenFreePassport.com or www.AllergyFreePassport.com.

These basic phrases have been translated to assist you with your gluten and allergen concerns and key preparation requests that may be required in foreign-speaking countries.

It is recommended that you present the appropriate card to the wait staff and/or chef at your selected eating establishment in the foreign-speaking country to communicate your special dietary requirements. It may also be helpful to print extra copies of the cards in the event that the restaurant staff or chef want to keep them for future reference!

The translation cards in the French, German, Italian and Spanish languages are excerpted from the award-winning *Multi-Lingual Phrase Passport*, Winner of the Best Language Guide and Best Travel Guide Award. As part of the *Let's Eat Out!* book series, this first-of-its-kind guide includes over 1,200 phrases as described in the Appendix.

Visit www.GlutenFreePassport.com or www.AllergyFreePassport.com for international travel resources including:

- Free downloadable pocket-sized translation cards—Traveling section

- Company listings for laminated translation cards available for purchase—Traveling section

- Food allergen and gluten-free labeling regulations around the world—Reference Center

- Hundreds of listings of global associations— Reference Center

- Store listings by country across the globe with gluten and allergen-free products—Reference Center

Sample Downloadable Translation Cards

English	Italian Translation
I need to special order my meal due to my food allergies.	Soffro di allergie alimentari, quindi devo ordinare cibi particolari.
I am allergic/intolerant/ hypersensitive to:	Ho un'allergia/intolleranza/ ipersensibilità a:
corn	granturco
dairy	latticini
eggs	uova
fish	pesce
gluten	glutine
milk	latte
nuts	noci
peanuts	arachidi
shellfish	crostacei
soy	soia
wheat	frumento
I cannot eat these foods because I will become ill.	Non posso mangiare questi cibi, perché potrebbero farmi stare male.
I have/am experiencing:	Soffro di/mi trovo in:
an emergency	un'emergenza
anaphylactic shock	shock anafilattico
an allergic reaction	reazione allergica
food allergies	allergie alimentari
celiac / coeliac disease	celiachia
lactose intolerance	intolleranza al lattosio
Thank you for your help.	Grazie per la cortesia.

Allergen-Free Italian Language Translation Card

Excerpted from the award-winning *Multi-Lingual Phrase Passport*—part of the *Let's Eat Out!* book series. Available at www.AllergyFreePassport.com

English	French Translations
I cannot eat the smallest amount of gluten which is wheat, rye or barley.	Je ne peux pas absorber la moindre quantité de gluten, qu'il provienne du blé, du seigle ou de l'orge.
I am allergic/intolerant/ hypersensitive to:	Je suis allergique/je ne tolère pas/je suis hypersensible:
gluten	au gluten
wheat	au blé
wheat flour	à la farine de blé
bread	de pain
breading	de chapelure
bread crumbs	de miettes de pain
pasta	de pâtes
soy sauce	de sauce au soja
I cannot eat these foods because I will become ill.	Je ne peux pas manger ces aliments parce que ça me rendrait malade.
Is this food dusted with wheat flour prior to cooking?	Est-ce que cet aliment est fariné à la farine de blé avant d'être cuit?
Is this food fried in the same fryer as items fried with breading?	Cet aliment est-il cuit dans la même friteuse que des aliments enrobés de chapelure?
I have a condition called celiac / coeliac disease.	Je souffre de la maladie coeliaque.
Thank you for your help.	Merci pour votre aide.

Excerpted from the award-winning *Multi-Lingual Phrase Passport*
For more information please visit: www.GlutenFreePassport.com
©2009 AllergyFree Passport®, LLC. All rights reserved.

Gluten-Free French Language Translation Card

Excerpted from the award-winning *Multi-Lingual Phrase Passport*—part of the *Let's Eat Out!* book series. Available at www.GlutenFreePassport.com

14

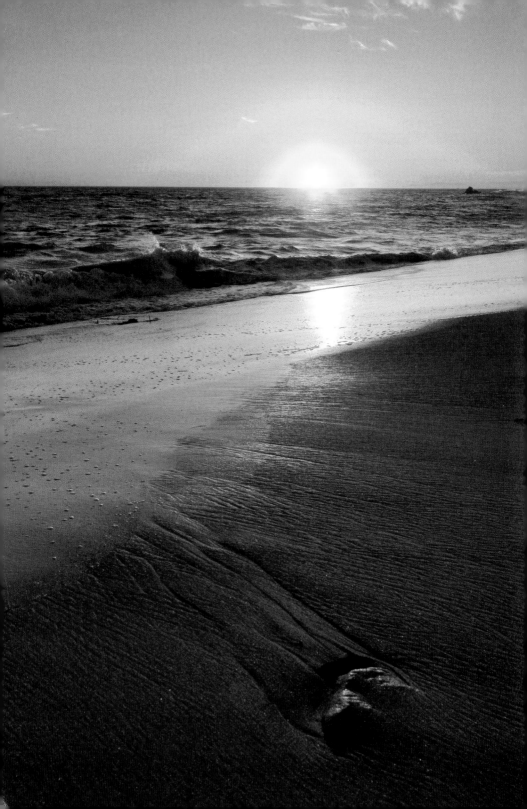

Throw your dreams into space like a kite,
and you do not know what it will bring back,
a new life, a new friend, a new love, a new country.
—Anais Nin

Appendix
Additional Gluten and Allergen-Free Resources

Appendix Overview

The following materials reflect additional educational resources including:

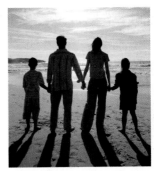

- Passport guides from the *Let's Eat Out!* series

- GlutenFree Passport® and AllergyFree Passport® solutions

- Global market research trends

- On-line educational resources

- Contact information

These resources are designed to further enhance safe gluten and allergen-free eating experiences for both guests and restaurants around the corner and around the world!

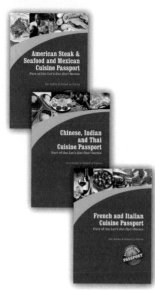

Passport Guides from *Let's Eat Out!* Series

Cuisine-Specific Passports

As part of the award-winning *Let's Eat Out!* series, R & R Publishing has also produced 3 pocket-size cuisine guides or "passports" in varying formats such as print and electronic. The cuisines are conveniently grouped into the following combinations for your convenience:

- *American Steak & Seafood and Mexican Cuisine Passport*

- *Chinese, Indian and Thai Cuisine Passport*

- *French and Italian Cuisine Passport*

These guides allow you to scan the menu at any restaurant, quickly identify the safest choices and ask the right questions to avoid the 10 most common allergens hidden in food preparation. As detailed in cuisine chapters 4–10, each passport provides sample menus, 50-plus menu dish descriptions, preparation techniques, quick reference guides and questions to ask to ensure safe meals anywhere you may be.

Multi-Lingual Phrase Passport

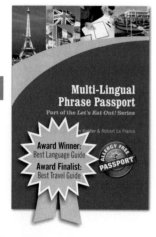

R & R Publishing has also produced a pocket-size translation phrase guide titled the *Multi-Lingual Phrase Passport* as part of the *Let's Eat Out!* series in varying formats such as print and electronic.

Winner of the Best Language Guide Award and Best Travel Guide Award, this innovative resource provides over 1,200 translations integral to international travel while managing celiac / coeliac, food allergies and special diets. The phrases include translations from the English language to the French, German, Italian and Spanish languages for reference while visiting foreign speaking countries.

A variety of dining requests, ingredients, food preparation techniques, common food allergens, breakfast dishes and health conditions are detailed to assist you in communicating gluten and allergen-free needs. All phrases have been translated by a professional translation service and quality assurance tested by native speakers to ensure phrase accuracy and applicability based upon contemporary cultural idioms.

Additional educational products are also in development to compliment the series and further facilitate safe eating around the corner and around the world. Visit www.GlutenFreePassport.com or www.Allergy FreePassport.com for more details.

GlutenFree Passport® and AllergyFree Passport® Solutions

In addition to creating the internationally acclaimed *Let's Eat Out!* series, GlutenFree Passport® and AllergyFree Passport® deliver innovative gluten and allergen-free client solutions on a worldwide basis. As global health education consulting firms, the unique team of authoritative experts, leading consultants and pioneering researchers has extensive expertise across the culinary, hospitality, travel, healthcare and product industries.

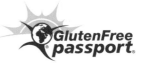

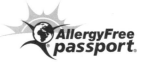

The mission of GlutenFree Passport® and Allergy-Free Passport® is to drive change worldwide for gluten and allergen-free lifestyles.

Our vision is two-fold:

1. Empower individuals with the knowledge to safely eat outside the home, while managing celiac / coeliac disease, food allergies & special diets

2. Educate businesses to recognize and expand their offerings to address special dietary needs

The uniquely qualified team designs and implements educational products and business services to increase the number of:

- Individuals who safely dine out and travel with special diets

- Restaurants that offer gluten and allergen-free meals as part of their standard services

- Travel, hospitality and food service providers to cater to guests with special needs

- Manufacturing companies that offer gluten and allergen-free products

As pioneers in the special diet community, with global knowledge and local expertise, our team offers knowledge resources, training services, food products and tailored solutions.

GlutenFree Passport® and AllergyFree Passport® also promote awareness of celiac / coeliac disease, food allergies and special diets worldwide.

Global Market Research Trends

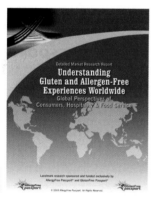

Sponsored by GlutenFree Passport® and AllergyFree Passport®, the global market research entitled *Understanding Gluten and Allergen-Free Experiences Worldwide: Global Perspective of Consumers, Hospitality & Food Service* provides industry-leading insights about special diet lifestyles. This cutting edge research details quantitative and qualitative analysis of thousands of consumer and business experiences across the globe. The three-dimensional research initiative presents market trends and best practices specific to eating out expectations, product preferences and quality of life considerations.

Focusing on consumers living with celiac / coeliac, food allergies and special diets and the businesses that serve them, this break-through research also encompasses comparisons between consumer and industry perspectives as well as future strategic advancements. Endorsed by associations worldwide, the empirical market research data helps to drive change for gluten and allergen-free lifestyles throughout the global community.

For a complimentary executive research summary and/or to purchase the detailed research findings, visit www.GlutenFreePassport.com or www.Allergy FreePassport.com.

On-Line Educational Resources

GlutenFreeOnTheGo.com

The world's largest on-line directory of gluten-free eating establishments, www.GlutenFreeOnTheGo. com offers verified places trusted by loyal and repeat gluten-free guests. Millions of consumers rely on www. GlutenFreeOnTheGo.com, with open access, to find quality establishments that cater to gluten-free needs including pizzerias, bakeries, restaurants, hotels, resorts and more! It also affords businesses with the opportunity to showcase their capabilities to this targeted customer segment across the globe.

GlutenFree OnTheGo
www.GlutenFreeOnTheGo.com

GlutenFreePassport.com and AllergyFreePassport.com

As two of the world's leading health consulting firms, GlutenFree Passport® and AllergyFree Passport® have developed significant educational resources associated with special diet lifestyles. Complimentary resources for consumers and businesses include proven eating out approach materials, worldwide labeling considerations, prevalence, snack guidelines, airlines, travel tips and translation chef cards.

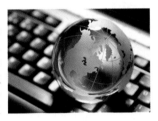

Links to hundreds and hundreds of up-to-date gluten and allergen-free books, publications, research organizations, stores, products, associations and businesses are also available by visiting:

www.GlutenFreePassport.com

www.AllergyFreePassport.com

Contact Information

If you would like to be included in the mailing list for GlutenFree Passport® and/or AllergyFree Passport®, obtain information on innovative educational services or have feedback, please contact the consulting firms via phone or electronically at info@GlutenFree Passport.com or info@AllergyFreePassport.com

North America
27 N. Wacker Drive, Suite 258
Chicago, IL 60606-2800
Telephone 1-312-952-4900

Europe
28 Old Brompton Road, Suite 72
South Kensington, London SW7 3SS
Telephone 44 0800 011 2542

Australia/New Zealand
56 The Corso, Level 1
Manly NSW 2095 Australia
Telephone 61 1800 451 637

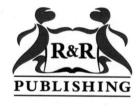

To inquire about special printings, volume discount pricing and foreign rights for the award-winning *Let's Eat Out!* book series, please contact R & R Publishing, LLC. via info@rnrpublishing.com or visit www. RnRPublishing.com for more details.

A